Vernacular Medicine in Colonial India

Conceptualised in opposition to 'orthodox' medicine, homoeopathy, a western medical project originating in eighteenth-century Germany, was reconstituted as vernacular medicine in British Bengal. India went on to become the home of the largest population of users of homoeopathic medicine in the world. Combining insights from the history of colonial medicine and the cultural histories of family in British India, Shinjini Das examines the processes through which western homoeopathy was translated and indigenised in the colony as a specific Hindu worldview, an economic vision and a disciplining regimen. In tracing the localisation of German homoeopathy in a British Indian province, this book analyses interactions between Calcutta-based homoeopathic family firms, disparate contributors to the Bengali print market, the British colonial state and emergent nationalist governments. The history of homoeopathy in Bengal reveals myriad negotiations undertaken by the colonised peoples to reshape scientific modernity in the subcontinent.

Shinjini Das is a Wellcome Trust Research Fellow at the Faculty of History, University of Oxford. She received her PhD from University College London and has previously held a postdoctoral fellowship funded by the European Research Council at the University of Cambridge.

Vernacular Medicine in Colonial India

Family, Market and Homoeopathy

Shinjini Das
University of Oxford

CAMBRIDGE
UNIVERSITY PRESS

CAMBRIDGE
UNIVERSITY PRESS

University Printing House, Cambridge CB2 8BS, United Kingdom

One Liberty Plaza, 20th Floor, New York, NY 10006, USA

477 Williamstown Road, Port Melbourne, VIC 3207, Australia

314-321, 3rd Floor, Plot 3, Splendor Forum, Jasola District Centre, New Delhi - 110025, India

79 Anson Road, #06-04/06, Singapore 079906

Cambridge University Press is part of the University of Cambridge.

It furthers the University's mission by disseminating knowledge in the pursuit of education, learning and research at the highest international levels of excellence.

www.cambridge.org
Information on this title: www.cambridge.org/9781108430692
DOI: 10.1017/9781108354905

First published 2019
First paperback edition 2020

A catalogue record for this publication is available from the British Library

Library of Congress Cataloging in Publication data
Names: Das, Shinjini, 1982– author.
Title: Vernacular medicine in colonial India : family, market, and homeopathy / Shinjini Das.
Description: Cambridge, United Kingdom ; New York, NY : Cambridge University Press, 2019. | Includes bibliographical references and index.
Identifiers: LCCN 2018033427 | ISBN 9781108420624 (hardback)
Subjects: | MESH: Homeopathy – history | Colonialism – history | Marketing of Health Services – history | Family Health – history | Health Policy – history | History, 19th Century | History, 20th Century | India
Classification: LCC RX71 | NLM WB 930 | DDC 615.5/32–dc23
LC record available at https://lccn.loc.gov/2018033427

ISBN 978-1-108-42062-4 Hardback
ISBN 978-1-108-43069-2 Paperback

For my loving parents,

Samar Das and Urmimala Ghosh

Contents

Illustrations

Acknowledgements

This book has been the product of my journey spanning several places and institutions. I humbly acknowledge the numerous debts, intellectual and otherwise, which I have accumulated. The dissertation which forms the backbone of this book was conceived, as a set of fledgling research ideas, at the Centre for Studies in Social Sciences, Calcutta (CSSSC). Gautam Bhadra first directed me to explore the depths of the vernacular archive that in many ways defined the course of my research. Generous funding from the Wellcome Trust Centre for the History of Medicine at University College London (UCL) enabled me to pursue my doctoral studies in London. Support from the UCL Graduate School further helped me undertake research-related travels in Kolkata and in London. A European Research Council (ERC)-funded collaborative fellowship at the Centre for Research in Arts Social Science and Humanities at the University of Cambridge gave me an intellectual home after my PhD years. While developing my postdoctoral research, this fellowship allowed me the time and support needed to undertake revisions to transform the dissertation into a monograph. The very final touches to the manuscript were given while holding a postdoctoral research fellowship at the Faculty of History at the University of Oxford.

My interest in history has been relentlessly stoked by my wonderful teachers. I remain grateful to my supervisors, Sanjoy Bhattacharya and Guy Attewell, for their faith in this project and for their comments on drafts of the dissertation. I have abiding debts to my teachers Rajat Kanta Ray and Subhas Ranjan Chakraborty at Presidency College, Calcutta, who first inspired me to think critically. Interactions with Bhaskar Chakrabarty, Shireen Maswood, Sukla Sanyal and Hari Vasudevan at the University of Calcutta aroused my inquisitiveness for first-hand research. The experience of pursuing the Research and Training Programme at the CSSSC has been stimulating. Exposed to a milieu of interdisciplinary teaching and research, I have learnt enormously from the courses offered by Gautam Bhadra, Partha Chatterjee, Rosinka Chaudhuri, P. K. Dutta, Udaya Kumar and Janaki Nair. I would like to particularly thank Sibaji Bandopadhyay and Tapati Guha-Thakurta for their support and interest in my work. At UCL, where I began my research, I learnt much from Roger Cooter's engagement with my work.

Over the years many have enriched this project. I sincerely thank my commissioning editor Lucy Rhymer, and the anonymous referees at Cambridge University Press, for their valuable thoughts and suggestions from which the manuscript benefitted greatly. I feel privileged that Joya Chatterji, Christopher Pinney and Partha Chatterjee very kindly read the doctoral thesis. Their insights and incisive comments have helped me reframe the book. Following a serendipitous encounter at the Department of History and Philosophy of Science in Cambridge, Jim Secord, with his characteristic generosity, guided me through the process of writing this book. My work is richer for having been read by Jim. James Poskett, Jonathan Saha, Kate Nichols, Ruth Jackson and Andrew McKenzie-McHarg have generously read various parts of the manuscript without complaint and have learnt more details about colonial homoeopathy in India than they ever wished to know! Over the last few years, in conferences and beyond, I have had the opportunity to discuss my ideas with scholars at various locations. Needless to say, these enriching experiences have shaped my work considerably. I remain indebted to David Arnold, Moinak Biswas, Dipesh Chakrabarty, Erica Charters, Anirban Das, Faisal Devji, Martin Dinges, Simon Goldhill, Ruth Harris, Mark Harrison, Sarah Hodges, Shruti Kapila, Michael Ledger-Lomas, Madhumita Mazumdar, Harish Naraindas, Eleanor Newbigin, Samiksha Shehrawat, Otto Sibum and Richard Staley for the delightful conversations we have had. I especially thank Simon Schaffer and Sujit Sivasundaram for their intellectual kindness.

Research for this book was carried out in Calcutta and London, at the British Library, Wellcome Library, the West Bengal State Archives, West Bengal Secretariat Library, National Library, Bangiya Sahitya Parishad, Rammohan Library and the archive of the CSSSC. The efficient guidance and assistance I received from the archivists, librarians and staff in these repositories – Asim Mukhopadhyay and Swati Bose at the National Library, Abhijit Bhattacharya and especially Kamalika Mukherjee at the CSSSC – made research much easier. Beyond the realms of these formal archives, informal collections at various familial holdings have proved critical for my research. I thank Amitabha Bhattacharya, Procheta Majumdar, Mahendra Singh and Subhash Singh for their help. Without the amazing support and patience of Durgashankar Bhar my research would not have taken the course it did.

Aspects of this work appeared in the journals *Modern Asian Studies*, 49, 6 (November 2015), *Medical History*, 56, 4 (October 2012) and in *Medical Pluralism in India and Germany*, edited by Martin Dinges (Franz Steiner Verlag, Stuttgart, 2014). I thank the editors and the reviewers for their most helpful suggestions.

I have been privileged to meet with wonderful fellow researchers and academic colleagues, who have enriched me and my work. Between Calcutta, London and Cambridge, I have benefitted greatly from the intellectual companionship of Gareth Atkins, Amelia Bonea, Upal Chakrabarti, Sejuti Dasgupta, Rohit De, Rajarshi Ghose, Cristina Inclan, Bodhisattva Kar, Nayanika Mathur, Ishan Mukherjee, Brian Murray, Kate Nichols, Pratyay Nath, Surabhi Ranganathan, Utsa Ray, Shrimoy Raychaudhari, Sukanya Sarbadhikary, Uditi Sen, Anwesha Sengupta, Partha Pratim Shil, Mishka Sinha and Sanjukta Sunderason. I continue to learn from their commitment to academia and to their own work.

I am obliged to my friends Apurbo Podder and Richard Blakemore for helping me with the crucial electronic formatting of the manuscript that exceeded my expertise. Sumati Dwivedi proofread the penultimate draft and offered crucial editorial suggestions. My friends beyond academia have provided much-needed warmth and refuge when work seemed overwhelming. I thank Sreeparna Chatterjee, Debopriya Basu, Debolina Sen, Banojyotsna Lahiri, Manish Basu and Dwaipayan Bera for being there whenever I reached out.

A work which interrogates the politics of 'family ties' could not, ironically, have been possible without the constant support of my own family. I fondly remember the care and warmth I have received from Sarmila and Pronob Guha since I was a child. I thank Rinki Deb Roy, Pradip Bhowmick, Amitabha and Joyasree Debroy for their unwavering encouragement. My late grandparents Bela Ghosh and Probodh Chandra Ghosh would have been thrilled to see this book in print. I remain grateful to my grandmother, a history teacher herself, for those childhood stories that made knowing the past sound so exciting. In the course of writing this book, it has been a pleasure witnessing my sister Sreecheta metamorphose into an independent woman. It is comforting to know that even as our lives and professional paths diverge, she is there for me as she always was.

My parents have had more faith in me than I ever did myself. Besides being a doting father, Samar Das shared with me his conviction that books were a man's greatest friend, and that words, ideas and art can indeed change the world – Baba, wish you were here. My mother Urmimala Ghosh, a fiercely independent mind, has been my pillar of strength all along – from her I have learnt that beyond every obstacle, there is a new beginning. This book is dedicated to their love.

From the time this project was no more than a set of inchoate ideas in my head, Rohan Deb Roy has walked with me every step of the way as I developed this book. He has inspired, encouraged and criticised me in equal measure – and above all has kept me sane with his humour-laden take on life. Without him, there would not have been a book.

Needless to say, the responsibility for inadequacies and error remains mine alone.

Note on Translation and Transliteration

All translations from Bengali are mine unless otherwise noted.

I have devised and followed my own code of transliteration, keeping in mind that many of the non-English terms mentioned here appear in at least three, if not more, South Asian languages: Bengali, Hindi and Sanskrit. To mark their specificities in words, texts and names of people and places, I have abided by the following general rules:

1. Diacritics have not been used.
2. Non-English terms are italicised and put in quotes when they appear for the first time. Also, a translation is provided following their usage in the main text, following the first appearance. If it is a significant historiographic concept, it is footnoted in its first usage.
3. Names of non-English monographs and articles are translated and provided in the text when they appear first. They are provided in parentheses in the footnote when they only appear in the latter. Further, the translations of non-English monographs are attached with the Bibliography at the end.
4. The final 'a' has been done away with while transliterating Bengali terms, unless it is pronounced; hence, Brihat, Samaj, Paribar and Kayastha, Vaisya, Amiya. However, for widely prevalent terms like ayurveda I have retained the spelling that is used in standard historiography.
5. In general, for the Bengali terms I have followed the standard norms of Sanskrit transliteration and not their phonetic use in Bengali. Thus, Paricharak and not Poricharok, Svasthya and not Swastha, Sahitya and not Sahityo. An exception is made in the use of the term 'swadeshi' and the widely prevalent translation has been retained.
6. For the most part, I have used 'b' instead of 'v' while transliterating Bengali terms; hence Baidya, Bhishak and Byabshayee.
7. In transliterating the names of books that are written in Sanskrit, I have followed the standard rules of Sanskrit transliteration. Hence, *Purana, Mahabharata* and *Ramayana*.

Introduction: 'A Growing Scandal under British Rule'

Families, Market and the Vernacular

Tucked away in a corner of one of the busiest roads of north Calcutta, and distinguished by its colonial-style architecture, stands a rather grand, old, porticoed building. The area, the erstwhile Baithakkhana Bazar in BowBazaar, is now part of the more recently christened Bipin Behary Ganguly Street near Sealdah station. For over a century, this locality has been a traditional hub for myriad commercial activities in the city. Among the jostling crowd of banks, mercantile offices and rows of jewellery shops, the building in question, the headquarters of the Hahnemann Publishing Company (HAPCO), is remarkable for the kind of pharmaceutical commerce it has housed without interruption since the early 1910s. HAPCO is one of the biggest dealers, manufacturers and publishers of homoeopathic medicine in India since the early years of the twentieth century. Its location would not, perhaps, seem strikingly unusual if one recognises the building next door as the premises of Basumati Sahitya Mandir, publishers of the iconic newspaper and magazine *Basumati*. Established in 1881 at Beadon street, *Basumati* shifted its base to Bowbazar in the early twentieth century. *Basumati* regularly carried advertisements for the HAPCO.

Climbing up the narrow, musty staircase of HAPCO, one is ushered into a busy world of medics, booksellers, compounders and clerks, working together in a massive pillared hall decorated with an impressive number of large, greying portraits of European physicians. The final preparation and large-scale packaging of drugs take place in several wings of the building, while across-the-counter sale of drugs and publications is carried out in others. Heavy cartons of medicine are continuously being sent out for shipment across the country. One is immediately struck by the old-world charm of the place, juxtaposed with the inevitable inflections of modernity in the form of computers, huge glass cabinets and other present-day instruments. Once permitted into the inner quarters of the building, one cannot but note its original design as a typically opulent residence of Old Calcutta, with rooms arranged along long verandas, across three storeys and around a quadrangular, cobbled courtyard at the centre. The top floor houses the office of the current proprietor, Dr Durga Shankar Bhar, grandson of HAPCO's founder Prafulla Chandra Bhar and the custodian, among other things, of a substantial private collection of early twentieth-century publications by the firm, primarily in the Bengali language. Arranged systematically but with restricted access for visitors, the collection, for Dr Bhar, is a precious documentation at once of his own family and the history of modern science in Bengal. The interior of the building soon begins to generate a sense of the ways in which cultivation of a vernacular scientific ethos is tied to practices of Bengali commerce. Using homoeopathy as a point of departure, this book explores how medicine, family and markets were interconnected in colonial Bengal.

Homoeopathy, a western medical project originating in eighteenth-century Germany, was reconstituted as vernacular medicine in British Bengal. Conceptualised in opposition to the prevalent notions of 'orthodox' medicine, homoeopathy was a distinct therapeutic ideology popularised since the 1790s in Germany by the reputed physician Friedrich Christian Samuel Hahnemann of Saxony (1755–1843), popularly known as Hahnemann. Put simply, homoeopathy was a novel German therapeutic paradigm that propounded the *Law of Similars* expressed in the Latin phrase *Similia Similibus Curantur* ('like cures like'). According to this *Law*, only those substances could be the cure for any disease, which were capable of producing a similar set of symptoms in a healthy person. Further, for the medications to be most effective, they needed to be administered in miniscule or infinitesimal doses. Borrowing from extant German ideas of *geist* – 'spirit' or vitalism – Hahnemann also developed the theory of 'vital force', which he defined as 'life itself'. Illness was caused by the disruption of the immaterial, spirit-like 'vital force' that animated the human body. How did homoeopathy, so distinctive a philosophy of medicine, endure as a credible genre of scientific medicine among large sections of an alien society in India, despite opposition from the British colonial regime? In mapping the vernacularisation of a western heterodoxy, I analyse the disparate ways in which the historical understanding of homoeopathy and family informed one another in the late nineteenth and early twentieth centuries in Bengal.

Along with phrenology, magnetism, mesmerism, herbalism, hydropathy, naturopathy and chiropractic, homoeopathy was considered a European medical and scientific heterodoxy. The colonial trajectories of these so-called heterodoxies have mostly remained underexplored in histories of the British Empire. So too have their relationships with the intellectual traditions, ideologies and aspirations of the colonised.

Relatively little is known about the colonial careers of these nineteenth-century, sectarian, medico-scientific doctrines, whose status was hotly debated in Europe itself.[1] Of all the so-called European heterodoxies, homoeopathy (along with naturopathy) is now officially recognised as one among the significant 'indigenous' medical systems of India, commanding the second largest government-supported infrastructure after modern biomedicine. Today, along with Ayurveda, Yoga and Naturopathy, Unani and Siddha, Homoeopathy is part of the Department of AYUSH set up by the government of India in 2003 to oversee the modernisation and development of various forms of 'indigenous medicine'.

In addition to being the initial launching ground for colonial rule in India, Bengal witnessed the early advent of a vibrant and enduring print market around the 1850s. The second city of empire for over a hundred years, until 1911, and a growing metropolis of millions, Calcutta witnessed the foundation of the very first western-style Medical College in South Asia. Other early institutions were also established here, such as the Calcutta Medical Physical Society, and the short-lived Native Medical Institution, the latter dedicated primarily to the study of traditional medicine. Leading historians of colonial public health in India have discussed Bengal's importance as the testing ground for many pioneering imperial medical policies and experiments, including dissection and sanitary governance.[2] A recent turn in studying the history of medicine through vernacular sources has established Bengal as a crucial region for interactions between colonial state medicine, and medicine practised by non-government (including indigenous) actors.[3] It is, therefore, a particularly suitable location for the study of colonising

[1] There are a few exceptions where practices such as mesmerism, naturopathy or Christian Science have been studied in the context of colonial South Asia. For an account of mesmerism in British India, see Alison Winter, 'Colonizing Sensations in Victorian India' in *Mesmerized: Powers of Mind in Victorian Britain* (Chicago: University of Chicago Press, 2000), pp. 187–212; and Waltraud Ernst, 'Colonial Psychiatry, Magic and Religion: The Case of Mesmerism in British India', *History of Psychiatry*, 15, 1 (2004), 57–68. For accounts of naturopathy and Christian healing, respectively, see Joseph Alter, *Gandhi's Body: Sex, Diet and Politics of Nationalism* (Philadelphia: University of Pennsylvania Press, 2000), pp. 55–82; and David Hardiman, 'A Subaltern Christianity: Faith Healing in Southern Gujrat' in David Hardiman and Projit Bihari Mukharji (eds.), *Medical Marginality in South Asia: Situating Subaltern Therapeutics* (Abingdon: Routledge, 2012), pp. 126–51.

[2] See David Arnold, *Colonising the Body: State Medicine and Epidemic Disease in Nineteenth-Century India* (Berkeley: University of California Press, 1993); and Mark Harrison, *Public Health in British India: Anglo-Indian Preventive Medicine, 1859–1914* (Cambridge: Cambridge University Press, 1994).

[3] Projit Bihari Mukharji, *Nationalising the Body: The Medical Market, Print and Daktari Medicine* (London and New York: Anthem Press, 2009); Ishita Pande, *Medicine, Race and Liberalism in British Bengal: Symptoms of Empire* (London and New York: Routledge, 2010).

aspects of western medicine, as well as resistance to it. Existing articles on the history of homoeopathy in the Indian subcontinent have acknowledged the early advent, sustained practice and deeply entrenched social ties of homoeopathy in Bengal.[4] Although the earliest known instance of homoeopathic practice in India is believed to be the Transylvanian physician Honigberger's treatment of Raja Ranjit Singh in Punjab in the 1830s,[5] previous authors have unequivocally described Bengal as the 'domicile for homoeopathy' in the nineteenth century, suggesting also that 'from Bengal homoeopathy spread up the Ganges valley'.[6] In the early decades of the nineteenth century, Calcutta was also the home to a number of non-British, European practitioners of homoeopathy. The presence of these practitioners gave a fillip to the practice of homoeopathy in the region, foremost among them Drs Berigny and Tonerre of French origin, Dr Salzer of Vienna and the Transylvanian Dr Honigberger, who moved to Calcutta for some years (after attending Ranjit Singh in Punjab).[7] Bengal remained at the heart of transactions of homoeopathic ideas, texts and people, not only between India and Europe but also between different regions of India.

The arrival of homoeopathy in Bengal, as elsewhere in India, is inextricably related to the colonial expansion of the British Empire since the early nineteenth century. The earliest promoters of homoeopathy were the English missionaries[8] or the 'amateurs, in the civil and military services' of the colonial state.[9] The short-lived Calcutta Native Homoeopathic Hospital of the 1850s furnishes us with tangible evidence for the British amateur and missionary interests in the early propagation of homoeopathy.[10] Established by Major General Sir J. H. Littler, the

[4] S. M. Bhardwaj, 'Homoeopathy in India' in Giri Raj Gupta (ed.), *The Social and Cultural Context of Medicine in India* (Delhi: Vikas Publishing House, 1981), pp. 31–54; and David Arnold and Sumit Sarkar, 'In Search of Rational Remedies: Homoeopathy in Nineteenth-century Bengal' in Waltraud Ernst (ed.), *Plural Medicine, Tradition and Modernity, 1800–2000* (London and New York: Routledge, 2002), pp. 40–1.

[5] J. M. Honigberger, though not a committed homoeopath, is said to have treated Raja Ranjit Singh, the ruler of Punjab, with homoeopathy shortly before his death in 1839. For an account of Honigberger's encounters with Ranjit Singh and the latter's treatment, see S. M. Bhardwaj, 'Homoeopathy in India', pp. 34–6.

[6] S. M. Bhardwaj, 'Homoeopathy in India', pp. 50–1. Also see Gary J. Hausman, 'Making Medicine Indigenous: Homoeopathy in South India', *Social History of Medicine*, 15, 2 (2002), 306.

[7] S. M. Bhardwaj, 'Homoeopathy in India', pp. 36–7.

[8] Instances of Dr Mullens of the London Missionary Society distributing cheap homoeopathic remedies in Bhowanipore can be found in Sarat Chandra Ghose, *Life of Dr. Mahendralal Sircar*, 2nd edition (Calcutta: Hahnemann Publishing Company, 1935), pp. 32–3.

[9] F. C. Skipwith, 'Homoeopathy and Its Introduction into India', *Calcutta Review*, 17 (1852), 52.

[10] S. M. Bhardwaj, 'Homoeopathy in India', p. 33.

hospital was run by English and European doctors. Early Indian patrons of homoeopathy in other parts of India as well, such as the Raja of Tanjore who set up a homoeopathic hospital in the 1840s, did so under the direction and supervision of English physicians. The Tanjore hospital was built under the supervision of a retired English surgeon from Madras, Samuel Brooking.[11] English, moreover, provided vital linguistic mediation in accessing the various currents of European homoeopathic thoughts for the literate Bengali *'bhadralok'* in the nineteenth century.[12] Yet, the historical trajectory of homoeopathy is distinct from the state-imposed, dominant medical practices variously and collectively referred to as 'western medicine', 'imperial medicine', 'colonial medicine', 'allopathy' or 'state medicine'. Especially in the nineteenth century, homoeopathy did not enjoy straightforward legislative patronage, nor overt infrastructural support from the colonial state. A series of regional Medical Registration Acts passed in the 1910s fundamentally questioned the legal status of practitioners of all kinds of non-official medicine. But even prior to these legislations, since the mid-nineteenth century, the state-endorsed apparatus of 'western' medicine – including the pioneering Calcutta Medical College, as well as the British Indian Medical Service – were meticulous in excluding practitioners associated with homoeopathy from their ranks. Although it was not an immediate beneficiary of state support, the history of homoeopathy in India remained deeply entangled with the priorities and prejudices of the colonial state. Homoeopathy featured recurrently in bureaucratic correspondence on the definitions and scope of 'legitimate' and 'scientific' medicine. It figured invariably in colonial anxieties related to medical malpractice, particularly in discussions of 'quackery' or 'corruption' and was

[11] Ibid.

[12] The term *bhadralok*, literally meaning 'respectable people', is a generic term widely used in Bengal to refer to the English-educated, though not necessarily affluent, middling to upper stratum of society. The historical research on the category *bhadralok* has been immense. Works by S. N. Mukherjee and John McGuire suggest that the term *bhadralok* referred both to a class of aristocratic, landed Bengali Hindus and to those of humbler origins. It included men who 'rose from poverty to wealth' in business and occupations involving shipping, indigo plantations and so on, as well as large shopkeepers, retail businessmen and workers in government and commercial houses, teachers, native doctors, journalists and writers. See, for instance, S. N. Mukherjee, *Calcutta: Essays in Urban History* (Calcutta: Subarnarekha, 1993); and John McGuire, *The Making of Colonial Mind: A Quantitative Study of the Bhadralok in Calcutta, 1875–1885* (Canberra: Australian National University, 1983). Also see Joya Chatterji, *Bengal Divided: Hindu Communalism and Partition, 1932–1947* (Cambridge: Cambridge University Press, 1994), pp. 3–13. Referring primarily to the salaried section of this class, Partha Chatterjee calls the *bhadralok* the mediators of nationalist ideologies and politics. See Partha Chatterjee, *The Nation and Its Fragments: Colonial and Postcolonial Histories* (Princeton, NJ: Princeton University Press, 1993), pp. 35–75.

frequently condemned as a 'growing scandal' proliferating within the enlightened British imperial rule.

Despite such anxieties, the relationship between homoeopathy and the colonial state was not one of straightforward governmental denunciation. It was, instead, a more dynamic history of negotiations, derivations and manipulations. Despite the colonial state, homoeopathy endured as a credible genre of 'scientific medicine' among large sections of Bengali literate society since the mid-nineteenth century.[13] Throughout the long nineteenth century, and across Indian society, a plethora of cultural practices proliferated in the name of homoeopathy. These included the consumption of infinitely diluted sweet potions, debating theories of vitalism, translating and reading key German texts, ingesting and experimenting with local vegetation in the hope of preparing home-made drugs, and observing ritualistic codes of moral regimentation in daily life. I map the paradoxical production and dissemination of homoeopathy by large sections of the intelligentsia as an unorthodox European science, peculiarly suited to Indian culture, tradition and constitution. Indeed, homoeopathy was simultaneously heralded by different social groups as a western, rational, progressive science, as well as a faith-based, indigenous spiritual practice; often accused of quackery, and yet upheld as a genre of radical and unorthodox cure; valorised as a symbol of the exotic, and at the same time embraced as a marker of the accessible, everyday and intimate. Because of this uniquely liminal and indeterminate aura, homoeopathy thrived as a ubiquitous ingredient of modernity in colonial and post-colonial India. Recent ethnographic research by Stefan Ecks on drug consumption in post-globalisation Calcutta reconfirms homoeopathy's liminal identity, caught between being simultaneously hypermodern and spiritual.[14]

But how does one write the history of such a liminal category? And how does homoeopathy lend a useful lens through which to study the institution of colonial family? It is impossible to retrace homoeopathy's South Asian trajectory without being sensitive to the question of the colonial archive. Homoeopathic medicine's intimate entanglement with the institution of 'family' in Bengal unfolded before me through a close reading of the (un)available sources. From the official state archives, I could only get fragmented, disorderly, yet suggestive glimpses of homoeopathy's

[13] For a historiographic overview of the complex relation between history of medicine and history of science, which throws light on the evolving understanding and connotations of 'science' with regard to 'medicine', see John Harley Warner, 'History of Science and Sciences of Medicine', *Osiris*, 10 (1995), 164–93.

[14] Stefan Ecks, *Eating Drugs: Psychopharmaceutical Pluralism in India* (New York University Press, 2013), p. 110, 194.

thriving sociocultural past. In the state sources, homoeopathy comes into focus and fades out of them mostly through allegations of rampant malpractice and the consequent governmental concerns of controlling, policing and regulating. Having lost the trail of many interesting archival clues in state repositories, I was reminded of what has been recently described as 'archival aporia' in reference to the relation between the colonial archive, and slippery or uncomfortable categories, such as sexuality.[15] Following conceptualisation of the colonial archives as 'fleeting configurations of epistemological and political anxieties rather than sites of pure erasure or misrepresentations', the elision of homoeopathy from state archives has been read 'along the grain'.[16] In regarding the archive exclusively 'not as a space of knowledge retrieval but (also) as that of knowledge production', I note the indifferent, ambivalent, hesitant and shifting attitude of the state towards homoeopathy over the years.[17]

It is no surprise, then, that in my pursuit of the cultural history of a category that the state archive largely occludes, I was compelled to trace the 'creation of documents and their aggregation into archives as a part of everyday life outside the purview of the state', as suggested by Arjun Appadurai.[18] Since most nineteenth-century sources on Bengali homoeopathy could be traced back to a handful of Bengali publishing houses, by concentrating on them, I was able to uncover an extremely rich repository of sources retained by a range of north Calcutta-based commercial houses deeply involved in the business of homoeopathy. While some have ceased to operate (such as Berigny and Company, M. Bhattacharya and Company and B. K. Pal and Company), a handful of these, particularly the Hahnemann Publishing Company and Majumdar's Homoeopathic Pharmacy, which now operates as a drug-chain named J. N. M. Homoeo Sadan, are still functional. These firms maintain a (mostly disorderly) collection of their published resources. Interviewing the present descendants-cum-owners of these commercial houses proved rewarding. Even the current descendants of the erstwhile concerns like M. Bhattacharya and Company, which was sold off as recently as 2009 to corporate giant Emami, could contribute generously to my research by sharing anecdotes, memories and publications of their former 'family business'. Together, they revealed a whole world of family archives: a network of north

[15] Anjali Arondekar, *For the Record: On Sexuality and the Colonial Archive in India* (Durham: Duke University Press, 2009), pp. 1–3.

[16] Ann Laura Stoler, *Along the Archival Grain: Epistemic Anxieties and Colonial Common Sense* (Princeton, NJ: Princeton University Press, 2010), pp. 1–17.

[17] Ann Laura Stoler, 'Colonial Archives and the Art of Governance', *Archival Science*, 2, 1–2 (2002), 87.

[18] Arjun Appadurai, 'Archive and Aspiration' in Joke Brouwer and Arjen Mulder (eds.), *Information Is Alive* (Rotterdam: V2 Publishing/NAI Publishers, 2003), p. 16.

Calcutta-based Bengali homoeopathic entrepreneurs in conversation as much with the depths of Bengali *'mofussil'*, the interiors of urban middle-class domesticity, as with European medico-scientific journals.[19] More than performing an 'extractive function', such unique archival spaces appeared as 'ethnographic sites' that fundamentally shaped my research.[20] The very survival and availability of a plethora of materials signify the power of such familial archives as 'an aspiration rather than a recollection'[21] – as the 'material site of a collective will to remember'.[22] The vital leads provided by the family archives were then systematically followed up, and complemented with research at the more predictable vernacular and English language repositories in Kolkata and in London. Apart from the relatively 'respectable' English or Bengali language health journals, there was a vast repertoire of manuals and cheap tracts, even of the *'Battala'* genre, that discussed homoeopathy and indicated its wide dissemination.[23]

These different kinds of texts, especially those published by the familial firms, imagined an idealised social constituency for Bengali homoeopathy. The desired social base was chiefly the middle to upper class, Hindu, primarily urban, literate classes, including women. While highlighting homoeopathy's urban stronghold, publications, particularly in the form of advertisements, also illustrated its reach beyond the bigger cities of Calcutta, Dacca, Chattagram or Patna. Indeed, advertisements by leading family firms often insisted on a large-scale circulation of drugs and texts into the depths of rural Bengal. Numerous villages and especially *mofussil* locations feature in urban discussions as spaces in need of homoeopathic benevolence, and where homoeopathy was in high demand. Places like Bankipore, Khagra, Murshidabad, Bhagolpur, Burdwan, Ranaghat, Munger and others surfaced regularly in advertisements, indicating a robust circulation of homoeopathy in households and dispensaries beyond the urban enclaves. By the early years of the twentieth

[19] The term *mofussil* originates from the Urdu ('mufassil', variant of 'mufassal', meaning 'divided'). In Indian historiography, it is widely used as a term relating to the suburban areas. It broadly referred to the regions of British India outside the three East India Company capitals of Bombay, Calcutta and Madras; hence, parts of a country outside an urban centre. It is believed to sometimes carry a negative resonance.

[20] Ann Laura Stoler, 'Colonial Archives and the Art of Governance', p. 87.

[21] Arjun Appadurai, 'Archive and Aspiration', p. 16. [22] Ibid., p. 17.

[23] *Battala*: a commercial name originating from a giant banyan tree in the Shovabazar and Chitpur area of Calcutta, where the printing and publication industry of Bengal began in the nineteenth century. Though it was increasingly ridiculed by the rising literary gentry for its questionable taste and production quality, *Battala* literature managed to survive in the publication industry until the end of the nineteenth century. A number of scholars have written on the history, productions and impact of the *Battala* publications. For an exhaustive history of *Battala*, see Sripantha, *Battala* (Calcutta: Ananda, 1997). For the most recent exploration of *Battala* print culture, see Gautam Bhadra, *Nyara Battalay Jay Kawbar* (Kolkata: Chhatim Books, 2011).

century, amateur lower-class practitioners in the *mofussil*, peddling poorly produced homoeopathic texts, appear as a cause of concern for reputed Calcutta-based homoeopathic firms. Beyond the records of the Calcutta firms, I also note the spurt of growth in homoeopathic dispensaries across the Bengal countryside, beginning in the 1920s. Dispensaries were usually charitable institutions built through the philanthropic efforts of the state or of the local elites to provide cheap medicine to the masses. A recent work has shown that, despite the Hindu, upper-caste background of most of the practitioners, the clientele of dispensaries in Bengal belonged to diverse social and religious groups including those described as Muslims or tribals, as well as members of the 'lower orders'.[24]

Perusal of the family archive further reveals a set of entrenched cultural and moral foundations that defined homoeopathy and made it popular in Bengal. It was claimed that homoeopathy offered cheap therapeutics (in terms of cost of drugs, homoeopathic publications and physician's fees), which made it accessible even to the financially disadvantaged. Besides, the principle of infinitesimal doses and the gentle nature of the homoeopathic drugs also helped homoeopathy claim a sharp contrast to some intrusive nineteenth-century allopathic procedures, such as blistering, leeching, bleeding and cauterising. But the most persistent feature that cries out of the archive is homoeopathy's promise to promote self-help, to ensure ordinary Indian householders and lay people became autodidacts, capable of administering western medicine. By claiming that homoeopathy was a cheap, affordable, gentle and painless mode of therapeutics that could be mastered by ordinary men and women, its advocates implicitly promoted a distinct vision of egalitarian medicine beyond the growing strictures of western professionalisation. Furthermore, along with committing themselves to the treatment of imperial public health categories and epidemic diseases (such as cholera, malaria, plague, smallpox and venereal diseases), homoeopaths pledged that they were able to heal even quotidian, individualised and chronic ailments. Indeed, Bengali publications indicate that individualised, symptom-based treatment of each patient was a prominent homoeopathic motto, apparently derived from Hahnemann's dictum to 'treat the patient, not the disease'. This even offered a new mode for treating public health categories, like smallpox or cholera, through self-medication.

[24] Projit Bihari Mukharji, 'Structuring Plurality: Locality, Caste, Class and Ethnicity in Nineteenth Century Bengali Dispensaries', *Health and History*, 9, 1 (2007), 99–101.

As I draw attention to the value of these colonial family archives, I focus on the intricate, double-edged interface between medicine and family in Bengal. On the one hand, the homoeopathic firms, as family businesses, recurrently projected a distinctive business ideology in the rich corpus of materials they published. The extensive body of journals, manuals, advertisements, pamphlets, monographs, letters and biographies published by these concerns reveals a specific business culture which was promoted around homoeopathy. Asserting their own familial, intergenerational presence, the protagonists of these concerns self-consciously encouraged their business, and indeed the homoeopathic profession itself, to thrive upon informal networks of friendship, kinship and affect. Their entrepreneurial practices prescribed a deliberate overlap between their business ethics, and the familial virtues of intimacy and paternalism. Modelling 'enterprise' on 'family', they emphasised the cultivation of wilful permeable boundaries between the realms of the familial and the entrepreneurial, and between the private and the public, in ensuring homoeopathy's proliferation. Professional relations, too, were understood through the metaphor of family. At the same time, intergenerational, patriarchal lines of inheritance were carefully marked out.

On the other hand, beyond the commercial operations, family was also written about as the quintessential locus where homoeopathy was to be preached, practised and eventually (re)produced. Homoeopathy came to be posited as an efficient disciplining mechanism to cure colonial domesticity of its various ills – even as a remedy to revitalise the foundations of the ailing Indian joint-family system. Beyond the mere materiality of drugs, homoeopathic science was projected and perceived as a way of living, capable of producing the ideal family for the nation. Thus, families acted both as the agent and the site that produced, nurtured and sustained homoeopathy. Rather than understanding 'family' as an unchanging and given entity, this work is sensitive to the diverse interests, commercial, cultural and ideological that shaped the notion of ideal family over the colonial period.

A focus on the Bengali entrepreneur families, and especially their family archives, has enabled my examination of the histories of institutionalisation beyond the immediate patronage from the state. The concept of 'alternative' medicine is revisited here, as I have distanced myself from studies that depict homoeopathy, or any other apparently non-state medical idea, as always and already 'alternative'.[25] I have drawn on the works

[25] Scholars often label homoeopathy an 'alternative' practice without adequately problematising such acts of labelling. See, for instance, Ursula Sharma, 'Contextualising Alternative Medicine: The Exotic, the Marginal and the Perfectly Mundane',

of scholars such as Roberta Bivins, who insists that labels such as 'alternative' and 'mainstream' be historically nuanced – that their mutual relationship be understood as relative, evolving and contextual.[26] Strict delineations between such labels, Bivins contends, often emanate from a decidedly 'western and twenty-first century perspective' and are guilty of 'engendering a view distinctly orthodox-medico-centric'. Moreover, recent histories have urged us to be more attentive to the newer meanings of 'orthodoxy' and 'alternative' in relation to colonial power dynamics. They point out that as much as colonial medicine was bolstered by notions of enlightenment science, it was, nonetheless, resisted and contested at several quarters in the colonies.[27] Thus, the understandings inherent in expressions such as 'alternative', 'scientific medicine', 'quackery', 'legitimate medicine' and 'medical registration' with regard to homoeopathy in colonial Bengal were shifting and ambiguous. While exploring the makings of 'scientific' medicine at different moments and contexts, especially with relation to colonial law, this work also distances itself from histories that investigate and debate the 'real' scientific merits of homoeopathy.[28] Rather than assuming an already marginalised status for homoeopathy, my work traces the resilience of the category in various registers, especially in the colonial family archives, beyond the official state repositories.

Vernacular Medicine in Colonial India explores the interactions between Calcutta-based homoeopathic family firms, sporadically dispersed rural/*mofussil* practitioners, the British colonial state and the emergent nationalist governments, to study the cultural production of homoeopathy as a 'vernacular science' in Bengal primarily between 1866 and 1941. The

Anthropology Today, 9, 4 (1993), 15–18. For a more sophisticated and historically grounded reading of homoeopathy, which nonetheless recognises its alternative status, see Naomi Rogers, *An Alternative Path: The Making and Remaking of the Hahnemann Medical College and Hospital of Philadelphia* (New Brunswick, NJ: Rutgers University Press, 1998).

[26] Roberta Bivins, *Alternative Medicine? A History* (Oxford and New York: Oxford University Press, 2007), p. 4, 38.

[27] Ibid., p. 30, 36. The contested and limited reach of western orthodoxy has been highlighted and discussed by several prominent scholars of South Asian history. See, for instance, David Arnold, *Colonising the Body: State Medicine and Epidemic Disease in Nineteenth Century India* (Berkeley: University of California Press, 1993), pp. 3–4, 61–115.

[28] H. L. Coulter, *Homoeopathic Science and Modern Medicine: The Physics of Healing with Microdoses* (Berkeley: North Atlantic Books, 1981). See also by the same author, Divided Legacy Vol III: The Conflict between Homoeopathy and the American Medical Association: Science and Ethics in American Medicine: 1800–1900 (Berkeley: North Atlantic Books, 1982); Peter W. Gold, S. Novella, R. Roy, I. Bell, N. Davidovitch, A. Saine, 'Homoeopathy – Quackery or a Key to the Future of Medicine?', *Homoeopathy*, 97 (2008), 28–33.

first private family firm, Berigny and Company's Calcutta Homoeopathic Pharmacy, was established in 1866. In 1941, under the imperatives of regional nationalist political parties, homoeopathy was formally legitimised as 'scientific medicine' and the State Faculty of Homoeopathic Medicine was established. This complex narrative of homoeopathy's vernacularisation has been woven around three central issues: the family, the market and the vernacular. The interactions between these three themes have been explored over five chapters, which examine in turn homoeopathic business practices (Chapter 1), medical biographies (Chapter 2), popular scientific translations (Chapter 3), quotidian health management (Chapter 4) and familial negotiation with colonial law (Chapter 5).

Homoeopathy and the South Asian Family

Commentators on bourgeoisie modernity have awakened us to the centrality of family in the making of modern regimes of power. The category 'family' has been identified as singularly fundamental to the operations of the modern state, indeed as one of its foundational 'ideological apparatuses'.[29] In his seminal 1971 essay, Louis Althusser identified such state apparatuses as crucial to governance, since in them 'the ruling ideology is heavily concentrated'.[30] Ensuring 'governance without the direct intervention of law', an apparatus such as the 'family' was shown to be crucial in producing 'willing compliance' in the 'reproduction of the existing relations of production'.[31] For Foucault too, as his lectures from the 1970s make clear, the apprehension of population as an entity in modern social order had the effect of transforming the significance of the family from serving as a model or analogy of the state to a 'privileged instrument for the government of the population'.[32] In modern regimes of power, 'family' was rendered the crucial 'segment' through which population could be accessed, regulated or, most importantly, disciplined. It contributed to the process of the modern state's imperatives of 'constitution of a *savoir* of government' that was 'inseparable from that of a knowledge of all the processes related to population in its larger sense'.[33] Gilles Deleuze

[29] Louis Althusser, 'Ideology and Ideological State Apparatuses', *Lenin and Philosophy, and Other Essays*, Trans. Ben Brewster (London: New Left Books, 1971), p. 127.
[30] Ibid., p. 150. [31] Ibid., pp. 153–7.
[32] Michel Foucault, 'Governmentality' in Graham Burchell, Colin Gordon and Peter Miller (eds.), *The Foucault Effect: Studies in Governmentality* (Chicago: University of Chicago Press, 1991), p. 100.
[33] Ibid., pp. 100–1.

and Felix Guattari's *Anti Oedipus* too, received wide attention for its criticisms of the bourgeois family.[34] Arguing that the structures of the modern nuclear family and that of the capitalist economy mirror one another, the book suggests how the nuclear family accepted and even relished capitalist social relations.[35] From this perspective, family is the agent of capitalist production and social oppression.

To unpack the role of family in modern society, some of these thinkers have further highlighted the significance of understanding it as a historically mutating institution. Scholarship on the Foucauldian analysis of family note that Foucault's purpose was to emphasise the genealogy of family, and to undermine 'any all-encompassing or transhistorical account of the institution'; to contest its status as a 'quasi natural formation or a bedrock of unassailable values'.[36] Following Foucault, and especially his thoughts on family in his lectures on 'Psychiatric Power' and in the *History of Sexuality*, these works contend that as with Foucault's genealogy of the psychiatric hospital or the prison, his thoughts on the family should also be read as revealing family's novelty and contingency, and most importantly its formation through power struggles. They argue for 'family' to be treated as a continuously contested fiction that masks its own becoming, pointing out that historical scholarship should reveal the constructed and political nature of familial institutions and its abiding and shifting investments in various power relations.

Since the 1990s, these two strands of conceptual understandings – the disciplinary role of family and the genealogical understanding of family – have informed several colonial histories, especially those exploring the power of colonial state and its politics of knowledge production and control. In his influential book, Bernard Cohn initiated discussions on a number of variegated modalities through which the colonial state established its cultural hegemony and political control.[37] In contrast to the 'brutal and spectacular' operations of the state, these 'cultural technologies of rule'[38] included the investigative modality, historiographic modality, observational/travel modality, survey modality, enumerative

[34] See Ian Buchanan and Adrian Parr (eds.), *Deleuze and the Contemporary World* (Edinburgh: Edinburgh University Press, 2006), p. 161–163. Also see Timothy Laurie, Hannah Stark, 'Reconsidering Kinship: Beyond the Nuclear Family with Deleuze and Guattari', *Cultural Studies Review*, 18,1 (2012), 19–39.
[35] Ibid.
[36] See Chloe Taylor, 'Foucault and Familial Power', *Hypatia: A Journal of Feminist Philosophy*, 27,1 (2012), 201–17. See also Leon Rocha and Robbie Duschinsky (eds.), *Foucault, the Family and Politics* (Basingstoke: Palgrave Macmillan, 2012), pp. 19–38.
[37] Bernard Cohn, *Colonialism and Its Forms of Knowledge: The British in India* (Princeton, NJ: Princeton University Press, 2002).
[38] Nicholas B. Dirks, 'Foreword' in Bernard Cohn, *Colonialism and Its Forms of Knowledge*, p. ix.

modality, museology modality as well as a surveillance modality.[39] It has been amply demonstrated how familial practices of the colonised people remained central to such 'ethnographic knowledge of the colonial state'.[40] Ann Laura Stoler's *Carnal Knowledge and Imperial Power: Race and the Intimate in Colonial Rule* demonstrates the extent to which the 'intimate' was a recurrent concern for the European colonial administration in Indonesia.[41] Examining not just sexual relations, but also 'parenting, pedagogy, and paternalism', her work conclusively shows how 'the microsites of familial and intimate space'[42] were related to the macro-political spaces of colonial governance.[43] My own account of embodied practices of homoeopathy as tools for corporeal and moral regulation of domesticity aims to contribute to the literature analysing what has been described as the 'medico-familial mesh'.[44]

The other conceptual parameter, that of exploring the genealogy of family, has also inspired significant scholarship that has commented on the making of the colonial family. Depending on the difference of their approaches, these works on the making of the colonial family can be classified into distinct strands of historiographic interventions. The first of these strands, heavily dominated by scholars writing on Bengal, has looked at the 'ideological deployment of the family ... in the politics of nation-building'.[45] In conceptualising colonial modernity, these historians critically analyse the ways in which 'family' or 'home' attained a 'special compensatory significance in the modernity that Indian

[39] Bernard Cohn, *Colonialism and Its Forms of Knowledge*, pp. 5–11.
[40] Nicholas B. Dirks, 'Foreword', p. ix. Also see, Bernard Cohn and Nicholas B. Dirks, 'Beyond the Fringe: The Nation State, Colonialism, and the Technologies of Power', *Journal of Historical Sociology*, 1, 2 (June 1988), 224–9.
[41] Ann Laura Stoler, *Carnal Knowledge and Imperial Power: Race and the Intimate in Colonial Rule* (Berkeley: University of California Press, 2002).
[42] Ibid., p. 19.
[43] For a recent work that studies such relation between colonial governance and the intimate and the familial also see Kathleen Wilson, 'Re-thinking the Colonial State: Family, Gender and Governmentality in Eighteenth Century British Frontiers', *American Historical Review*, 116, 5 (2011), 1294–322. For a discussion of sociocultural surveillance by the colonial state over domesticity, sexuality, morality and reproduction in British India, see Sarah Hodges, *Reproductive Health in India: History, Politics, Controversies* (Hyderabad: Orient Longman, 2006); Charu Gupta, *Sexuality, Obscenity and Community: Women, Muslims and the Hindu Public in Colonial India* (Delhi: Permanent Black, 2005); and Srirupa Prasad, *Cultural Politics of Hygiene in India, 1850–1940: Contagions of Feeling* (Basingstoke: Palgrave Macmillan, 2015).
[44] Foucault refers to the term in the context of medicalisation of families. See Leon Rocha and Robbie Duschinsky (eds.), *Foucault, the Family and Politics*, pp. 19–38.
[45] The phrase is used by Indrani Chatterjee in referring to the historiographic trend that analysed the politics of the nationalist envisioning of family. See Indrani Chatterjee (ed.), *Unfamiliar Relations: Family and History in South Asia* (New Brunswick: Rutgers University Press, 2004), pp. 4–5.

nationalists experienced in the context of imperial domination'.[46] Reflecting on the Bengali valorisation of 'home' (*griha*) and 'women' (*grihalakshmi*), Partha Chatterjee, Tanika Sarkar, Dipesh Chartabarty and Sumit Sarkar have analysed the nationalist discourse around Bengali domesticities as sites of 'reform', 'recluse' and as a 'spiritual domain', in terms of either patriarchy or capitalism or both.[47] I have traced the recurrent interventions of authors advocating homoeopathy in the nationalist literatures on Bengali domesticity. Homoeopathy was projected not only as a form of medicine, but also an ethical and moral regimen of Hindu life, capable of producing ideal, self-sufficient, nationalism-inspired domesticities, specifically in the form of Hindu joint families.

Another distinct set of South Asian studies on 'family' questions, problematises and breaks away from the very assumption of family as a rigid, enclosed and private domain.[48] These scholars have demarcated the 'simple conjugal family' as a historically contingent 'site of desire' – more of a nationalist male aspiration than a reality.[49] Committed to the idea that 'family needs to be historicized and understood within an embedded set of local practices', these works focus on the potentially fluid structures or contours of the institution over time, and on the traffics between notions of the household, family, public and private relations. The blurred and flexible boundaries of 'family' were constituted through the frequently intersecting lens of law, labour (servants, dependants, prostitutes), sexuality and governance.[50] Through explorations into the business ethics of the family-based homoeopathic concerns, I trace the

46 Dipesh Chakrabarty, 'Family, Fraternity, Salaried Labor' in *Provincializing Europe: Postcolonial Thought and Historical Difference* (Princeton, NJ: Princeton University Press, 2000), p. 215.

47 See Partha Chatterjee, 'Nationalist Resolution of the Women's Question' in Kumkum Sangari and Sudesh Vaid, (eds.), *Recasting Woman: Essays in Indian Colonial History* (New Brunswick, NJ: Rutgers University Press, 1989), pp. 233–53; Tanika Sarkar, 'The Hindu Wife and the Hindu Nation: Domesticity and Nationalism in Nineteenth Century Bengal', *Studies in History*, 8, 2 (1992), 224; Dipesh Chakrabarty, 'Difference-Deferral of (A) Colonial Modernity: Public Debates on Domesticity in British Bengal', *History Workshop Journal*, 36, 1 (1993), 1–34; Sumit Sarkar, 'Kaliyuga, Chakri, and Bhakti: Ramakrishna and His Times', *Economic and Political Weekly*, 27, 29 (18 July 1992), 1549–50.

48 Indrani Chatterjee (ed.), *Unfamiliar Relations: Family and History in South Asia*, 2004, pp. 3–45.

49 Ibid., p. 5.

50 See Indrani Chatterjee, 'Gossip, Taboo and Writing Family History' in Indrani Chatterjee (ed.) *Unfamiliar Relations*, pp. 222–60; Durba Ghosh, *Sex and the Family in Colonial India: The Making of Empire* (Cambridge: Cambridge University Press, 2006); Bhawani Raman, 'The Familial World of the Company's Kacceri in Early Colonial Madras', *Journal of Colonialism and Colonial History*, 9, 2 (2008), www.muse.jhu.edu/article/246576 (last accessed 11 August 2018); Swapna Banerjee, *Men, Women and*

consistent invocation of the metaphor of 'family' in organising business as well as professional relations. I thereby map the importance attached by homoeopathic entrepreneurs to a flexible, commodious understanding of business, akin to an extended family bound by paternalistic ties of affection, trust and loyalty.

Others have also examined the gradual delineation of 'family', under colonialism, into a rigidly defined economic unit. Exploring the intersections of law, marriage, inheritance, property and economy, these works explore the crystallisation of family as a normative property-holding unit in the face of colonial legal interventions.[51] Historians working specifically with the archive of law have been underlining how the personal law privileged certain male patriarchal relations within the joint family by making distinctions between 'inheritance' and 'maintenance'.[52] Several of these works have studied the colonial rigidification of notions of the Hindu joint family as based solely on male descent and inheritance, which can be contrasted with earlier practices of a more loosely and eclectically organised Indian extended family. These burgeoning studies together are illuminating the patriarchal, hierarchical and authoritative nature of the Hindu family.

Domestics: Articulating Middle-Class Identity in Colonial India (Delhi and New York: Oxford University Press, 2006). Moreover, with their emphasis on the fluidities of structures and experiences, these studies further speak to some of the concerns raised with regards to transcontinental experiences of families from the perspective of 'new imperialist histories'. See Elizabeth Buettner, *Empire Families: Britons and Late Imperial India* (New York: Oxford University Press, 2004); and Esme Cleall, Laura Ishiguro and Emily Manktelow (eds.), 'Imperial Relations: Histories of Family in the British Empire', *Journal of Colonialism and Colonial History*, 14, 1 (2013), www.muse.jhu.edu/article/503247 (last accessed 11 August 2018).

51 Malavika Kasturi, *Embattled Identities: Rajput Lineages and the Colonial State in Nineteenth Century North India* (Delhi: Oxford University Press, 2002); Rachel Sturman, 'Property and Attachments: Defining Autonomy and the Claims of Family in Nineteenth Century Western India', *Comparative Studies in Society and History*, 47, 3 (2005), 611–37; Radhika Singha, 'Making the Domestic more Domestic: Colonial Criminal Law and the Head of the Household, 1772–1843', *Indian Economic and Social History Review*, 33, 3 (1996), 309–43.

52 See, for instance, Leigh Denault, 'Partition and the Politics of the Joint Family in Nineteenth-Century North India', *Indian Economic and Social History Review*, 46, 1 (2009), 27–55; Rachel Sturman, *Government of Social Life in Colonial India: Liberalism, Religious Law and Women's Rights* (Cambridge: Cambridge University Press, 2012); Rochona Majumdar, *Marriage and Modernity: Family Values in Colonial Bengal* (Durham: Duke University Press, 2009); Eleanor Newbigin, *The Hindu Family and the Emergence of Modern India: Law, Citizenship and Community* (Cambridge: Cambridge University Press, 2013); Mytheli Sreenivas, 'Conjugality and Capital: Gender, Families, and Property under Colonial Law in India', *Journal of Asian Studies*, 63, 4 (2004), 937–60; and Narendra Subramanian, *Nation and Family: Personal Law, Cultural Pluralism and Gendered Citizenship in India* (Stanford University Press, 2014).

Focusing on economic and entrepreneurial practices concerning families, some of these scholars are particularly committed to the study of the political economy of family and its constitution through intimate ties between the 'commercial' and the 'domestic'. In a recent exploration of such history, Ritu Birla has investigated the unique kinship-based operations of the Marwari 'family firms' and their governance in colonial India through a special Anglo-Indian legal construct, the Hindu Undivided Family (HUF).[53] Birla adds to the 'new research on the historical meanings of family in India' by addressing a significant discourse on the joint family, 'one emerging not in debates on domesticity, but in an archive of economy'.[54] C. A. Bayly's work on the transition of north Indian society in the late eighteenth century also studied, in considerable depth, north Indian merchant families.[55] Dwelling on the central roles of caste, religion, right marriage, piety and credit in the operations of these intermediary merchant households in their 'profit making enterprise', Bayly hinted at the role of these 'family firms' in the contemporary formations of Hindu families.[56] Beyond South Asia, resonances of this approach can be found in the significant work of Catherine Hall, who analysed the makings of familial values through a close study of Victorian business families in England.[57] Taken together, these works seek to foreground the role of capital (in most cases mercantile capital) in constituting and conceptualising familial practices, ethos and values. Similarly, the familial investments and operations of the homoeopathic commercial concerns I study here negotiated with law in asserting the legitimacy of homoeopathic medicine in Bengal. A traffic between entrepreneurial ethos and familial values enabled the discursive constitution of rigidly patrilineal Hindu families.

Bringing each of these various strands of research into conversation with one another, this book offers the following contributions to the historiography of the South Asian family. First, the homoeopathic archive reveals a number of distinct understandings of family and its functions.

[53] Ritu Birla, *Stages of Capital: Law, Culture and Market Governance in Late Colonial India* (Durham: Duke University Press, 2009).

[54] Ibid., p. 15.

[55] Christopher Bayly, *Rulers, Townsmen and Bazaars: North Indian Society in the Age of British Expansion, 1770–1870* (Cambridge: Cambridge University Press, 1983). The introduction to this book makes it clear that a third level of argument for the book is to study the 'view of the north Indian merchant family and the trading institutions from the inside. The aim is to show how economic organization was inseparable from the family firm's identity as a body of pious and credit worthy Hindus', p. 8.

[56] Ibid., see particularly the chapter on 'Merchant Family as Business Enterprise', pp. 394–426.

[57] Catherine Hall and Leonore Davidoff, *Family Fortunes: Men and Women of the English Middle Class, 1780–1850* (Chicago: University of Chicago Press, 1987).

There was the vision of an idealised, romanticised joint family for the nation nurtured through nationalistic aspirations of reform, harmony and spiritualism. Joint families were imagined to be selfless, affective, capacious and paternalistic spaces that were based on multiple and heterogeneous kinship networks. The family firms, which modelled themselves on the joint family, represented a flexible, commerce-based kinship network loosely organised around the metaphor of an extended family reliant on alliance, loyalty and affection beyond immediate blood relations. At the same time, there coexisted more nucleated families headed by the protagonists of the family firms, which thrived on rigid patrilineal ideas of male descent and inheritance.

Second, this coexistence (of the idealised joint family, the firms modelled on joint families and the nucleated family of the owners of family firms) complicates any narrative of simple, linear and seamless transition from joint family to nuclear family engendered by colonial modernity. There is an element of irony in the same groups of men simultaneously mythifying an egalitarian joint-family ideal, and also adhering to emerging notions of strict patrilineal descent. Indeed, the romantic ideal of the selfless, egalitarian Hindu joint-family was being celebrated in popular print at the precise historical moment that the significance of individual male authority in the joint-family system was being asserted. Often the same group of men, like the entrepreneur-physicians discussed here, ended up advocating the egalitarian joint-family ideal, as well as the nucleated family based on patrilineal descent. A close focus on the patriarchal, inheritance-based operations of the family firm reveals the ways in which colonial family was increasingly animated by sovereign notions of power symbolised by individuation of power at the top.[58]

Finally, the disciplinary function of the colonial family is also highlighted in the ways in which homoeopathy was posited as an embodied ideal for regulating everyday domestic corporeal practices. Thus, with a focus simultaneously on the commercial operations of family firms, as well as the ideological valorisation of Indian family, this study uses the history of homoeopathy to demonstrate family as one of the enduring sites where the disciplinary as well as the sovereign, repressive as well as reproductive notions of power converge. It reveals both the disciplinary functions of family, as well as some of the historical processes involved in the making of the colonial Bengali family.

[58] Chloe Taylor makes this analysis following upon Foucault's lectures on 'Psychiatric Power'. Taylor demonstrates an irony in these lectures: while Foucault so often argued that we theorise power as sovereign when in fact it is disciplinary, in the case of family he makes the reverse claim: we think of family as disciplinary, when it is actually sovereign. See Chloe Taylor, 'Foucault and Familial Power', pp. 203–5.

Family in Bengal could simultaneously pose as the agent producing and disseminating homoeopathy, and as the site where this so-called European heterodoxy was best nurtured and preserved. The category 'family' with its multiple connotations could constitute an institution capable of sustaining a burgeoning science over a period of time. Through their sustained investments in print, drug, pedagogy and knowledge, families could indeed provide the institutional refuge to a fledgling science along with or perhaps ahead of colleges, hospitals or formal associations.

Swadeshi Homoeopathy and the Market

Closely connected with the theme of family business is the question of medical marketplaces. The distinct archiving of Bengali homoeopathy by the Bengali entrepreneur families, their investments and leading role in publications, the large-scale networks of drug distribution, the range of homoeopathic domestic health manuals as well as the intermittent interventions by the imperial state together indicate a conspicuous market for homoeopathy engendered by familial commerce. Studies on 'medical marketplaces' have proliferated since the 1980s, especially in relation to the role and position of non-orthodox health practices within a society.[59] Ever since the concept was floated in the 1980s by Roy Porter and Harold Cook to make sense of preprofessional medicine,[60] the idea of 'medical markets' has been analysed and reinterpreted from various perspectives, whether in relation to historicising the patient or the role of commerce in history of medicine, or in relation to the identity of non-orthodox, indigenous medicine.[61] In their edited volume on the theme of medical markets, Mark Jenner and Patrick Wallis express regret that the term is being slowly reduced to a descriptive commonplace, and propose that it

[59] For a critical overview of this topic, see Mark Jenner and Patrick Wallis (eds.), *Medicine and the Market in England and Its Colonies, c. 1450–c. 1850* (Basingstoke: Palgrave Macmillan, 2007).

[60] Roy Porter, 'The Patient's View: Doing Medical History from Below', Theory and Society, 14 (1985), 188; by the same author, *Health for Sale: Quackery in England, 1660–1850* (Manchester: Manchester University Press, 1989); and Harold Cook, *The Decline of the Old Medical Regime in Stuart London* (Ithaca: Cornell University Press, 1986).

[61] Pratik Chakrabarti, 'Medical Marketplaces Beyond the West: Bazaar Medicine, Trade and the English Establishment in Eighteenth Century India' in Mark Jenner and Patrick Wallis (eds.), *Medicine and the Market in England and Its Colonies, c. 1450–c. 1850*, pp. 196–215; Maarten Bode, *Taking Traditional Knowledge to Market: the Modern Image of the Ayurvedic and Unani Industry, 1980–2000* (Hyderabad: Orient Longman, 2008); and Madhulika Banerjee, *Power, Knowledge, Medicine: Ayurvedic Pharmaceuticals at Home and in the World* (Hyderabad: Orient Blackswan, 2009).

needs renewed scholarship for specific contexts. They have argued against any 'generalized image of the medical market or medical marketplace' and have urged scholars to begin thinking in terms of markets involving particular 'medical goods and services'.[62] Developing on Jenner and Wallis' contention, historians of South Asia have more recently cautioned against the egalitarian image of plurality and harmonious coexistence that is often projected onto the notion of 'medical marketplace', and have instead alerted us to the hierarchies and power inherent in the medical market.[63]

Building upon these insights, I have studied the discursive constitution of a discrete market involving homoeopathic boxes, drugs, manuals, journals and medical biographies in Bengal. The result of my explorations brings to life a vivid cultural history of Bengali commercial enterprise beginning in the late nineteenth century. In comparison with the early nineteenth century's 'age of enterprise' and the early twentieth century beginnings of *swadeshi*-inspired native business ventures, sporadic commercial endeavours in late nineteenth-century Bengal have mostly escaped historical attention.[64] Indeed, important social and intellectual histories of the Bengali *bhadralok* have emphatically highlighted the landed rentier interests, along with Bengali obsessions with *chakri* or salaried jobs as markers of education and culture. It has been observed that these trends were opposed to the development of any sustained Bengali commercial industry in this period.[65] In contrast, the multitude of homoeopathic business firms, which this work studies, marks this same period as part of the development of Bengali entrepreneurial commerce. While other scholars have talked about an 'ideology of education' that animated the *bhadralok* in this period, I explore the thoughts and practices of a distinct group of entrepreneur-physicians about an 'ideology of wealth' accumulated through enterprise, which encompassed ideas of respectability, national self-sufficiency as well as scientific progress.[66]

62 Mark Jenner and Patrick Wallis (eds.), *Medicine and the Market in England and Its Colonies, c. 1450–c. 1850*, p. 16.

63 See Projit Bihari Mukarji and David Hardiman (eds.), *Medical Marginality in South Asia: Situating Subaltern Therapeutics*, 2012, pp. 28–30. Also see Waltraud Ernst, *Plural Medicine, Tradition and Modernity, 1800–2000*, 2002, p. 4–5.

64 Shekhar Bandopadhyay (ed.), *Bengal: Rethinking History: Essays in Historiography* (Delhi: Manohar Publishers, 2001), pp. 18–19.

65 See, for instance, Tithi Bhattacharya, *Sentinels of Culture: Class, Education and the Colonial Intellectual in Bengal* (New York: Oxford University Press, 2005), pp. 28–30, 42–55; Sumit Sarkar, 'Kaliyuga, Chakri and Bhakti: Ramakrishna and His Times' in *Writing Social History* (Delhi: Oxford University Press, 1997), pp. 186–214.

66 Tithi Bhattacharya, *Sentinels of Culture: Class, Education and the Colonial Intellectual in Bengal*, pp. 26–34.

In addition to the critical interventions summarised here on the subject of the medical market, historians of colonial markets have argued for the need to understand market as a non-autonomous domain, asserting the underpinnings of culture and politics in the process of economic exchanges.[67] Manu Goswami has critiqued the conventional understandings of economy as a restricted domain of business and production. Her work suggests porosity and interrelatedness between the notions of the economic, the political and the cultural in relation to nationalism.[68] Emerging reflections on the medical market are similarly inclined to explore the mutual enmeshing of the market with other institutions such as the state, family and religion. Speaking to these concerns, this book also unfolds the role of a distinct market which indigenised homoeopathy. It presents a tapestry of intersecting ideas about quotidian domesticity, Hindu nationalism and the consumption of homoeopathy that blurs and complicates any rigid distinctions between the figures of the 'patient', 'physician', 'producer', 'consumer', 'author' and 'reader'. With a heightened emphasis on economic self-sufficiency and indigeneity, the practitioners of homoeopathy often valorised it as an essential means of ensuring individual welfare as well as a collective national good. They extended the ethic of production to contend that every household, with the support of select nationalist enterprises, could be a potent centre for the production of indigenous items for everyday consumption, including medico-scientific products.

This inclusive and participatory model of the medical market, with its emphasis on ethically charged and ubiquitous domestic production of knowledge and drugs, was often upheld as the blueprint for the nation. Indeed, such a blurred distinction between market and domesticity, along with advocacy for the qualities of self-reliance, enterprise, nationalism, Hindu-ness and indigeneity, resonated deeply with early twentieth-century '*swadeshi* nationalism'. *Swadeshi*, literally meaning 'indigenous', was a specific strand of Indian nationalist ideology that focused on confronting colonial rule by developing the Indian economy. It advocated the boycott of British products and the strengthening of indigenous production processes.[69] The homoeopathic ideas examined here, thus, fit in with the more recent historiography of *swadeshi* that seeks to understand the

[67] Sudipta Sen, *Empire of Free Trade: East India Company and the Making of the Colonial Marketplace* (Pennsylvania: University of Pennsylvania Press, 1998), pp. 8–12.

[68] Manu Goswami, 'From Swadeshi to Swaraj: Nation, Economy, Territory in Colonial South Asia, 1870–1907', *Comparative Studies in Society and History*, 40, 4 (1998), 631–2.

[69] The origin and the progress of the *swadeshi* movement in the political heartland of Bengal, following the partition of Bengal in 1905, have been detailed in Sumit Sarkar, *Swadeshi Movement in Bengal, 1903–1908* (Calcutta: People's Publishing House, 1973).

phenomenon as 'Hindu nationalism's linkage of an indigenist cultural politics with a "productionist" vision'.[70] The productionist vision of homoeopathy further shared *swadeshi* nationalism's critique of British rule as a 'superimposed, parasitical and unnatural global structure of exchange relations', and in opposition, upheld the nation as a 'natural unit of productive activity and the genuine substance of wealth'.[71] Indeed, in advocating the importance at once of indigenous firms and of the home-based production of drugs, the homoeopathic authors resonated with the *swadeshi* ideals that later converged with Gandhian political rhetoric around homespun cloth and national sovereignty.[72] Besides alluding to homoeopathy's indigenisation through the medical market, the phrase '*swadeshi* homoeopathy' captures this overlapping ethos of indigenous production, domesticity and self-sufficiency shared both by homoeopathy and *swadeshi* ideology.[73]

Recent scholarship, rather than envisioning *swadeshi* nationalism as an insulated 'episode' associated with the partition of Bengal between 1905 and 1911, has situated its ideology within an enduring economistic critique of colonial capital. This critique, extant since the late nineteenth century, contributed to the consolidation of the notion of a nationalist economy.[74] Published in the year of the first partition of Bengal and the beginning of the Swadeshi movement in 1905, the eminent homoeopathic entrepreneur-physician Mahesh Chandra Bhattacharya's book *Byabshayee* (*Businessman*), for example, detailed how the author developed his views on the importance of indigenous capital to produce essential items of quotidian consumption including medicines. Bhattacharya mentioned in the book that his ideas on indigenous capital have been developed since the 1880s. The book continued to be published by the homoeopathic enterprise M. Bhattacharya and Company over the first quarter of the twentieth century, with the

70 Andrew Sartori, 'The Categorical Logic of a Colonial Nationalism: Swadeshi Bengal, 1904–1908', *Comparative Studies of South Asia, Africa and the Middle East*, 23, 1 & 2 (2003), 274.

71 Ibid., p. 275.

72 See Christopher Bayly, 'The Origins of Swadeshi: Cloth and Indian Society' in Arjun Appadurai (ed.), *The Social Life of Things* (Cambridge: Cambridge University Press, 1986), pp. 311–13.

73 In his analysis of Indian technological development around the turn of the twentieth century, David Arnold too refers to the important impetus *swadeshi* ideologies provided for small-scale enterprises relying on technology. See David Arnold, *Everyday Technology: Machines and the Making of India's Modernity* (Chicago and London: University of Chicago Press, 2013), pp. 95–120.

74 Manu Goswami, 'From Swadeshi to Swaraj: Nation, Economy, Territory in Colonial South Asia, 1870–1907', pp. 609–36.

fourth edition appearing in 1921. Bhattacharya's career reinforces studies that question the characterisation of *swadeshi* as an isolated phase of nationalist thinking in the first decade of the twentieth century. Indeed, the Bengali homoeopathic firms that were first established in the 1880s or even earlier need to be understood as important predecessors to the highly publicised *swadeshi* indigenous pharmaceutical initiatives, such as the foundation in 1893 of Bengal Chemical Pharmaceutical Works (BCPW) by the noted scientist Prafulla Chandra Roy.[75] Although autonomous homoeopathic drug manufacturing was initiated only around 1917 (pioneered by the Hahnemann Publishing Company), these nineteenth-century firms were involved in the final preparation, mixing of mother tinctures, dilution and packaging of their imported products at least since the 1880s, as evidenced by the pharmacopoeias they published.[76]

Existing works on *swadeshi* have focused almost exclusively on the writings of the acclaimed nationalist intellectuals of the time. They have drawn upon the works of the 'great political economists of Congress'[77] including Dadabhai Naoraji, R. C. Dutt, M. G. Ranade and G. V. Joshi, or revolutionary extremists like M. N. Roy,[78] as well as the avowed nationalist social thinkers/reformers like Aurobindo Ghosh, Bipin Chandra Pal, Satishchandra Mukherjee and even the iconic Rabindranath Tagore.[79] My focus is on a distinct section of the Bengali *bhadralok*, usually ignored in conventional histories of *swadeshi* nationalism.[80] Beyond the realm of the high intelligentsia, *swadeshi* ideals were also espoused by a distinct group of homoeopathic entrepreneur-physicians like Rajendralal Dutta, Batakrishna Pal, Jitendranath Majumdar and Mahesh Chandra Bhattacharya, who offered a quotidian interpretation of *swadeshi* nationalism, framed around the production and consumption of indigenous medicine. Their writings upheld and

[75] For a comprehensive history of BCPW, see Pratik Chakrabarti, 'Science and Swadeshi: The Establishment and Growth of the Bengal Chemical and Pharmaceutical Works' in Uma Dasgupta (ed.), *Science and Modern India: An Institutional History, 1784–1947* (Delhi: Pearson Education, 2010), pp. 117–42.

[76] See, for instance, Mahesh Chandra Bhattacharya, *The Pharmaceutics' Manual: A Companion to the German and American Homoeopathic Pharmacopeia* (Calcutta: M. Bhattacharya and Company, 1892).

[77] Andrew Sartori, 'The Categorical Logic of a Colonial Nationalism: Swadeshi Bengal, 1904–1908', p. 274.

[78] See Kris Manjapra, *M. N. Roy: Marxism and Colonial Cosmopolitanism* (London, New York and New Delhi: Routledge, 2010).

[79] See Andrew Sartori, 'The Categorical Logic of Colonial Nationalism', pp. 271–82.

[80] The role of P. C. Roy and the BCPW has been noted in isolation. See Pratik Chakrabarty, *Western Science in Modern India: Metropolitan Methods, Colonial Practices* (Delhi: Permanent Black, 2004), pp. 219–52.

popularised homoeopathy as the ideal 'indigenous' remedy for a nation suffering from the ills of colonialism, prioritising it over ayurveda.

Ironically, categories such as '*swadeshi*' and 'indigenous' were shaped by colonial cosmopolitanisms. Histories of colonial cosmopolitanism emphasise how nationalism and cosmopolitanism often entailed one another in the South Asian context.[81] A case study of homoeopathy elucidates the ways in which the logic of importation of commodities was accommodated within the parameters of *swadeshi* ideology. Such logic was not confined to the abstract idea of German therapeutics. Instead, as I elaborate here, it can be found in the dynamics of circulation of an entire range of commodities, ideas and practices, including drugs, authoritative figures, journals, brands and expertise, extending between various parts of Bengal, British India, Britain and North America. Therefore, understanding *swadeshi* nationalism within the dichotomous schemes of 'the inner versus outer, the local versus global, the spiritual versus secular or the indigenous versus the Western' is problematic.[82] In revealing the historical processes through which German homoeopathy was constituted as 'indigenous' or '*swadeshi*' in British India, this study responds to David Arnold's important caution against the problems of excessive reliance on 'frameworks grounded in sharp western/indigenous divides'.[83] Following this line of argument, rather than considering 'vernacular medicine' as preordained, this book seeks to understand the historical specificities through which certain ideas and practices associated with homoeopathy were rendered distinct, delineated and celebrated as a form of 'vernacular medicine' in colonial Bengal.

Making Medicine Vernacular

The concept 'vernacular' seems especially relevant in unpacking homoeopathy's history in South Asia. It is a useful concept emerging out of current historiography, especially in analysing the sociocultural life of western ideas in India. It is particularly productive in making sense of the processes through which homoeopathy, whose 'scientific' status in

[81] Sugata Bose and Kris Manjapra (eds.), *Cosmopolitan Thought Zones: South Asia and the Global Circulation of Ideas* (Basingstoke: Palgrave Macmillan, 2010), pp. 2–3.

[82] Kris Manjapra, *M. N. Roy: Marxism and Colonial Cosmopolitanism*, p. 5.

[83] David Arnold and Sumit Sarkar, 'In Search of Rational Remedies: Homoeopathy in Nineteenth-Century Bengal' in Waltraud Ernst (ed.), *Plural Medicine, Tradition and Modernity, 1800–2000*, 2002, p. 54. Also see Gary J. Hausman, 'Making Medicine Indigenous: Homoeopathy in South India', pp. 303–22.

Europe was highly contested, castigated and unsure, succeeded in coexisting with orthodox western medicine, and in asserting its scientific claims in colonial India through cultural and legal negotiations.[84]

The idea of the 'vernacular' is also related to processes of linguistic translation of western concepts – in this case western medicine – into Indian languages. As one reads through the archive of Bengali health writings, the term catches the eye quite frequently, used by physician-authors claiming to translate science 'into our own vernaculars' for a 'vernacular audience'. *Vernacular Medicine in Colonial India* deals with the purposeful mandate the 'homoeopathic families' gave themselves, of translating 'science' for the good of the nation. As such, it delves deep into questions of linguistic translation of western science and medicine and the associated debates over language, culture and politics. Drawing upon an emerging, rich historiography of imperial science translation, it addresses itself to issues such as 'fidelity to sources' versus 'impulses of popularisation', 'wholesale transliteration' versus 'coining of new vernacular terms' and the contested issue of 'equivalence' in relation to South Asian homoeopathy.[85] These issues are mired (as I show especially in Chapter 3) in larger questions around the hierarchic status of languages, traditions and issues of power and class, not only between English and Indian vernacular languages but also between various social groups accessing the vernacular (in this case, the Bengali language).

'Translation' ought to be understood as a complex process far beyond the 'simple transfer of words or texts from one language to another'; but instead, as a 'translingual act of transcoding cultural material – a complex act of communication'.[86] A recent reflection on the future directions of history of science has contended that the processes of circulation and material interaction of ideas and texts through changing contexts are important and need further scholarly attention.[87] Over the years, divergent strands of South Asian scholarship have studied the relationship

[84] For a similar study of Tibetan medicine's various identities, and an insightful discussion around the criminalisation and acceptability of post-colonial Tibetan medicine both in Tibet and in the United States, see Vincanne Adams, 'Randomised Control Crime, Postcolonial Sciences in Alternative Medicine Research', *Social Studies of Science*, 32, 5/6 (2002), 659–90.

[85] See Marwa Elshakry, 'Knowledge in Motion: The Cultural Politics of Modern Science Translation in Arabic', *Isis*, 99, 4 (2008), 701–30; and Lydia Liu (ed.), *Tokens of Exchange: The Problem of Translation in Global Circulations* (Durham: Duke University Press, 2000).

[86] Douglas Howland, 'Predicament of Ideas in Culture: Translation and Historiography', *History and Theory*, 42, 1 (2003), 45.

[87] James Secord, 'Knowledge in Transit', *Isis*, 95, 4 (2004), 654–72.

between science, medicine and colonialism.[88] In the process, intercultural encounters have been studied with a myriad of emphases, on themes of assimilation,[89] exchange and dialogue,[90] circulation and contact zones.[91] Currently, historians have begun exploring 'translation' in its wider meaning as a significant perspective from which to understand the cultural valence of western science and medicine in South Asia. Existing literature has suggested how translations often reconceptualised and transformed the appeal of western scientific categories in colonial India.[92] Through an analysis of Hindu ritualised symbols and emergent Hindu domesticity, this work is in particular conversation with histories that interrogate the interactions between translation and Hindu religious revivalism.[93]

Recent works on what has been termed 'vernacular translation' look into the processes of vernacularisation of 'distinct categories and discrete concepts' through translation.[94] Saurabh Dube's important work on biblical translations among the catechists in central India, as well as the work of Juned Shaikh[95] on the translation of Marx's writings among the Bombay labourers reveal such dynamics of vernacularisation in the repackaging of particular understandings of concepts like 'Christianity' or 'class' as 'historically contingent, distinctly Indian'.[96]

88 For an overview of the debate over the command of science on the Indian psyche, and of the divergent strands of historiography on science and colonialism in South Asia, see Mark Harrison, 'Science and the British Empire', *Isis*, 96, 1 (2005), 56–63.

89 David Arnold, *Science, Technology and Medicine in Colonial India* (New Cambridge History of India III: 5) (Cambridge, Cambridge University Press, 2000).

90 Pratik Chakrabarti, *Western Science in Modern India: Metropolitan Methods, Colonial Practices*, 2004.

91 Kapil Raj, *Relocating Modern Science: Circulation and the Construction of Knowledge in South Asia and Europe, 1650–1900* (Basingstoke and New York: Palgrave Macmillan, 2007).

92 See Gyan Prakash, 'Translation and Power', *Another Reason: Science and the Imagination of Modern India* (Princeton, NJ: Princeton University Press, 1999), pp. 49–85; and by the same author, 'Science "Gone Native" in Colonial India', *Representations*, 40, Special Issue: Seeing Science (Autumn 1992), 153–78. Also see Shruti Kapila, 'The Enchantment of Science in India', *Isis*, 101, 1 (2010), 120–32.

93 See Marwa Elshakry, *Reading Darwin in Arabic, 1860–1950* (Chicago and London: University of Chicago Press, 2013), pp. 7–10; also see Amitranjan Basu, 'Emergence of a Marginal Science in a Colonial City: Reading Psychiatry in Bengali Periodicals', *Indian Economic and Social History Review*, 41, 2 (2004), 135–36. For a discussion of the Bengali reconstitution of homoeopathy with Hindu undertones through the writing of medical biographies, see Shinjini Das, 'Biography and Homoeopathy in Bengal: Colonial Lives of a European Heterodoxy', *Modern Asian Studies*, 49, 6 (2015), 1760–8.

94 Saurabh Dube, 'Colonial Registers of a Vernacular Christianity: Conversion to Translation', *Economic and Political Weekly*, 39, 1 (2004), 164.

95 Juned Shaikh, 'Translating Marx, Mavali, Dalit and the Making of Mumbai's Working Class', *Economic and Political Weekly 1928–1935*, 46, 31 (2011), 65–72.

96 Saurabh Dube, 'Colonial Registers of a Vernacular Christianity', p. 163.

Vernacularisation of homoeopathy, likewise, is traced in this book through manifestly religio-cultural idioms of Hinduism in Bengal.

In one sense, therefore, 'vernacularisation' in relation to homoeopathy was a linguistic process. In their self-proclaimed efforts to translate homoeopathic science into the 'vernacular' for a 'vernacular' audience, homoeopathic authors were implicated in what has been characterised as a linguistic exercise of the 'will to vernacular'.[97] In mapping the operations of the Bengali homoeopathic authors around a specific locale and language, my work speaks to Sheldon Pollock's understanding of the vernacular as a wilful exercise or choice of a language around precise 'geo-cultural spaces' and 'socio-textual communities'.[98] However, as discussed already, vernacular translations of homoeopathy can hardly be understood without taking into account homoeopathy's strong cultural underpinnings. These underpinnings, while frequently imposing local values and religious symbolisms, helped homoeopathy strike deeper roots within Indian social worlds.

But what was the vernacular? The category 'vernacular' in South Asian historiography is no longer understood as necessarily a purely linguistic identity. In the print market dealing with homoeopathy in Bengal, the vernacular remained an inherently relational and flexible label. In this context, the status of vernacular could shift, even to the extent that English as much as Bengali or Marathi could act as the medium for articulating vernacular homoeopathy, once it was encoded with culturally specific words, meanings and contexts. It might be more pertinent to regard the 'vernacular' in colonial Bengal, as Partha Chatterjee has recently contended, as a 'style and sensibility' rather than an inflexible label describing any particular language.[99]

Ritu Birla's work on the colonial production of 'the market' delineates the caste, community and kinship-based operations of Marwari 'family firms' as examples of 'vernacular capitalism', which was at loggerheads with the contractual codes of a capitalist market.[100] Her work traces the colonial legal rendering of 'vernacular commerce' as 'indigenous' or 'pre-

[97] Sheldon Pollock, 'The Cosmopolitan Vernacular', *Journal of Asian Studies*, 57, 1 (1998), 8–9. Also see by the same author, 'Cosmopolitan and Vernacular in History', *Public Culture*, 12, 3 (2000), 605.

[98] Sheldon Pollock, 'The Cosmopolitan Vernacular', *Journal of Asian Studies*, 57, 1 (1998), 8–9.

[99] See Partha Chatterjee and Raziuddin Aquil (eds.), *History in the Vernacular* (Ranikhet: Permanent Black, 2008), pp. 1–19.

[100] Ritu Birla, *Stages of Capital: Law, Culture and Market Governance in Late Colonial India*, 2009, pp. 3, 9–14.

modern' modes of capital, in so far as the practitioners of caste and kinship-based enterprises were considered 'insiders to the colonial economy but outsiders to the modern market ethics'.[101] Projit Bihari Mukharji related vernacularisation to an ongoing process of nationalisation 'whereby a loose affective community is given a more concrete shape as a nation'.[102] Positioning nationalisation and vernacularisation as virtually coterminous ideas, he contended that vernacularisation of western medicine helped actualise the nation through 'nationalisation of the body'.[103]

Building on these insights, this book acknowledges the strong inflections of language, indigeneity, culture, affect and nationalism, but hesitates in conflating the 'vernacular' fully with any one of them. Indeed, along with tracing processes of vernacularisation, this study goes a step further to reflect on what the 'vernacular' is. Rather than assuming it to be always and already present, it looks into the ways in which 'vernacular' was (re)constituted through colonial encounters. In pursuing this question, I draw on works that understand vernacularity as a rather slippery idea that is not 'pure, systemic, temporally primordial or territorially bounded'.[104] Of special relevance to me are studies that have hinted at the possibility of analysing the vernacular as a 'cultural artefact in its own right'[105] – a complex field that is forged when elements of both the 'elite' and the 'popular' are assimilated and 'remade into something else'.[106] In exploring the making of Kannada language and the intricate relation between vernacular poetry and polity, Sheldon Pollock, too, situates the 'vernacular' in between the 'mutually constitutive interaction of the local and the global'.[107] Others have analysed the 'vernacular' as a realm signifying that 'in-between space of solidarities of various non-state authorities', a space of consolidation between the national and the imperial/global.[108] Resonances of such formulations, albeit in vastly different registers,

[101] Ibid., p. 3.
[102] Projit Bihari Mukharji, *Nationalizing the Body: The Medical Market, Print and Daktari Medicine* (London, New York and Delhi: Anthem Press, 2009), p. 33; also see pp. 22–3.
[103] Ibid., pp. 28–9.
[104] Kajri Jain, *Gods in the Bazaar: Economies of Indian Calendar Art* (Durham: Duke University Press, 2007), pp. 13–16.
[105] Mary E. Fissell, *Vernacular Bodies: The Politics of Reproduction in Early Modern England* (Clarendon: Oxford University Press, 2004), pp. 6–7.
[106] Ibid., p. 6. Mary Fissell refuses to conflate vernacular knowledge with either 'trickle down science' or 'popular', which is often reduced to mean 'of the poorer classes'.
[107] Sheldon Pollock, 'The Cosmopolitan Vernacular', *Journal of Asian Studies*, 57, 1 (1998), 9.
[108] Bhaskar Mukhopadhyay, *Rumours of Globalisation: Desecrating the Global from Vernacular Margins* (London: C. Hurst and Co., 2013), pp. 3–5.

can be found in recent works on the making of knowledge about the African 'primitive'.[109] Helen Tilley regards 'vernacular science' as an in-between field, as a 'subgenre of research' that is produced through the interactions between 'native knowledge' and 'colonial science'. The term 'vernacular' in these works seems to refer to the outcome of 'translations between different epistemologies and ways of knowing'.[110]

Therefore, *Vernacular Medicine in Colonial India* explores the co-constitution of the worlds of the vernacular, the family and homoeopathy. It maps both the colonial vernacularisation of homoeopathy in Bengal, as well as the processes that constituted the vernacular itself in the colonial period. It examines the makings of a vernacular field around homoeopathy through the multifarious functions of familial capital. In the course of these explorations, it further highlights the dynamic potentials and shifting manoeuvres of the family-based enterprises in response to the challenges posed by the colonial state and market, over a period of time. It shows the complicity of the caste, religion and kinship-based practices of the homoeopathic families with the profit-based operations of the market. While shaping the production of such a vernacular field, family-based elite enterprises in collusion with the state, with the prejudices based on existing social identities (such as caste, religion and kinship) and with the market, marginalised various suburban, lower middle-class or semi-literate practitioners as illegitimate voices.

Homoeopathy could simultaneously project itself as being imported yet indigenous, western but also traditional, secular as well as deeply religious; and could claim to be equally conversant with the world of metropolitan science as with local cultural practices. Straddling these various identities, homoeopathy in Bengal constituted a vernacular field that was facilitated by homoeopathy's historic enmesh with the category 'family' in Bengal. An intimate and intricate entanglement with the institution of family subjected Bengali homoeopathy to diverse currents of interests, which included the imperatives and apprehensions of colonial governance, medical bureaucracy, Hindu revivalist endeavours (especially around the domestic space), profiteering motivations of private commercial firms, regional print markets, nationalist enterprises of narrating and

[109] Helen Tilley, 'Global Histories: Vernacular Science and African Genealogies; or Is the History of Science Ready for the World', *Isis*, 101, 1 (2010), 110–19.
[110] Ibid., pp. 110, 117–19.

historicising the nation, as well as the developmentalist electoral manifestoes of the nationalist parties in the province from the late 1920s. Through its negotiations with this wide spectrum of interests, homoeopathy could embody a range of politico-cultural meanings and liminal identities. These negotiations enabled homoeopathy to consolidate a complex 'vernacular' field of operation, which in turn sustained it.

1 A Heterodoxy between Institutions

Bureaucracy, Print-Market and Family Firms

> 'It is now an acknowledged fact that the number of homoeopaths, either good, bad or indifferent is a legion in India and there has been a network of homoeopathic pharmacies ... all over our country ... Harmony [between them] should be the basic principle upon which true friendship and good business can last and flourish.'[1]

> 'All householders are businessmen in a sense. But in general, by businessmen one understands the traders.'[2]

> 'To a businessman, honest, dutiful and efficient employee [*sic*] is more precious than the son. Many entrepreneurs trust such employees more than their own son.'[3]

In August 1882, the *Indian Medical Gazette* published a lengthy editorial article titled 'Medical Practice in Calcutta'.[4] The article contemplated the status of western state medicine in the city as well as the main hindrances to its wider dissemination. The *Indian Medical Gazette*, an unofficial mouthpiece of the Indian Medical Service, mostly comprised of contributors variously involved in the colonial state's public health endeavours. Its editorial, penned by the influential Kenneth Macleod, Professor of Surgery at the Calcutta Medical College and the Chairman of the Calcutta Health Society, was in many ways voicing the anxieties of the imperial state and its medical bureaucracy. Macleod particularly raised an alarm about the messy nature of the medical market in Calcutta that allowed for an extensive sphere of unregulated practices to flourish. The article brought to life a world of medical relief sharply polarised

1 'Editorial: New Year's Retrospection and Introspection', *The Hahnemannian Gleanings*, 4, 1 (February 1933), 10–11.
2 Jitendranath Majumdar, *Arther Sandhan (Pursuit of Wealth)*, 3rd edition (Calcutta: Sisir Publishing House, 1932), p. 115.
3 Mahesh Chandra Bhattacharya, *Byabshayee (Businessman)*, 1st edition (Calcutta: M. Bhattacharya and Company, 1905), p. 72.
4 Kenneth McLeod, 'Medical Practice in Calcutta', *Indian Medical Gazette*, 17 (August 1882), 213–17.

between the qualified practitioners and those whom the state summarily deemed unqualified. Even in 1882, Calcutta, the second city of the empire and a bustling metropolis of a million people, could boast of only about 100 qualified practitioners duly trained in state-endorsed western medicine. These practitioners received their degrees either from Europe or from the newly instituted medical schools in India, including the pioneering Calcutta Medical College established in 1835. Macleod's real worry, however, was with the extensive sphere of the so-called unqualified practitioners, of whom he remarked, 'there is a variety almost defying classification'.[5] This sphere ranged from practices which claimed to be more traditionally 'Indian', to those involving the most recently discovered patent drugs. Indeed, the vast population of unregulated and unqualified practitioners included medical college dropouts; a large number of 'quacks and impostors' among whom Macleod included several South Indian practitioners on Wellesley street claiming to be 'Professors of piles and fistula'; those dealing in specifics along with a large number of *hakims* and *kobirajes* 'who were very fluent with traditionary rules and maxims' and were 'the surviving representatives of the ancient medical creeds of Hindustan, and are doomed to early extinction'.[6] This editorial put forward one of the early pleas for a Medical Registration Act for India as the indispensable step towards the development of a colonial public health system.

For Macleod, a particularly annoying presence common to both the domains of qualified and unqualified practitioners was the significant number of homoeopathic practitioners in Calcutta. In his account, homoeopathy curiously featured in the realms of both the qualified and the unqualified, the state and the traditional. The editor marvelled at the popularity and rising demand for homoeopathy in colonial homes. He was amazed that the natives would frequently resort, interchangeably, to qualified Indian practitioners of state medicine and to the homoeopaths. The sheer range of homoeopathic practitioners baffled him – there were duly qualified practitioners of state medicine who chose to practice homoeopathy, as well as failed students of medical colleges, and in addition, a very large number or amateur homoeopaths with flourishing practices. The colonial medical bureaucracy was trying to solve, to borrow Macleod's phrase, 'the mystery of homoeopathy' – to make sense of the thriving market for homoeopathy and the various networks through which it circulated.[7] It was also grappling with the reasons for homoeopathy's rising popularity among the natives of India. Macleod's article proposed several possible explanations, which revealed the medical

[5] Ibid., p. 216. [6] Ibid., p. 216. [7] Ibid., p. 215.

establishment's prejudicial bias against colonised peoples. The reasons cited by Macleod ranged from the 'imaginative and unpractical minds' of Indians, and 'the milder and more passive nature of the Hindoos' to the 'transitionary state of India as regards medical science and practice'.[8]

Beyond the anxieties of the colonial medical bureaucracy, the entrenched presence of homoeopathy was being felt in other aspects of Bengali life. By the turn of the twentieth century, the figure of the homoeopath recurred vicariously in the rich domain of Bengali fiction. Homoeopathy featured in myriad genres of Bengali literature, including a series of colonial farces, written as social commentaries on the deplorable state of medical relief in the region. But how, indeed, can one solve 'the mystery of homoeopathy'? While the twin worlds of colonial administration and vernacular literature grappled with the figure of the homoeopath with mixed emotions of anxiety, resentment and humour, how was the European heterodoxy[9] being popularised in the province? How did the homoeopaths come to acquire a position of value and trust in colonial homes in Calcutta?

To answer this question, I studied a range of intergenerational Bengali business concerns which, from around the 1860s, began sustained investments involving homoeopathy. By the latter half of the nineteenth century, these printing and publication establishments ensured a steady circulation of popular scientific writings on homoeopathy in the regional print market. As they facilitated publications, as well as the establishment of numerous pharmacies across the city of Calcutta and beyond, these firms asserted their authority in the overlapping domain of medical knowledge and commerce. Publications by these commercial firms specifically projected the domestic space of the Bengali household as the ideal site where the western heterodoxy could proliferate. While the government expressed anxiety over the lack of organisation in its practice, Bengali homoeopathy was being uniquely institutionalised around these firms asserting themselves as 'families'. The distinct process of

[8] Ibid.

[9] There has been endless debate around the nomenclature of so-called alternative medicine, and all terms such as 'alternative', 'complementary', 'heterodox', 'fringe medicine', 'unorthodox medicine', 'sectarian medicine' have been understood as problematic one way or the other, especially in the discourses of universalising state medicine or modern biomedicine. Recently, it has been argued that 'heterodoxy' is a relatively more useful term to describe these forms of healing, since at least it does not assume either a hierarchy or a specific geography and can therefore include medical systems from any culture. Besides, homoeopathy is widely regarded as a classic heterodox medicine of the late eighteenth century, which even helped define understandings of medical orthodoxy in the West. See Roberta Bivins, 'Histories of Heterodoxies' in Mark Jackson (ed.), *The Oxford Handbook of Medicine* (Oxford University Press, 2011), pp. 579–80. The use of the descriptive term 'heterodoxy' is not used here to indicate any assumptions of marginalised status.

homoeopathy's institutionalisation is explored by focusing on the publications generated by the protagonists of six such leading homoeopathic business enterprises in late nineteenth-century Calcutta.

The literature published by the pharmaceutical companies illustrated a sustained engagement with three apparently distinct and unrelated themes. They reflected simultaneously on the importance, function and organisation of business, family and homoeopathic practice in late nineteenth and early twentieth-century Bengal. I focus on this entanglement to examine Bengali homoeopathy's intimate imbrication with the institution of family. The domains of the familial and the entrepreneurial appear blurred together in these texts, and norms involving family and business appear positively interchangeable and overlapping. Beyond the preliminary sections of this chapter on the state and the realm of Bengali fiction, we take our cue from the projected ethic and organisation of homoeopathic enterprises and investigate how 'family' itself was being construed as both an affective and a profitable institution, which nurtured Bengali homoeopathy.

A 'Growing Scandal … Under British Rule'

Since about the 1870s, along with ayurveda and other traditional practices like unani, homoeopathy invariably surfaced in anxious governmental discussions of medical malpractice in Bengal, being referred to as 'a growing scandal'.[10] After an initial phase of attempts at syncretism with the traditional medical cultures, which lasted until about the 1850s, the British government launched an extended phase of public health policies that all but delegitimised traditional therapeutics, as well as any other up-and-coming European heterodoxy such as homoeopathy.[11] Existing studies have remarked that there were renewed beginnings of official tolerance for 'indigenous' medicine around the First World War. Furthermore, a dyarchic system of government was instituted in 1919; more recent scholarship identifies this as a key moment that signalled a slow policy transition towards accepting and standardising practices other than western state medicine.[12]

[10] From the Coroner of Calcutta to the Secretary to the Government of Bengal, Judicial Department, Municipal Department Medical Branch, File Number A/15 2, Proceeding 46 (September 1887 [West Bengal State Archives, hereafter WBSA]).

[11] For efforts at supposed harmony and syncretism see Zhaleh Khaleeli, 'Harmony or Hegemony? The Rise and Fall of the Native Medical Institution, Calcutta; 1822–35', *South Asia Research*, 21 (2001), 77–104.

[12] Rachel Berger, *Ayurveda Made Modern: Political Histories of Indigenous Medicine, 1900–1955* (Basingstoke: Palgrave Macmillan, 2013), pp. 2–4.

Through the second half of the nineteenth century, homoeopathy thus emerged as a topic of frequent concern in the leading and widely circulating 'orthodox' journals like the *Indian Medical Gazette* and the *Lancet*. Equally, it featured in the writings of the physicians associated as faculty with the premier colonial institutions, such as the Calcutta University and the Calcutta Medical College. It also featured in the bureaucratic correspondence of the colonial medical officials. Much like Macleod's editorial quoted earlier, these various registers of the nineteenth-century colonial administration unanimously criticised homoeopathy's presence in the medical landscape of the time, often equating it with quackery. It was pointed out,

> We know little of this sphere of practice, but we suspect that a good deal of quacking goes on. Quacking is inseparable from dealing in occult agencies. We have met with two instances in which homoeopaths undertook, on prepayment of substantial fee, to cure cataract and cancer by infinitesimals.[13]

The state authorities questioned the very basis of the homoeopathic doctrine, conflating it with 'charlatanism', 'quackery' or as in the aforementioned instance, with the 'occult'. However, homoeopathy was put under the official scanner most frequently for the way it was practised. The notion of 'quackery' was therefore invoked in such official correspondence in at least two distinct ways: at times, it involved the outright rejection of homoeopathy as a rational doctrine; but more specifically, it included criticisms of the homoeopathic practitioners' lack of qualifications, training and competence. Thus, besides questioning the scientific basis of homoeopathy, the official registers complained more about the lack of formal institutional structure around nineteenth-century homoeopathy. In a later Chapter (Chapter 5), I will explore the twentieth-century colonial state's about-turn on its definition of scientific, recognised medicine, in response to growing nationalist politics around issues of public health.

But before this reversal of policy in the mid- to late nineteenth century, the leading, self-proclaimed 'orthodox' journals like the *Indian Medical Gazette* and the *Lancet* published articles that were mostly dismissive of the validity of the homoeopathic principle itself. The typical tone of these writings may be captured from a letter to the editor of the *Lancet* written in 1861, which argued,

> In all times there have been pretenders, who have persuaded a certain part of the public that they have some peculiar knowledge of a royal road to cure, which those of the regular craft have not. It is homoeopathy now; it was something else

[13] Kenneth McLeod, 'Medical Practice in Calcutta', *Indian Medical Gazette*, 17 (August 1882), 215–16.

formerly; and if homoeopathy were to be extinguished, there would be something else in its place.[14]

A culmination of such attitudes may be seen in the raging controversy surrounding the admission of Mahendralal Sircar to the medical faculty of the Calcutta University in 1878 following a decision of the University Senate. Dr Sircar, a reputed physician and the second MD to qualify from the Calcutta Medical College, had in 1867 ceremoniously declared his conversion to homoeopathy. Throughout this book, we will have detailed encounters with Sircar and his activities as a figure central to the publicisation of homoeopathy in Bengal. The other members of the medical faculty fought tooth and nail against Sircar's inclusion, arguing that 'they were unable to associate themselves as a Faculty of Medicine with a member who professes and practices homoeopathy'.[15] The medical establishment of Calcutta closed ranks and stood firm in their decision in the face of repeated petitions from Mahendralal Sircar justifying his inclusion into their ranks.[16] In the end, Dr Sircar was forced to resign. The decision of the faculty was widely appreciated in the contemporary leading journals. An article 'Homoeopathy and the University of Calcutta', published in the *Indian Medical Gazette* in 1878, celebrated the decision as the most appropriate step in 'maintaining the cause of scientific truth and purity in Bengal, unflinchingly against the faintest encouragement of or association with delusion or error'.[17]

From the 1880s on, the state was increasingly more concerned with the organisational and institutional aspect of homoeopathy, than its inherent (ir)rationality. Over the 1880s and 1890s, there was a swelling administrative anxiety over organisational irregularities pertaining to traditional medicine, as well as to European heterodoxies like homoeopathy.[18] There was also a growing colonial resentment with the informal networks of pedagogy through which homoeopathy appeared to circulate. These developments forced the state to contemplate an imperial legislation

[14] Anonymous, 'Letter to the Editor: Sir Benjamin Benjamin Brodie on Homoeopathy', *The Lancet*, 7, 1984 (7 September 1861), 238–9.

[15] See Arun Kumar Biswas, *Collected Works of Mahendralal Sircar, Eugene Lafont and the Science Movement, 1860–1910* (Kolkata: Asiatic Society, 2003), p. 232.

[16] Ibid., pp. 231–47.

[17] Anonymous, 'Homoeopathy and the University of Calcutta', *Indian Medical Gazette*, 13 (June 1878), 159.

[18] The story of the state's policing of homoeopathy needs to be positioned within the broader processes of the state's failure in controlling epidemics and its larger surveillance of all non-state practices, particularly the indigenous medicinal practices like ayurveda and unani. See Kavita Sivaramakrishnan, *Old Potions, New Bottles: Recasting Indigenous Medicine in Colonial Punjab (1850–1945)* (Hyderabad: Orient Longman, 2006), pp. 87–103.

which would streamline and standardise the non-state practices. The idea of introducing a Medical Registration Act on the model of the English Act was being actively debated in official circles. An article 'India: Registration of Medical Practitioners', published in 1888 in the *Lancet*, complained that it was no longer possible for the public to 'discriminate between the qualified and the unqualified' physicians.[19] Similarly, a typical letter to the editor of the journal *The Medical Reporter* in 1895 regretted that '[n]owadays a large number of vaidic [*sic*], homoeopathic and allopathic quacks have a magnificent field for the exercise of their powers, and many are their victims'.[20] Referring specifically to homoeopathy, these writings urged the government that 'there is no alternative to this vile injurious system until the Indian Government take due steps to stop it by medical Acts'.[21]

That homoeopathic malpractice remained a crucial reference for the debate around a Medical Registration Act is evident from medico-legal cases that adjudicated death allegedly caused by homoeopathic pills. An example at hand is the case involving the death of a Bengali woman, Shyrobee Raur, in the late 1880s. After lying dormant with the police department for a while, the case was brought before the coroner of Calcutta in May 1891 for a final verdict.[22] The coroner delved into the details of the jury's findings on the circumstances attending the death following the administration of a homoeopathic drug by a charitable dispensary. No one was found conclusively guilty.[23] Nevertheless, the coroner used the excuse of this death and the attending jury report to submit a detailed 'proposal for passing an Act for the registration of qualified medical practitioners, with a view to put down quacks'.[24] The witness accounts in the case, which were taken at the coroner's court in June 1887, recorded that the two accused men – the owner of the Bowbazar Charitable Dispensary, Behary Loll Mullick, and his assistant Jogendra Loll Bose, who had administered the drug to the deceased – lacked any formal training in medicine whatsoever.[25] However, on

19 Anonymous Correspondent, 'India', *The Lancet*, 131, 3365 (25 February 1888), 399–400.
20 Anonymous, 'Letter to the Editor, Correspondence: The Indian Systems of Medicine', *The Medical Reporter*, VI (16 August 1895), 125.
21 Ibid., p. 125.
22 From the coroner of Calcutta to the secretary to the government of Bengal, Medical Department, Municipal Department, Medical Branch, File Number A/15, Proceedings 1–5 B, May 1891 [WBSA].
23 Ibid.
24 From the coroner of Calcutta to the secretary to the government of Bengal, Judicial Department, Municipal Department Medical Branch, File Number A/15 2, Proceeding 46, September 1887 [WBSA].
25 Ibid.

enquiry, both revealed that they considered themselves trained in homoeopathy as they possessed experience of curing patients. They stated that they had acquired their homoeopathic training by reading relevant books.[26] The owner, Behary Loll Mullick, particularly emphasised that although he was a clerk in a merchant office, he was simultaneously 'a homoeopathic practitioner for the past 15 years'.[27]

The coroner's summary of the jury report, which was submitted to the secretary to the Judicial Department of the government of Bengal in June 1887, reveals that the jury unanimously held the opinion that,

> from what has been said by the witness from the Bowbazar Homoeopathic Charitable Dispensary that, there is much risk at present, for the public from the indiscriminate practice of medicine by persons who are not qualified sufficiently to do so – we think that the time has arrived when the public should be protected by a Legislative Enactment such as the Medical Registration Act now in force in England.[28]

While summarising the jury's opinion, the coroner further justified the importance of such a legislation by highlighting that the necessity of implementing a Medical Registration Act was inherent in the English Act itself. He argued that 'it might be fairly presumed that the interests of her Majesty's subjects in the vast Indian Empire were not excluded from those in the colony'.[29] The unregulated practice of homoeopathy as exemplified in the Shyrobee Raur case was referred to as an embarrassing 'scandal', as the coroner appealed for the 'gradual suppression of the growing scandal of men and women undertaking charlatanism and quackery so utterly unworthy of enlightened India under British rule'.[30]

Of Humour, Trust and Bengali Fiction

While the colonial state contemplated the appropriate legal measures to control homoeopathy, the latter continued to attract the interest of a variety of Bengali authors. This literary attentiveness to homoeopathy continued uninterrupted well into the twentieth century. It surfaced in myriad genres of literature by several writers, including the reputed nineteenth-century playwrights Dwijendralal Ray and Girish Chandra Ghosh, as well as the anonymous writers of short *Battala* farces.[31] At the turn of

[26] Ibid. [27] Ibid. [28] Ibid. [29] Ibid. [30] Ibid.

[31] *Battala* texts appeared from the numerous small presses huddled close together in the narrow lanes and bylanes of the Battala area, a part of the teeming 'native town' in north Calcutta. Despite being regularly ridiculed by the rising literary gentry, these small presses did a brisk trade in cheap ephemeral pamphlet literature, which enjoyed a large and popular readership in lower middle-class urban and rural homes. This comprised almanacs, popular religious mythologies, sensational romances and dramas, erotic

the twentieth century, fiction involving homoeopathy spanned the two worlds of respectable *bhadralok*, upper-class literature, and that of 'low' literature which targeted the less-privileged sections of society.[32] The figure of the homoeopathic physician appeared in dramas, as well as in short stories and novels written by widely read and esteemed Bengali authors such as Sarat Chandra Chattopadhyay, Rajshekhar Basu (Parashuram), Tarashankar Bandopadhyay and Saradindu Bandopadhyay.

At first reading, the figure of the homoeopathic physician in these various literary forms appears to resist any overarching stereotype. The homoeopaths are presented in various moulds ranging from honest, charitable, well-meaning village practitioners to fraudulent, corrupt physicians smuggling cocaine in the guise of homoeopathic globules. While some stories are set in obscure *mofussil* locations where the practitioner is shown struggling to find a niche for himself, others are placed in the Calcutta mansions of the elite, acting as revered physicians to the affluent urban bourgeoisie. However, several texts concerning homoeopathy belonged to the growing contemporary genre of farces. Extant work shows the importance of farce as an important literary genre addressing social malaise through exaggerated situations, caricatures and laughter.[33] Other genres that involved homoeopathy, such as plays, short stories and novels, also frequently invoke what Sudipta Kaviraj has termed the tradition of 'literary humour' in Bengali literature.[34] Cumulatively these fictions generated social criticism, presented through the medium of humour, which took on a multiplicity of forms including outright fun, ridicule, sarcasm, irony or satire. A central social issue addressed in these fictions was the pathetic condition of medical relief in Bengal, and the inaccessibility and/or the inefficiency of the therapeutic options available to the common man. Homoeopaths in these texts are frequently mocked, while homoeopathy is often used as a euphemism to discuss larger

poems and songs and the like. Several scholars have written on the history, productions and impact of the *Battala* publications. For an exhaustive history of *Battala*, see Sripantha, *Battala* (Calcutta: Ananda, 1997). For the most recent exploration of *Battala* print culture, see Gautam Bhadra, *Nyara Battalay Jay Kawbar* (Kolkata: Chhatim Books, 2011).

32 For a discussion of the hierarchical layers of Bengali print in the nineteenth century between 'high' and 'low' literature, see Anindita Ghosh, 'Revisiting the "Bengal Renaissance": Literary Bengali and Low-Life Print in Colonial Calcutta', *Economic and Political Weekly*, 37, 42 (2002), 4329–38.

33 For an account of 'farce' as an important literary genre, see Anindita Ghosh, 'Revisiting the "Bengal Renaissance": Literary Bengali and Low-Life Print in Colonial Calcutta', pp. 4333–4.

34 Sudipta Kaviraj, 'Laughter and Subjectivity: The Self-Ironical Tradition in Bengali Literature', *Modern Asian Studies*, 34, 2 (May 2000), 382.

problems associated with colonial modernity, including declining morality, excessive Anglicisation and the failing health of the Bengalis. Yet, in their repeated acts of reproaching the idiosyncrasies related to these practitioners, the authors hardly ever appear to condemn homoeopathy altogether. In fact, they seem at once to ridicule and celebrate homoeopathy. Their literary depictions exude an unmistakeable sense of approval, of endorsing homoeopathy as a ubiquitous object of value and trust. In several narratives, homoeopathy comes across as the lesser evil in an otherwise corruptible regime of colonial rule and modern medicine. The stories are a testament to homoeopathy's necessary and valued presence, especially within Bengali households, while it could also be laughed at. In sharp contrast to the state's agnosticism, Bengali fiction exhibited a palpable trust towards homoeopathy, which was nonetheless expressed chiefly through the mode of humour.

Late nineteenth-century fictions often illustrated an increasing faith in homoeopathy over competing genres of medicine within the domestic sphere. An anonymous 1875 farce, *Daktarbabu* (*The Physician*), elaborated the dilemma of a representative middle-class professional in choosing an appropriate remedy for his family.[35] The second scene detailed the thoughts of Nilkantha, one of the *bhadralok* protagonists of the farce, who after enumerating the various debilitating ailments plaguing his household resolved to turn to homoeopathy for help. In his words, 'the doctors and *kavirajes* have been of no help, so I will turn to homoeopathy this time'.[36] When discouraged from doing so, he turned to the readers to announce, 'whatever you might hold, I sincerely feel homoeopathy is hundred times better than *daktari* [vernacular term for western state medicine or allopathy]. Even if their drugs fail to cure, they at least never cause any harm. At the very least, they are good to taste, which is useful for children'.[37]

A similar agnosticism towards all forms of medicine, with a growing proclivity towards homoeopathy, was reflected in the satirical play *Kritanter Bangadarshan* (*Visit of the King of Hell to Bengal*) that was put up at the reputed Minerva Theatre Hall in early twentieth-century Calcutta.[38] In a satirical gesture towards the medical scene of contemporary Bengal, the drama depicted the arrival of the mythical Yama, or the Hindu deity of death, in Bengal with his trusted associate Chitragupta. Ironically enough, on his arrival Yama was immediately infected with malaria through one of his own employees, stationed in

[35] Anonymous, *Daktarbabu* (*The Physician*) (Calcutta: Jogendra Ghosh, 1875), pp. 5–10.
[36] Ibid. [37] Ibid., pp. 5–10.
[38] A detailed report on the play appeared in an editorial in a popular homoeopathy journal. See 'Editorial', *Homoeopathy Paricharak*, 1, 4 (July 1927), 226–7.

that region for the purpose of spreading the fatal disease. Yama vehemently turned down Chitragupta's suggestions of seeking medical relief from either a *kaviraj* or an allopath. He cited a long list of the near-innumerable pitfalls of using either ayurveda or allopathy. His bias in favour of homoeopathy became evident when he readily agreed to take medical aid from a homoeopath. Of homoeopathy, none other than Yama, the deity of death himself opined, 'if available please summon [a homoeopath] fast. Their drugs are good, no adulteration, moderate expense, no trouble gulping them, no fuss, and no façade of having supplementary food. Even if I am made to suffer flawed diagnosis, I will at least have sweet water to taste when I die'.[39]

In parallel with acknowledging homoeopathy as a viable option in an otherwise impoverished field of options for medical relief, these literary texts evinced a complementary engagement with the irregularities associated with this form of medicine. A central character of Dwijendralal Ray's play *Tryhasparsha ba Sukhi Paribar* (*Triangular Impact or the Happy Family*) was a homoeopath.[40] A man of dubious qualifications, he kept referring to English texts of absurd nomenclature by way of showing his grasp of the western 'science' of homoeopathy.[41] The drama depicted a humorous account of the ill-trained practitioner managing to infiltrate the household of the prosperous Calcutta elite as a trusted 'family physician'. In the course of the drama, he perpetrated various corrupt acts, including faking his own qualifications, as well as issuing a false death certificate in favour of his patron's wife, that led to the climax of the narrative. However, in a perverse sense his acts of medical fraud, in fact, help expose other rampant social evils like adultery and marital deception.

Homoeopathic physicians of similarly questionable character and qualifications were brought to life by other contemporary authors. The farce *Daktarbabu* depicted how a physician, Manmatha, violated the trust bestowed on him by a middle-class family as he intimately examined Hem, their daughter.[42] Girish Chandra Ghosh's drama *Haranidhi* (*Lost Gem*), similarly, recorded the fate of a character who was advised to turn to homoeopathy after his ill character was exposed, on the argument that it would be compatible with his deceitful temperament.[43] The drama *Manpyathy* was another farce staged in 1924, based on the

[39] Ibid., pp. 226–7.
[40] Dwijendralal Ray, *Trhyasparsha ba Sukhi Paribar* (*Triangular Impact or the Happy Family*), 2nd edition (Calcutta: Surdham, 1915).
[41] Ibid., pp. 19–21. [42] Anonymous, *Daktarbabu* (Calcutta, 1875), pp. 38–45.
[43] This is quoted in K. N. Basu, 'Homoeopathic Upadhi Samasya' (Problem of Homoeopathic Degrees), *Hahnemann*, 9, 10 (1926), 547.

1923 short story 'Chikitsha Sankat' ('Crisis of Treatment') by the famous humourist Rajshekhar Basu or Parashuram.[44] The story was later turned into a film, as Fig. 1.1 shows. The play *Manpyathy*, authored by the native landed elite the Maharaja of Kassimbazar, was inaugurated at his own residence in 1924 before being staged at various public theatres across Calcutta.[45] Both the short story and the stage adaptation captured the contemporary society's wariness of the alleged incompetence of various forms of medicine, including homoeopathy. While the play was a sarcastic comment on the general inefficiency of modern medicine, the figure of the homoeopath was shown to be full of idiosyncrasies relating to his art of diagnosis. He was depicted as being so obsessed with consulting western texts and studying his patient's symptoms that he failed to arrive at any conclusion regarding the possible medication. Engrossed in a bitter polemic against allopaths, he only recommended drugs to purge the body of 'allopathic poison', before demanding a staggering fee for such futile consultation.

Notwithstanding their dubious qualifications and idiosyncrasies, some characters comparable to the homoeopath in 'Chikitsha Sankat' were portrayed with great empathy. The character of Priyanath Mukherjee in Sarat Chandra's 1920 novel *Bamuner Meye* (*Daughter of a Brahmin*) and that of physician Srinath in Tarashankar Bandopadhyay's 1934 short story *Srinath Daktar* are unforgettable tragic heroes of Bengali literature who practised homoeopathy to their doom.[46] Amateurish, well-meaning and struggling, both were depicted as obsessed with the 'science' of homoeopathy in a strangely futile way. Srinath's burning passion to produce newer homoeopathic drugs by experimenting at home resulted in the unfortunate death of his wife.[47] Set in early twentieth-century rural Bengal, the character of Priyanath Mukherjee rendered by Sarat Chandra Chattopadhyay was a poor, rustic physician popular among his fellow villagers.[48] However, the villagers often avoided him because of his copy-book commitment to Hahnemann's canons, that sometimes got in the way of his pragmatism in diagnosis. They were shown preferring his daughter Sandhya, who dispensed homoeopathic drugs from home, as a complete amateur. At the climax of the novel, Priyanath was brutally implicated in a caste-

[44] Srish Chandra Nandi, *Monpyathy* (Kasimbazar: Publisher not cited, 1931).
[45] Srish Chandra Nandi, 'Dedication page', *Monpyathy* (Kasimbazar: Publisher not cited, 1931).
[46] See Sarat Chandra Chattopadhyay, 'Bamun er Meye' ('Daughter of a Brahmin'), *Sarat Sahitya Samagra*, Vol I (Kolkata: Ananda Publishers, 1920/1986), pp. 979–1013; and Tarashankar Bandopadhyay, 'Srinath Daktar', *Tarashankar er Galpaguchha* (Kolkata: Sahitya Samsad, 1934/1990), pp. 373–83.
[47] Ibid. [48] See Sarat Chandra Chattopadhyay, 'Bamun er Meye', pp. 979–1013.

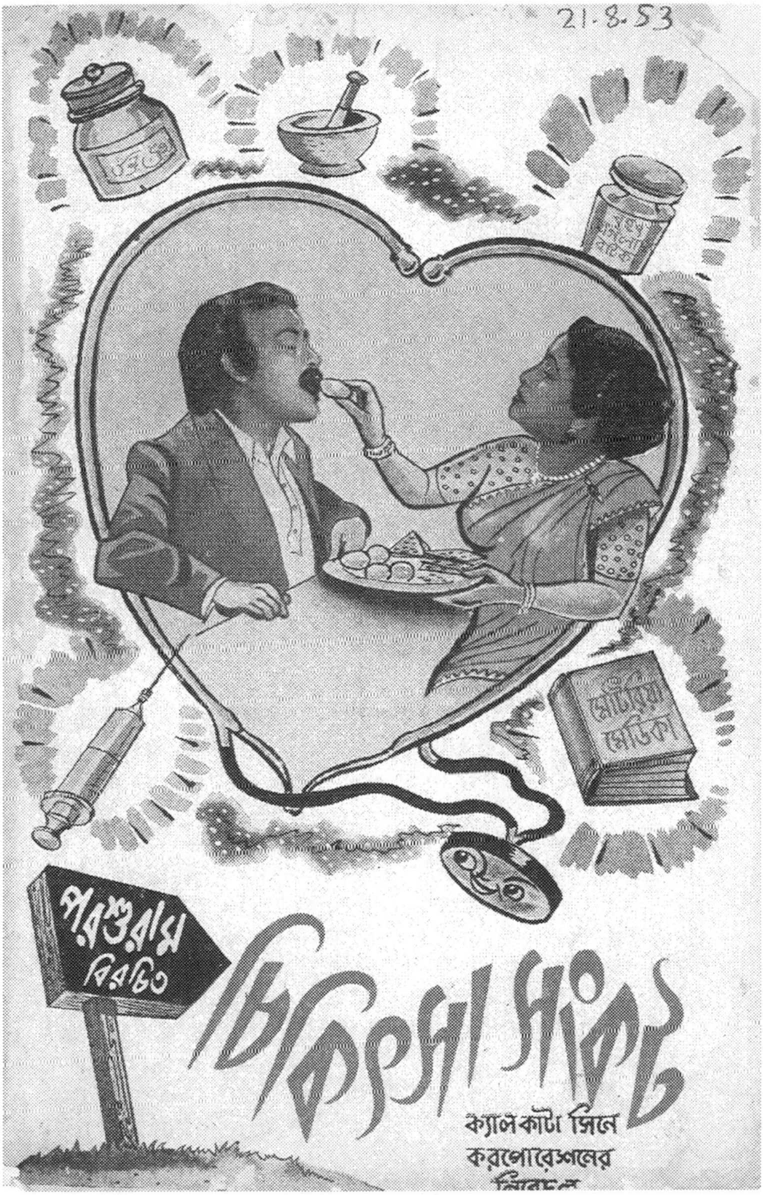

Fig. 1.1 Poster of a film adaptation of the story 'Chikitsha Sankat' ('Crisis of Treatment') by Rajshekhar Basu, produced by the Calcutta Cine Corporation in 1953. Reproduced from the collection of the Archives of the Centre for Studies in Social Sciences, Calcutta.

conflict in his village, which related to a secret illegal abortion with which the village landlord entrusted him.[49] However, implicit in the very act of requesting a secret abortion from Priyanath is an inherent trust – both in the character of the homoeopathic physician as well as in his therapeutics. Homoeopaths such as Priyanath were portrayed as harmless, ubiquitous figures who could be trusted with the inner, private and feminine aspects of society. The characters in the novel exhibit a deep-seated conviction in the homoeopathic physician's abilities to perform covertly, effectively and faithfully.

Such trust seemed to resonate with Yama's proclamation in the farce *Kritanter Bangadarshan* that homoeopathic drugs, even if not effective, can never be harmful. These practitioners prescribing the most gentle, sweet tasting, insignificant, white globules were somehow considered incapable of causing any significant social harm. They were considered the gentlest and most trustworthy characters, who could easily be victimised at the hands of the more powerful. In the early 1940s author Saradindu Bandopadhyay can be seen working with a well-entrenched understanding of the ubiquitous, trustworthy homoeopath when he introduced his famous Bengali detective series, starring the sleuth Byomkesh Bakshi, with the story *Satvanneshi* (*Searcher of Truth*).[50] The climactic revelation in the plot that the helpful, trusted, sweet-natured, amateur homoeopath Anukul *daktar* was in fact the leader of an infamous drug-peddling gang smuggling cocaine, was therefore meant to shock the readers.

The recurrence of the figure of the homoeopathic physician in myriad genres of Bengali fiction, thus, evoked the simultaneous effects of overt ridicule and covert appreciation. These fictional texts seem to castigate homoeopathy for its many slippages while equally celebrating it as a pervasive, ubiquitous and trustworthy practice. Frequently presented as humour, these stories were directed at exposing the everyday plight of colonial life. Homoeopathy remained at the centre of many of these plots as an object both of ridicule and value. Such depictions suggest revealing tensions as much in the status of homoeopathy in Bengal as in the genre of Bengali satirical prose itself, which often highlighted the importance of its subjects only by making fun of them.

[49] Ibid., pp. 1006–7.

[50] See Saradindu Bandopadhyay, 'Satvanneshi' ('Searcher of Truth'), *Byomkesh Omnibus*, Vol I (Calcutta: Ananda Publishers, 1932/2000), pp. 13–32.

The Competing Companies

Differing in approach from the conventional and coercive institution characterised by the colonial bureaucracy, the cause of homoeopathy was nonetheless being taken up by a range of commercial enterprises advertising themselves as trusted authorities on homoeopathy. These firms combined multiple roles in themselves: pharmacies dealing with the importing and selling of homoeopathic drugs, publishing houses for homoeopathic literature including journals, and often, also dispensaries staffed with physicians. Most advertised themselves as 'homoeopathic chemists, druggists, booksellers and publishers'.[51] I focus here on six protagonists prominent among such enterprises, and their firms: Berigny and Company owned by the physician Rajendralal Datta; the Pals of the famous Batakrishna Pal and Company, who owned the Great Homoeopathic Hall[52]; the Sircars headed by the famous physician Mahendralal Sircar; Pratap Chandra Majumdar along with his son Jitendranath Majumdar, who owned the Majumdar's Pharmacy; the M. Bhattacharya and Company, headed by Mahesh Chandra Bhattacharya; and finally, Prafulla Chandra Bhar and his sons, who owned the Hahnemann Publishing Company. These were among the most prominent business concerns dealing in homoeopathy. Situated at 12, Lalbazar Street and owned by Rajendralal Datta (1818–89) and his nephew Ramesh Chandra Datta, Berigny and Company's Calcutta Homoeopathic Pharmacy was reputedly 'the first and the oldest' homoeopathic pharmacy in India.[53] The Pharmacy was built by Rajendralal Datta in memory of the French homoeopath Dr Berigny (see Fig. 1.2), who practised in early nineteenth-century Calcutta and initiated Datta into homoeopathy. The name of Rajendralal Datta, who studied for some years at the Calcutta Medical College, deserves a special mention as he influenced several Bengali luminaries including Mahendralal Sircar to take up homoeopathy.[54]

In addition to publishing literature and supplying drugs, some of the homoeopathic firms were subsequently involved in establishing formal institutions like schools and colleges. This twentieth-century development will be explored in Chapter 5. Between them, these

[51] 'Advertisement of Lahiri and Company', *Indian Homoeopathic Review*, 21, 2 (February 1912), page number not cited.

[52] In some English advertisements of the period, the name was also spelt as Butto Krishto Paul.

[53] See Sarat Chandra Ghosh, 'Dr. T. Berigny', *Hahnemann*, 22, 4 (1939), 198.

[54] Others influenced by Rajendralal Datta's homoeopathic treatment are said to be the eminent social reformer Ishwarchandra Vidyasagar, and the scholar and leader Raja Radhakanta Deb.

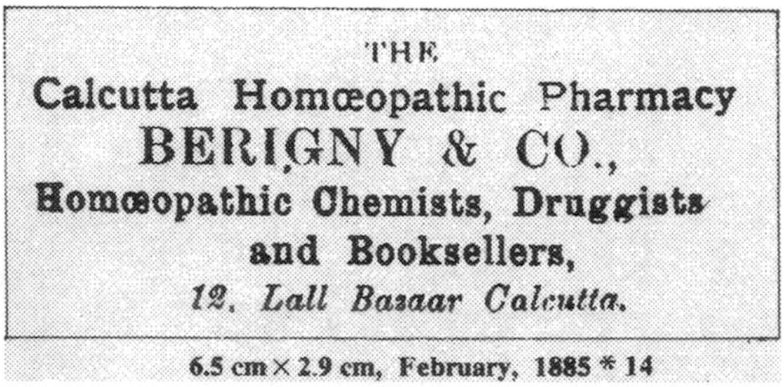

Fig. 1.2 Advertisement by Berigny and Company in English newspaper *The Statesman*, 1885. R. Ray Choudhuri, *Early Calcutta Advertisements, 1875–1925: A Selection from the Statesman* (Bombay: Nachiketa Publications, 1992), 400. Credit: *The Statesman*, Kolkata.

firms edited the most important journals dedicated exclusively to homoeopathy. Interestingly, as Fig. 1.3 suggests, most of these companies were run by physicians across generations. Early twentieth-century accounts of homoeopathy also highlight these physicians and their enterprise as crucial to the development of the doctrine not only in Bengal but in India more generally.[55] These accounts noted these enterprises as being invested in homoeopathy as a 'family'. Writing about the Majumdar family, author Sarat Chandra Ghosh noted, 'Dr. Pratap Chandra Majumdar is dead but will live long through his works and accomplishments. Dr. Jitendra Nath Majumdar is the eldest son of late Dr. P. C. Majumdar ... he is an eminent homoeopath and has kept up the traditions of his father and their house remarkably well.'[56]

However, these six concerns were in no way alone in a growing market for homoeopathic drugs and publications. The leading firms this book focuses on need to be situated within the plethora of other Bengali firms advertising themselves as 'dealers in homoeopathic drugs and books'. The purpose is to get a sense of the crowd of companies associated with homoeopathic business, and to note some of the normative codes of their business operation, as well as the material culture of their practice culled primarily from their extensive advertisements.[57] Lahiri and

[55] See, for instance, S. C. Ghosh, *Life of Mahendralal Sircar*, 1st edition (Calcutta: Oriental Publishing Company, 1909).
[56] S. C. Ghosh, *Life of Mahendralal Sircar*, 2nd edition (Calcutta: Hahenmann Publishing Company, 1935), pp. 67–72.
[57] Medical advertisements as an important aspect of the commercialised print culture around South Asian science and medicine is slowly being opened up as an area of study. For some initial explorations, see Madhuri Sharma, 'Creating a Consumer:

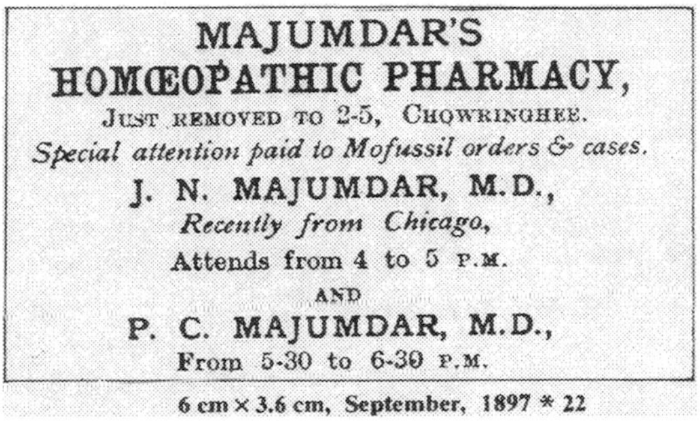

Fig. 1.3 Advertisement by Majumdar's Homoeopathic Pharmacy in the English newspaper *The Statesman*, 1897. R. Ray Choudhuri, *Early Calcutta Advertisements, 1875–1925: A Selection from the Statesman* (Bombay: Nachiketa Publications, 1992), 400. Credit: *The Statesman*, Kolkata.

Company (14 and 35, College Street), B. Datta and Company (Chitpur Road), Chatterjee and Company (121/1 Bowbazar Street), C. Ringer and Company (4, Dalhousie Square East), Carr and Company (36, Cornwallis Street), L. V. Mitter and company (1 Upper Circular Road), C. Kylye and Company (150, Cornwallis Street), Messrs K. Dutta and Company (21, Bowbazar Street), King and Company (Harrison Road), Sarkar and Banerjee (110, College Street), B. K. Pal and Company (12, Bonfield Lane), N. K. Majumdar and Company (Clive Street) were just a few of the range of companies that recurrently published their homoeopathic products.

In his *Life of Mahendralal Sircar* written in 1909, physician Sarat Chandra Ghosh noted the presence of around 200 such indigenous concerns doing 'excellent business' in and around Calcutta.[58] Thriving primarily along the hub of north Calcutta, most had branches all over the city and also in the *mofussil.* Lahiri and Company was a typical homoeopathic concern, owned by physician Jagadish Lahiri and later by his son, the physician Satyaranjan Lahiri. An advertisement for the Company, published in a book authored

Exploring Medical Advertisements in Colonial India' in Mark Harrison and Biswamoy Pati (eds.), *The Social History of Health and Healing in Colonial India* (New York: Routledge, 2009), pp. 213–28. However, the fragile condition of medical advertisements, due to poor preservation, makes it difficult to recreate the narrative around them.

[58] S. C. Ghosh, *Life of Mahendralal Sircar*, 1st edition (Calcutta: Oriental Publishing Company, 1909), p. 101.

by the founder Jagadish Lahiri in 1907, mentioned several other branches in addition to the main office in College Street.[59] Apart from the branches in Burrabazar and in Shobha Bazaar in the north of the city, there was also a Bhawanipore branch in the south, as well as in Bankipore and Patna which were advertised as the *mofussil* branches.[60]

There was a sense of stiff competition between these companies in trying to attract a large body of consumers. The western roots of homoeopathy were carefully played up in the way these firms marketed themselves and their products. But the chief index of competition remained quality – both of the drugs they dispensed and the books they published. The advertisements often made a strong case for the importance of 'trust' in selecting a pharmaceutical store, especially relating to homoeopathy.[61] Most of them emphasised the 'accurate' mode of preparation as crucial for the efficacy of the drugs. A few factors were represented in myriad advertisements as constitutive of the purity and authenticity of homoeopathic medicine. Since these firms engaged in the autonomous manufacture of drugs only much later (Hahnemann Publishing Company were one of the earliest manufacturers who began producing Indian pills around 1916), most of the late nineteenth-century advertisements emphasised the process of importation. The country of origin, the way these drugs were being imported, their freshness, local packaging by the companies, the credibility of the physicians involved in the final preparation, the potency of the drugs, their prices and how long the drugs lasted, all converged in the rhetoric around what constituted 'pure' and 'good quality' homoeopathic drugs.

As Fig. 1.4 reveals, the drugs were chiefly claimed to be imported from England, America or Germany. Each company vouched for the efficacy of their own products and as opposed to the ones imported by the rest. A typical advertisement of C. Ringer and Company in the journal *Krishak* read, '[i]f you really want your homoeopathic medicine to work, then refrain from using the cheap German variety and kindly use the fresh and genuine English medicine that is available in our store'.[62]

59 'Advertisement of Lahiri and Company', in Jagadish Chandra Lahiri, *Homoeopathy r Bipokkhe Apotti Khondon* (*Negation of Allegations against Homoeopathy*) (Calcutta: Lahiri and Company, 1907), page number not cited.
60 Ibid.
61 Batakrishna Pal, 'Preface', *Homoeopathic Mowt e Saral Griha Chikitsha* (*Simple Domestic Treatment According to Homoeopathy*), 7th edition (Calcutta: Great Homoeopathic Hall, 1926), page number not cited.
62 'Advertisement of C. Ringer and Company', in *Krishak*, 11, 1 (1910), page number not cited.

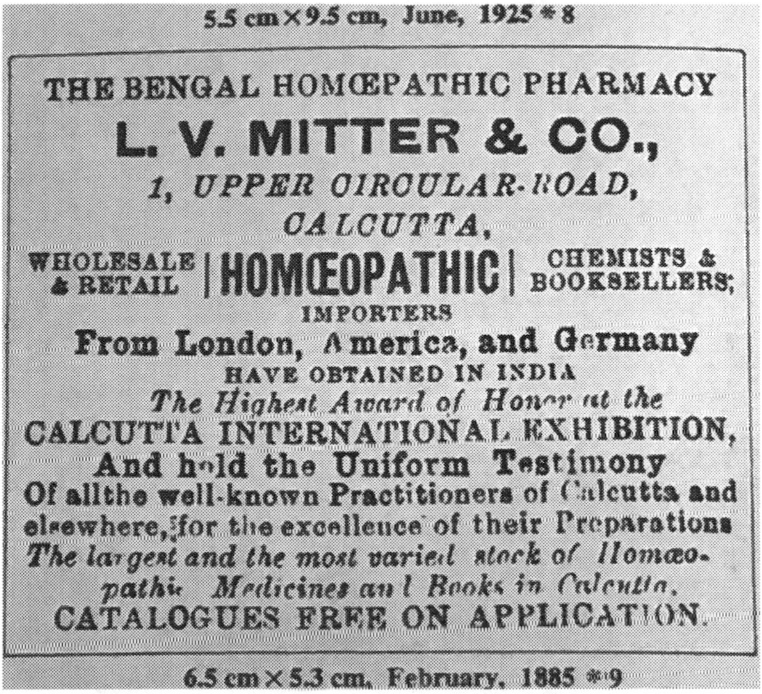
5.5 cm × 9.5 cm, June, 1925 * 8
THE BENGAL HOMŒPATHIC PHARMACY
L. V. MITTER & CO.,
1, UPPER CIRCULAR-ROAD,
CALCUTTA,
WHOLESALE & RETAIL
HOMŒOPATHIC
CHEMISTS & BOOKSELLERS;
IMPORTERS
From London, America, and Germany
HAVE OBTAINED IN INDIA
The Highest Award of Honor at the
CALCUTTA INTERNATIONAL EXHIBITION,
And hold the Uniform Testimony
Of allthe well-known Practitioners of Calcutta and
elsewhere, for the excellence of their Preparations
The largest and the most varied stock of Homœo-
pathic Medicines and Books in Calcutta.
CATALOGUES FREE ON APPLICATION.
6.5 cm × 5.3 cm, February, 1885 * 9

Fig. 1.4 Advertisement of L. V. Mitter and Co claiming to import the best homoeopathic drugs from London, America and Germany, in the English newspaper, *The Statesman*, February 1885. R. Ray Choudhuri, *Early Calcutta Advertisements, 1875–1925: A Selection from the Statesman* (Bombay: Nachiketa Publications, 1992), p. 400. Credit: *The Statesman*, Kolkata.

Invoking the supposedly reputed western firms that supplied medicine to these stores added weight to their campaigns. Thus the Great American Homoeopathic Store run by Carr and Company, and the Homoeopathic Medical Hall run by Messrs K. Dutta and Company, claimed to sell genuine American drugs imported from the firm Boericke and Tafel.[63] Meanwhile the College Street-based Maitra and Company claimed their drugs were imported from the reputed London firm Goolf and Sons, which was 'the suppliers of

[63] 'Advertisement of Carr and Company', in *Chikitsha Sammilani* New Series, 2, *1* (1912), page number not cited.

drugs to the London Homoeopathic Hospital and was the best homoeopathic pharmacy in London'.[64] Boericke and Tafel was described in a K. Dutta and Company advertisement as the 'great American homoeopathic chemists and the most eminent firm in the world'.[65] Claiming to import the 'original potency' drugs directly from Messrs Boericke and Tafel, another north Calcutta-based company named the Homoeopathic Serving Society advertised themselves as the suppliers of the longest-lasting homoeopathic drugs.[66] Arguing that drugs from their store would remain effective until the last drop or the last globule in each bottle, they claimed that 'it was not the case with drugs imported from any other company or those prepared in any other way'.[67]

Apart from the source of importation, the quality of the drugs was likewise argued to vary with the skill of the physicians who handled the final preparation. Companies regularly vouched for the expertise they offered in their pharmacies, as Fig. 1.5 suggests. Citing the experience and credibility of their physicians, a typical advertisement from the firm Sarkar and Banerjee challenged the potential buyers, saying 'on the first use itself one immediately gets to understand the difference between the available medicine in the market, and that of our own, prepared in a far superior way'.[68]

The companies asserted their importance in the realm of drug packaging as well. Most of the pharmacies owned by these companies sold drugs in several sets of self-contained boxes. The Homoeopathic Laboratory run by B. Datta and Company regularly put up elaborate descriptions of medical chests they had for sale.[69] The range was extensive, both in terms of the price and the size of the boxes. There were boxes priced between Rs 3 and Rs 100, containing twelve bottles of medicine to eighty bottles. The advertisements contained descriptions of boxes including their exact dimensions and the material used in their making.[70] In addition, different advertisements addressed various

[64] 'Advertisement of Maitra and Company' in Bipin Bihari Maitra, *Diseases of Children and Its Homoeopathic Treatment* (Calcutta: Maitra and Company, 1887), page number not cited.

[65] ' Advertisement of Messrs K. Dutta and Company', *Calcutta Journal of Medicine*, 10 (April 1882), page number not cited.

[66] 'Advertisement of Homoeopathic Serving Society', in *Homoeopathy Pracharak*, 1, 5 (1926), page number not cited.

[67] Ibid.

[68] 'Advertisement of Sarkar and Banerjee', *Bigyan*, 2, 9 (1913), page number not cited.

[69] 'Advertisement of Homoeopathic Laboratory', Basanta Kumar Dutta (ed.), *Datta's Homoeopathic Series in Bengalee*, 1, 1 (January 1876), page number not cited.

[70] Batakrishna Pal, 'Preface', *Homoeopathic Mowt e Saral Griha Chikitsha* (*Simple Domestic Treatment According to Homoeopathy*), 1926, page number not cited.

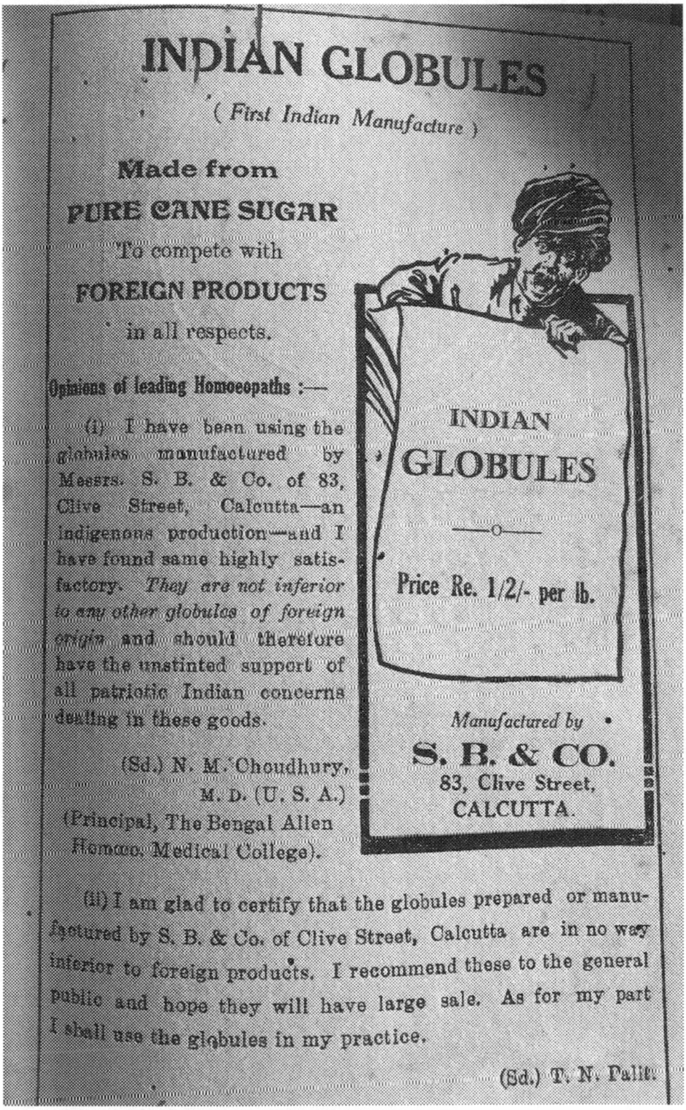

Fig. 1.5 Advertisement of India-made globules by S. B. and Company claiming excellence, *Hahnemannian Gleanings*, November 1935. Credit: Hahnemann Publishing Company Pvt Limited, Kolkata.

constituencies of consumers: householders, women, homoeopathic practitioners and cholera patients. Some companies even included information regarding the security of their homoeopathic chests, detailing arrangements for locking them with keys.[71]

Yet another index of self-promotion was the quality of the firms' publications. Most of these companies owned printing presses and published homoeopathic works authored by their owners as well as by other physicians associated with their firms. These publications included monographs, *materia medica*, stand-alone or serially published manuals and journals. B. Datta and Company, for instance, published a series of manuals: *Datta's Family Guide, Datta's Homoeopathic Series in Bengalee*, and *Datta's Series Griha Chikitsha.* The print run of a particular book counted as an obvious indicator of its popularity. Advertisements by Lahiri and Company included exhaustive lists of books authored by the owner physician Jagadish Chandra Lahiri and published by the company.[72] The name of each book was followed by quotations from generous newspaper reviews. An advertisement quoted the newspaper *Bangabasi*, praising the book *Griha Chikitsha* (*Domestic Treatment*) mentioning, 'this book has had five editions. This statistic is enough in itself. There is hardly any need for the authors of such books to hunt for further publicity as they have already justified the reputation of their publication'.[73]

Another important standard for judging the quality of the texts were the names of their original authors and places of publication. Books were regularly advertised as compilations from various important western authorities on the subject. As with the drugs, the quality of the books also relied on the names of the western authors whose works were being translated and compiled. I will be looking into the extensive practices, politics and impact of these homoeopathic translations in Chapter 3, I will note here, however, that accessing and translating authentic European texts remained a hallmark of the achievements of these local companies. Thus, the obituary of the second-generation owner of C. Ringer and Company, Dr Kishorimohan Bandopadhyay, described the company as a trendsetter in translating the works of eminent western scholars.[74] This obituary recited a list of books that

[71] 'Advertisement of Carr and Company', in *Chikitsha Sammilani* New Series, 2, 1 (1912), page number not cited.

[72] 'Advertisement of Lahiri and Company', in Jagadish Chandra Lahiri, *Homoeopathy r Bipokkhe Apotti Khondon* (*Negation of Allegations against Homoeopathy*) (Calcutta: Lahiri and Company, 1907), page number not cited.

[73] Ibid.

[74] Sarat Chandra Ghosh, 'Kishorimohan Bandopadhyay', *Hahnemann*, 23, 12 (1940), 728–9.

it claimed the company began translating long before others in the field. Some of them were *Farrington's Materia Medica*, *Hughes' Pharmacodynamics*, *Nash's How to Take the Case and Find the Similium*, *Hughes' Principles and Practice of Homoeopathy.*[75] Often, such books were advertised as more than a straightforward translation of any single English work. For instance, B. K. Pal and Company, while advertising one of its publications *Chikitsha Darpan* (*Mirror of Treatment*), especially underlined that it contained the views and experiences of 'not one, but a range of English physicians including Tanner, Johnson, Roberts, Bear and Herring'.[76] The company claimed that this made the book count as one of the best works of medicine in the Bengali language.[77] The links that the advertising companies maintained with international homoeopathic journals were also carefully drawn to the public's attention. Thus, favourable reviews of *Datta's Homoeopathic Series* in the London-based journals *The Homoeopathic World* and *Homoeopathic Review* were quoted extensively in the promotional advertisements of the series.[78]

As has already been suggested, the keen sense of competition between the companies hinged fundamentally on two issues: the quality of the drugs supplied through their pharmacies and the literature they published. Developing each of these aspects required the companies to be in regular contact with the West. Success in any enterprise involving homoeopathy apparently relied on the capacity to keep up with the latest developments in western therapeutic knowledge. A covert implication of all the advertisements was the service they were rendering in bringing these advanced western medical ideas to India. In an 1876 marketing drive, B. Datta and Company included reviews from the newspaper *Bharat Sangskarak* in their advertisement, which declared, 'Basanta Datta is not only involved in medical business with homoeopathy. He is deeply concerned about popularising this useful medical doctrine for the common people of this country.'[79] An editorial article of the journal *Hahnemann*, edited by B. Datta and Company, hence proclaimed,

[75] Ibid.

[76] 'Advertisement of Batakrishna Pal and Company', in Batakrishna Pal, *Homoeopathic Mowt e Saral Griha Chikitsha* (Simple Domestic Treatment According to Homoeopathy), 7th edition (Calcutta: Great Homoeopathic Hall, 1926), page number not cited.

[77] Ibid.

[78] Basanta Kumar Dutta (ed.), 'Review of Datta's Homoeopathic Series' in *Datta's Homoeopathic Series in Bengalee*, 5, 6 (May–June 1876), promotional advertisement at the end.

[79] Basanta Kumar Dutta (ed.), 'Review of Datta's Homoeopathic Series' in *Datta's Homoeopathic Series in Bengalee*, 3, 3 (March 1876), cover page.

Discovered in 1793, the homoeopathic doctrine is already far ahead of the other prevalent doctrines in the west. Not only one – almost all the civilised races are gracefully embracing this useful form of treatment. *Hahnemann* (the journal) is the Bengali messenger of homoeopathy . . . we can assert with pride and happiness that our efforts are bearing fruit. Homoeopathy is gaining popularity even among the fallen races of this conquered land.[80]

The companies claimed the credit not only of importing the latest medical innovations to India, but also of distributing them fairly beyond urban locations into the remote countryside. Most advertisements highlighted the firm's service to the consumers based in the *mofussils*: they diligently recorded how their drugs and books were sent in transit, and how the cost of extra postage, and advanced subscriptions, was received from their *mofussil* customers.[81] An advertisement for the Great American Homoeopathic Store read, 'we invite the attention of mofussil doctors to our stock of genuine homoeopathic medicines, indented direct from Messrs Boerike and Tafel, U.S.A'.[82]

Within this crowd of companies and their proprietors, the activities of Rajendralal Dutta, Batakrishna Pal, Mahesh Chandra Bhattacharya, Pratap Chandra Majumdar, Mahendralal Sircar and Prafulla Chandra Bhar stand out. With their regular investments in homoeopathic publications and drugs over generations, these protagonists remained central in the production and dissemination of homoeopathic knowledge in Bengal. Between them, they edited and published the most widely circulating and enduring homoeopathic journals, including *Indian Homoeopathic Review* (edited and published by the Majumdars), *Homoeopathic Herald* and *Homoeopathy Chikitsha* (published by M. Bhattacharya and Company), *Hahnemann* and *The Hahnemannian Gleanings* (published by Hahnemann Publishing Company). Most important among these was the *Calcutta Journal of Medicine*, edited and published by Mahendralal Sircar and his son Amritalal Sircar, uninterruptedly from 1867 to at least 1913. In its heyday under Mahendralal, limited copies were sent for sale in London as is evident from Mahendralal's diary entries of 22 January 1874.[83] Besides, the Sircars were associated with some of the most prominent pharmacies dealing in homoeopathic drugs. In their publications, these entrepreneurs frequently endorsed one another as conducting the most credible

[80] 'Editorial: Hahnemann er Borsho Bridhhi' ('Growth of Hahnemann over the Years'), *Hahnemann*, 3,1 (Baishakh 1885), 4.

[81] 'Advertisement of Datta's Homoeopathic Series', in *Datta's Homoeopathic Series in Bengalee*, 1, 1 (January 1876), page number not cited.

[82] 'Advertisement of The Great American Homoeopathic Store', in *Indian Homoeopathic Review*, 19 (October 1910), page number not cited.

[83] Arun Kumar Biswas (ed.), *Gleanings of the Past and the Science Movement: In the Diaries of Drs. Mahendralal and Amritalal Sircar* (Kolkata: Asiatic Society, 2000), p. 16.

business around homoeopathy. For instance, an editorial article in the journal *Hahnemannian Gleanings* published by the Hahnemann Publishing Company identified the 'Hahnemann Publishing Company (of Prafulla Chandra Bhar), the Economic Pharmacy (Mahesh Bhattacharya) and one or two other pharmacies' as the 'pioneers of introducing neat, genuine and rightly prepared homoeopathic remedies ... in India'.[84] It contrasted the position of these reputed pharmacies with the numerous smaller ones that indulged in various forms of practices which were 'tantamount to a pure professional misconduct'.[85] Emphasis was also laid on the pitfalls of unnecessary rivalry between one another. The secret to successful business was shown to be reliance on mutual help and collaboration. The same editorial further noted, '[h]armony should be the basic principle upon which true friendship and good business can last and flourish. Selfishness, greed, enmity, rivalry and mutual vilification do away with and undo that which it took years to build up'.[86]

'One Cannot Accumulate Wealth Without Trade and Business'

Printing and publishing comprised a central aspect of the enterprises led by the six foremost homoeopathic protagonists. Along with homoeopathy, most of these firms also indulged in publications on themes not exclusively related to medicine. A frequently visited theme by these entrepreneur-physicians in their non-medical publication was the importance of business.[87] In addition, the owners of these enterprises published a number of biographies and a few autobiographies. These detailed their thoughts and ideologies, which emphasised the utility of generating wealth. They were unanimous in underlining the necessity of business and entrepreneurship in earning money. Through their twin emphases on wealth and business, these texts promoted a culture and ethic of entrepreneurship. In his book '*Byabshayee*' (literally meaning *Businessman*) Mahesh Chandra Bhattacharya suggested a distinct hierarchy of professions, observing, '[o]ne can never be rich without doing business. One gets to earn the most through business. Next (in hierarchy) is the income through industry, then agriculture, then salaried service or *chakri*. The least income is incurred through begging'.[88] Jitendranath

[84] 'Editorial: New Year's Retrospection and Introspection', *The Hahnemannian Gleanings*, 4, 1 (1933), 4.
[85] Ibid., p. 7. [86] Ibid., p. 11.
[87] Jitendranath Majumdar, *Arther Sandhan* (*Pursuit of Wealth*), 1932, p. 116.
[88] Mahesh Chandra Bhattacharya, *Byabshayee* (Businessman), 1905, p. 8.

Majumdar (who sometimes published as J. N. Majumdar) also noted in his text *Arther Sandhan* (*Pursuit of Wealth*), 'one cannot accumulate wealth without engaging in trade and business'.[89]

The texts charted the importance of wealth at various levels of social life. First was the exclusively individualistic domain of the maintenance and well-being of the household. Narrating the life and achievements of his physician father, Jitendranath Majumdar recounted how Pratap Chandra Majumdar was forced to spend almost the whole of his 'princely income' on the marriage of his daughters as well as the education of his sons and sons-in-law, all of whom studied in England or in America.[90] He noted with regret that familial obligations exhausted nearly all of his father's savings and deterred him from engaging in substantial acts of charity.[91] As a consequence, at his death, the famous physician could barely leave anything more than his immovable assets. Jitendranath noted how his father would often recall his initial brushes with poverty in early life, concluding that 'wealth is the most desired thing in life!'[92]

The importance of wealth was also discussed in relation to social respectability. Such texts often reflected upon the links between independent enterprise, however small, and social respect. Contrary to the dominant historiographical understanding of the late nineteenth-century association between education, salaried jobs and respectability, these authors registered an emphatic case for enterprise as an ideal way to garner social respect.[93] At the very beginning of his instructive 1905 monograph *Byabshayee* (*Businessman*), which ran into several editions,[94] Mahesh Chandra Bhattacharya engaged in a long discussion of business and social status. He lashed out against the Bengali perception that business had lower social status.[95] Bhattacharya referred to laws and customs from ancient *shastras* to argue that the traditional trading and business castes, i.e. the Baisyas, historically commanded prestigious social standing. He contended that, far from considering business socially denigrating, both the ancient lawmaker Manu and the Hindu Puranas considered the Baisyas (the traditional business caste) socially at par even

[89] Jitendranath Majumdar, *Arther Sandhan* (*Pursuit of Wealth*), 1932, p. 116.
[90] J. N. Majumdar, 'Dr. Pratap Chandra Majumdar MD', *Hahnemann*, 23, 8 (1940), p. 451.
[91] Ibid. [92] Ibid., pp. 452–3.
[93] See Srish Chandra Talapatra, *Mahesh Chandra Charitkatha* (*Life of Mahesh Chandra*) (Calcutta: Economic Press, 1946), pp. 120–1.
[94] *Byabshayee* was written and first published by Mahesh Chandra Bhattacharya in 1905. It had at least four later editions, the last one being published in 1921. The prefaces to the various editions proclaimed that the purpose of the tract was to introduce potential beginners to the fundamentals of business and entrepreneurship.
[95] Mahesh Chandra Bhattacharya, *Byabshayee* (*Businessman*), 1905, pp. 2–6.

with the Brahmins in certain contexts.[96] He pointed out, further, that conventional synonyms for 'businessman' in the Bengali language, including '*mahajan*', '*uttamarna*' and '*sadhu*', were all epithets indicating respect in society.[97] Indeed, the biography of protagonist Batakrishna Pal titled *Sadhu Batakrishna Pal* (*The Saintly Batakrishna Pal*) dwelt extensively upon the etymology of the epithet '*sadhu*'.[98] His biographer invoked precolonial Bengali authoritative texts such as the *Mangal Kabyas* and the iconic mythic merchant figure of Chand Saudagar from *Manasa Mangal.*[99] He pointed out that the rich Gandhabanik businessmen in medieval times were traditionally referred to as '*sadhu*' or 'saint'.[100] The biography characterised Batakrishna as belonging to the same Gandhabanik trading caste as the venerated Chand Saudagar, arguing that in ancient and medieval Bengal the epithet 'sadhu' was reserved for successful businessmen. Further, the author expressed his understanding of the contemporary connotation of the word 'sadhu' in the Bengali vocabulary, arguing that it stood for pious, religious men of impeccable character, who dedicated their lives to spiritual salvation or social good.[101] He insisted that these associations with the word encompassed past references to great businessmen who had shown remarkable integrity of character, honesty and dignity in conducting business.[102]

Advocating the importance of enterprise, Mahesh Chandra Bhattacharya suggested a distinct hierarchy between income from landed, agrarian properties and that from business. He expressed deep respect for the erstwhile class of landed gentry – the *zamindars* and *talukdars* – and appreciated their benevolence in patronising men of knowledge and letters through the gift of tax-free or '*brahmottar*' lands.[103] At the same time, he resisted the idea of acquiring landed property for himself. His biography noted his standard reply to all well-wishers advising him to buy landed assets: 'buying

[96] Ibid., pp. 3–4. [97] Ibid.

[98] Gopal Chandra Mukhopadhyay, *Sadhu Batakrishna Pal* (*The Saintly Batakrishna Pal*), Vol II (Calcutta: Butto Krishto Paul, 1919), pp. 243–8.

[99] *Mangal Kabyas*, or 'Poem of Benediction', is a genre of Hindu narrative poetry, didactic and religious, composed roughly between the fifteenth and the eighteenth centuries, notably comprising narratives of indigenous deities of rural Bengal. The *Mangal Kabyas* are typically dedicated to promoting the worship of particular deities: mostly local, Bengali folk deities like Manasa, Candi or Dharma Thakur. For recent work on this body of texts, see David Curley, *Poetry and History: Bengali Mangal Kabya and Social Change in Precolonial Bengal* (Delhi: Chronicle Books, 2008). Here, the particular reference in Pal's biography is to the story *Mansamangal*, which revolves around the snake goddess Manasa.

[100] Ibid., pp. 244–7. [101] Ibid. [102] Ibid., p. 248

[103] Srish Chandra Talapatra, *Mahesh Chandra Charitkatha* (*Life of Mahesh Chandra*), 1946, pp. 16–17.

a zamindari will turn my son into an indolent, extravagant rich man. That will be tantamount to committing a sin as a parent. I would rather leave my business-firm for him. If he is hardworking and honest the store will earn him enough to live a comfortable life'.[104]

In the context of formulating an ideology and ethic of business, some of these texts drew their readers' attention to the Bengali obsession with salaried jobs and hinted that it had grave implications. Mahesh Chandra was worried that even the leaders of the society secretly aspired for their own children to become lawyers or judges, or at the very least clerks, even at low salaries.[105] Initiating an elaborate discussion on the relative advantages of business over salaried jobs or '*chakri*', he primarily focused on the unlimited possibilities of expansion that business offered, as opposed to the security of a job.[106] Bhattacharya pointed out that while income from '*chakri*' tended to diminish drastically in old age, return from business could increase substantially with age if it were in the hands of competent successors or good employees.[107] Jitendranath Majumdar's book *Arther Sandhan* (*Pursuit of Wealth*) dealt with similar concerns and made a compelling case for entrepreneurship against salaried jobs.[108]

Beyond the individual, the texts asserted the importance of enterprise as a larger socio-political commitment – as a way to serve society and the nation. For instance, a biography of Batakrishna Pal devoted an entire chapter to discussing the protagonist's anxieties over the failure of Bengalis to accumulate capital. Resonating with Bengali regionalism, these thoughts were, nonetheless, couched unmistakably in nationalist sensibilities. Titled 'Svajatipriyota' or 'Love for One's Race', this chapter dwelt upon Batakrishna's thoughts for the improvement of the Bengalis from their current fallen status in comparison with the British.[109] He expressed a conviction that the British were the most advanced race primarily because of their proliferating trade and business.[110] For him, British superiority in all spheres – political, scientific or intellectual – emanated from their fundamental power of wealth.[111] Batakrishna strongly asserted that generating wealth through business was the ideal way of self-assertion for any race and nation.[112]

[104] Ibid.
[105] Mahesh Chandra Bhattacharya, *Byabshayee* (*Businessman*), 1905, pp. 2–3.
[106] Ibid., pp. 8–12. [107] Ibid., p. 10.
[108] Jitendranath Majumdar, *Arther Sandhan* (*Pursuit of Wealth*), 1932, p. 132.
[109] Gopal Chandra Mukhopadhyay, *Sadhu Batakrishna Pal (The Saintly Batakrishna Pal)*, Vol II, 1919, pp. 256–61.
[110] Ibid., p. 257. [111] Ibid. [112] Ibid., p. 258.

Ideas of national self-assertion were almost always underpinned by a concern with the regional identity of the Bengalis. This is evident in the writings of Mahesh Chandra Bhattacharya and Jitendranath Majumdar. Mahesh Chandra noted in *Byabshayee*,

> So far only the Europeans were draining the wealth of this country through trade. Now the Marwaris and the Bhatias have joined them. They are buying off all the lands in and around Calcutta. The Bengalis are only concerned with their education, degree and with the ways of becoming teachers, lawyers, judges or doctors. They are oblivious about their future – about where they will live and what they will eat.[113]

Typically, these authors reflected on the mercantile prowess of the British, which earned them political mastery over distant shores.[114] Connecting economic self-sufficiency with the overall development of a nation, Batakrishna pointed out that races that managed to be self-sufficient in terms of food production were the only ones that could ensure development of their own nation (*'sva-desh'*) and own race (*'sva-jat'*).[115] Passionately he proclaimed,

> races which are unable to feed themselves and are forever hankering for food, are hardly any different from slaves. They are detestable lots. Such races are not only deficient in food but in almost everything. All kinds of vices get hold of such people and they become completely sapped of vitality.[116]

To him, the foremost duty of the monarch or the leaders of any nation was to address the issue of widespread hunger.[117] These thoughts resonate closely with the larger economic nationalist formulations, especially the goal of a self-sufficient economy, as histories of *swadeshi* nationalism have identified.[118] Manu Goswami convincingly traced a genealogy of *swadeshi* ideology to the twin 'processes of consolidation of a spatially bounded sense of territory and economy' since the late nineteenth century.[119] *Swadeshi* ideology was integrally bound up, she argued, with the 'colonial production of India as a bounded, coherent entity' and the emergent nationalist imaginings of a school of thinkers who 'urged to develop

[113] Mahesh Chandra Bhattacharya, *Byabshayee* (*Businessman*), 1905, p. 9.
[114] Gopal Chandra Mukhopadhyay, *Sadhu Batakrishna Pal* (*The Saintly Batakrishna Pal*), Vol II, 1919, p. 258.
[115] Ibid., pp. 258–9. [116] Ibid., p. 259. [117] Ibid., p. 259.
[118] See Manu Goswami, 'From Swadeshi to Swaraj: Nation, Economy, and Territory in Colonial South Asia, 1870 to 1907', *Comparative Studies in Society and History*, 40, 4 (1998), 609–36; and Andrew Sartori, 'The Categorical Logic of a Colonial Nationalism: Swadeshi Bengal, 1904–1908', *Comparative Studies of South Asia, Africa and the Middle East*, 23, 1&2 (2003), 271–85.
[119] Manu Goswami, 'From Swadeshi to Swaraj: Nation, Economy, Territory in Colonial South Asia, 1870 to 1907', pp. 624–5.

a specifically national developmentalist model to ground their critique of colonial rule and classical political economy'.[120] Such historical intertwining of ideas concerning economy, enterprise and nationalism, was reflected in the homoeopathic literature under discussion from the late nineteenth century.

Pursuing the theme of national self-sufficiency, Mahesh Bhattacharya urged the youth to engage in innovative and new enterprises.[121] He drew up an impressive list of suggestions in *Byabshaee* and devoted a substantial part of the tract to discussing a wide range of possible fields of investment.[122] These were meant for beginners equipped with business capital of various proportions, from meagre to large.[123] His lengthy discussion engaged with the potentials of business in various fields: the traditional fields for investment included order supply, publishing, opening factories for manufacturing different goods, and construction work.[124] But his list also included apparently unusual sectors of investment, including opening of auction houses, business involving astrological predictions, shoes, clocks and so on.[125] In that context, Bhattacharya further discussed the immense lucrative potentials of opening up homoeopathic dispensary-cum-pharmacies, in comparison with allopathic pharmacies in Calcutta and other big cities.[126]

These texts argued that a nation needed to produce its own essential necessities.[127] Resonating closely with the 'drain of wealth' theories put forward by the late nineteenth-century economic historians like R. C. Dutt and Congress ideologues like Dadabhai Naoraji, the authors spoke of the ideal of importing raw materials and manufacturing the necessities on one's own soil. Bhattacharya quipped that whenever a country managed to accomplish this, 'it is as praise worthy as it is profitable. Importing manufactured items is a matter of utmost shame as it involves national losses'.[128] He put a premium on business involving the everyday necessities of common people including groceries, oil and cloth.[129] Jitendranath Majumdar further added that investment in such quotidian necessities of the people inevitably ensured a profitable business.[130]

Although none of the protagonists of these texts proclaimed themselves *swadeshi* nationalists, their efforts were often appropriated within the framework of *swadeshi*-nationalist endeavours. On a visit to the premises

[120] Ibid., pp. 615–23.
[121] Srish Chandra Talapatra, *Mahesh Chandra Charitkatha* (*Life of Mahesh Chandra*), 1946, p. 47.
[122] Mahesh Chandra Bhattacharya, *Byabshayee* (*Businessman*), 1905, pp. 95–132.
[123] Ibid. [124] Ibid. [125] Ibid. [126] Ibid., pp. 104–5. [127] Ibid., pp. 83–4.
[128] Mahesh Chandra Bhattacharya, *Byabshayee* (*Businessman*), 1905, p. 83.
[129] Ibid., p. 84.
[130] Jitendranath Majumdar, *Arther Sandhan* (*Pursuit of Wealth*), 1932, p. 118.

of B. K. Pal and Company in 1911, Maharaja Sir Pradyot Coomar Tagore was said to have commented,

> I was highly impressed with what I saw. The business is entirely under Indian management and is by far the biggest concern of its kind in the whole of India. This is the right kind of Swadeshi enterprise and as such deserves commendation and encouragement.[131]

Enterprises in homoeopathy were often retrospectively described as embodying a strong *swadeshi* spirit. Referring to the 1880 pharmaceutical enterprise initiated by Rajendralal Dutta, one of his later biographies observed,

> In these days of swadesism we have heard much about Industrialism, of starting Cotton Mills and Steamer Service Companies, of National Education . . . in those days when nobody even dreamt of such things and when to do such things was hazardous enough to make one very unpopular . . . Rajendra Dutt practically organised such institutions quite single-handed.[132]

Another concern reflected in these tracts, related to their discussions of business, was the prevalent system of education in India. Mahesh Chandra, for instance, criticised the existing education system as 'purposeless' and therefore harmful for the country.[133] Bhattacharya was convinced of the futility of technical and commercial schools.[134] The disgust these authors had for formal pedagogic institutions extended even to the institutional dissemination of homoeopathic knowledge. According to Bhattacharya, one could hardly learn to become a good businessman by attending a school or by reading any book; he felt that apprenticeship to a successful businessman was the ideal way to learn good business.[135]

Emphasising the importance and fundamentals of business, Mahesh Chandra made a clear distinction between medical practice on one hand, and business involving medicine on the other. In his view, specialised knowledge of medicine was useful in such a business, but one did not need to be a physician. In his autobiography, he cited himself as an

[131] Gopal Chandra Mukhopadhyay, *Sadhu Batakrishna Pal* (*The Saintly Batakrishna Pal*), Vol II, 1919, p. 80.

[132] S. C. Ghose, 'Homoeopathy and Its First Missionary in India', *The Hahenemannian Gleanings*, 3, 8 (September 1932), 337.

[133] Srish Chandra Talapatra, *Mahesh Chandra Charitkatha* (*Life of Mahesh Chandra*), 1946, p. 79.

[134] This was a conviction shared by P. C. Ray, the eminent nationalist chemist. See Pratik Chakrabarti, 'Science and Swadeshi: The Establishment and Growth of the Bengal Chemical and Pharmaceutical Works' in Uma Dasgupta (ed.), *Science and Modern India: An Institutional History, 1784–1947* (Delhi: Pearson Education, 2010), pp. 117–42.

[135] Mahesh Chandra Bhattacharya, *Byabshayee* (*Businessman*), 1905, p. 57.

example, saying that he consciously steered away from learning medicine until an age to be able to focus solely on the business aspect of it. It is not surprising, therefore, that some of the entrepreneurial families simultaneously invested in fields other than medicine. For the Bhattacharyas, the Pals and for the family of Rajendralal Datta, enterprise focused on homoeopathic drugs; although it was the chief portion of their business, it coexisted with other entrepreneurial efforts. The Dattas, for instance, owned shipping companies and other business concerns, chief among which was the Dutt's Lintzee and Company.[136]

Business as Family, Family as Business

Along with articulating the more abstract significance of enterprise, the non-medical texts published by our protagonist firms focused also on the concrete approaches and ways in which commercial establishments functioned. Efficient management of firms emerged as a persistent theme in these texts. Labour recruitment and management was the foremost matter for discussion. These texts seemed to blur any rigid distinction between a presumably private domain of 'family' and public domain of 'business'. They insisted on strategically replicating within the sphere of business the personal, intimate ties of affection usually associated with families. The ideal form for a business, which generated the maximum revenue, was projected as one functioning through kinship networks and modelled on familial ties. While discussing labour management in particular, the homoeopathic publications promoted a flexible, commodious and porous understanding of family.

Batakrishna Pal, Jitendranath Majumdar and also Mahesh Chandra Bhattacharya underlined the importance of competent employees for the success of any business. They characterised ideal employers as paternalistic. It was argued that, '[t]o a businessman, an honest, dutiful and efficient employee is more precious than the son. Entrepreneurs ought to trust such employees more than their own son'.[137] Mahesh Chandra Bhattacharya attached considerable importance to the recruitment and training of employees and devoted a rather lengthy chapter of *Byabshayee (Businessman)* titled 'Karmachari' or 'Employee' to discussing these aspects.[138] He advocated recruiting one's own relatives or those belonging to one's own region or caste.[139] He felt that employers ought to overlook these considerations only in the exceptional case of

136 S. C. Ghose, 'Homoeopathy and Its First Missionary in India', *The Hahnemannian Gleanings*, 3, 8 (September 1932), 337–8.
137 Mahesh Chandra Bhattacharya, *Byabshayee (Businessman)*, 1905, p. 72.
138 Ibid., pp. 62–82. 139 Ibid., p. 65.

a candidate of extraordinary calibre.[140] Batakrishna Pal, too, abided by these criteria for recruiting employees; his biographer noted that distant relatives and those who were considered part of the broader kinship network invariably found preference in his company.[141] The author recounted that Batakrishna recruited many relatives and other men from his own caste background.

Protagonists such as Mahesh Chandra Bhattacharya and Batakrishna Pal attached a remarkable amount of importance to caste ties in the process of recruiting employees for their companies. A Brahmin by birth, Mahesh Chandra often chose other Brahmins as objects of his charities and also for recruitment in his company. His weakness for Brahmins as employees was widely known and even resulted in accusations of bias.[142] Batakrishna Pal's biographies note his deep loyalties to his caste, and his involvement in the Gandhabanik movement in early twentieth-century Calcutta.[143] In 1900, he was made the president of the committee that dealt with issues relating to the improvement of the Gandhabanik caste.[144] Batakrishna was also the publisher and distributor of the 1902 tract *Gandhabaniktattva* (*Theories relating to the Gandhabaniks*), which dealt with the history and lineage of his caste.[145]

Once employees were recruited, their management and maintenance was a major concern for most protagonists. The rhetoric of family was invoked recurrently and most powerfully to define the relationship between the employer and the employee. Indeed, business in such homoeopathic firms was organised in such a way as to resemble an extended joint-familial household, bound by ties of loyalty and affection. Batakrishna Pal's biography notes that the protagonist was diligent in looking after the well-being of the five-hundred-plus body of employees at B. K. Pal and Company, and paid minute attention to their diet and maintenance.[146] Brahmin cooks were appointed to look after their dietary needs. Mahesh Chandra's biography also noted how he looked after all his employees as if they were 'his own son'.[147]

140 Ibid.

141 Gopal Chandra Mukhopadhyay, *Sadhu Batakrishna Pal* (*The Saintly Batakrishna Pal*), Vol II, 1919, pp. 54–5.

142 Srish Chandra Talapatra, *Mahesh Chandra Charitkatha* (*Life of Mahesh Chandra*), 1946, p. 64.

143 Gopal Chandra Mukhopadhyay, *Sadhu Batakrishna Pal* (*The Saintly Batakrishna Pal*), Vol II, 1919, pp. 261–8. Gandhabaniks are a Bengali Hindu trading caste, who claim the status of Baisyas and who, as the literal translation of their caste name suggests, used to trade in perfumes and exotic spices.

144 Ibid., p. 262. 145 Ibid., Vol I, p. 64.

146 Mahesh Chandra Bhattacharya, *Byabshayee* (*Businessman*), 1905, pp. 93–5.

147 Srish Chandra Talapatra, *Mahesh Chandra Charitkatha* (*Life Mahesh Chandra*), 1946, p. 57.

It is revealing that Batakrishna Pal preferred using parts of his own residence as the premises of his firm. Thus, in the context of the homoeopathic firms, even the spatial and architectural distinction between the business and the household would sometimes collapse. At first, the various departments of B. K. Pal and Company were dispersed over different parts of north Calcutta.[148] Biographies of the protagonist noted how, eventually, Batakrishna built a huge palatial residence at Shobhabazar Street and found it convenient to move the head offices of his various departments there, including the branch offices of his homoeopathic pharmacy, Great Homoeopathic Hall (see Fig. 1.6).[149] The Hahnemann Publishing Company also continued to function in a similar way since the early twentieth century. The Bowbazaar complex of HAPCO still houses the office and the pharmacy, concurrent with serving as the residence of the Bhars for a long time.[150]

The personalised affection of the protagonist entrepreneurs for their employees was especially emphasised in their publications. Mahesh Chandra's life story mentioned that although he was professionally quite strict, yet in cases of ill health or other trouble, he took personal care of the employees, helping them either with cash or in kind.[151] The projected interpersonal relations in the firms suggested a veritable moral economy of care, warmth and love. To examine an instance of how the texts construed a mandate of familial care, let me refer to the case of an employee named Atul from Mahesh Chandra's biography. Atul was described as having contracted plague in the year 1902–3.[152] The biography reminded its readers of the abiding stigma

[148] By the turn of the twentieth century, B. K. Pal and Company was a reputed Calcutta-based entity, which in addition to homoeopathic medicine, had branched out into various other departments, including the import and distribution of allopathic medicine. But the company's humble nineteenth-century beginnings as a homoeopathic family firm is noted in Batakrishna's biography. Although an in-depth historical study of Batakrishna's diverse entrepreneurial activities remains to be written, for some preliminary exploration, see Nandini Bhattacharya, 'Between the Bazaar and the Bench: Making of the Drug Trade in Colonial India, ca. 1900–1930', *Bulletin of the History of Medicine*, 90, 1 (April 2016), 61–91.

[149] Gopal Chandra Mukhopadhyay, *Sadhu Batakrishna Pal* (*The Saintly Batakrishna Pal*), Vol II, 1919, pp. 168–9.

[150] As narrated by Dr Durgashankar Bhar, the current owner of Hahnemann Publishing Company and grandson of the founder Prafulla Chandra Bhar, in an interview conducted in the same residential-cum-commercial building in late August 2009.

[151] Srish Chandra Talapatra, *Mahesh Chandra Charitkatha* (*Life of Mahesh Chandra*), 1946, p. 57.

[152] Ibid., pp. 59–60.

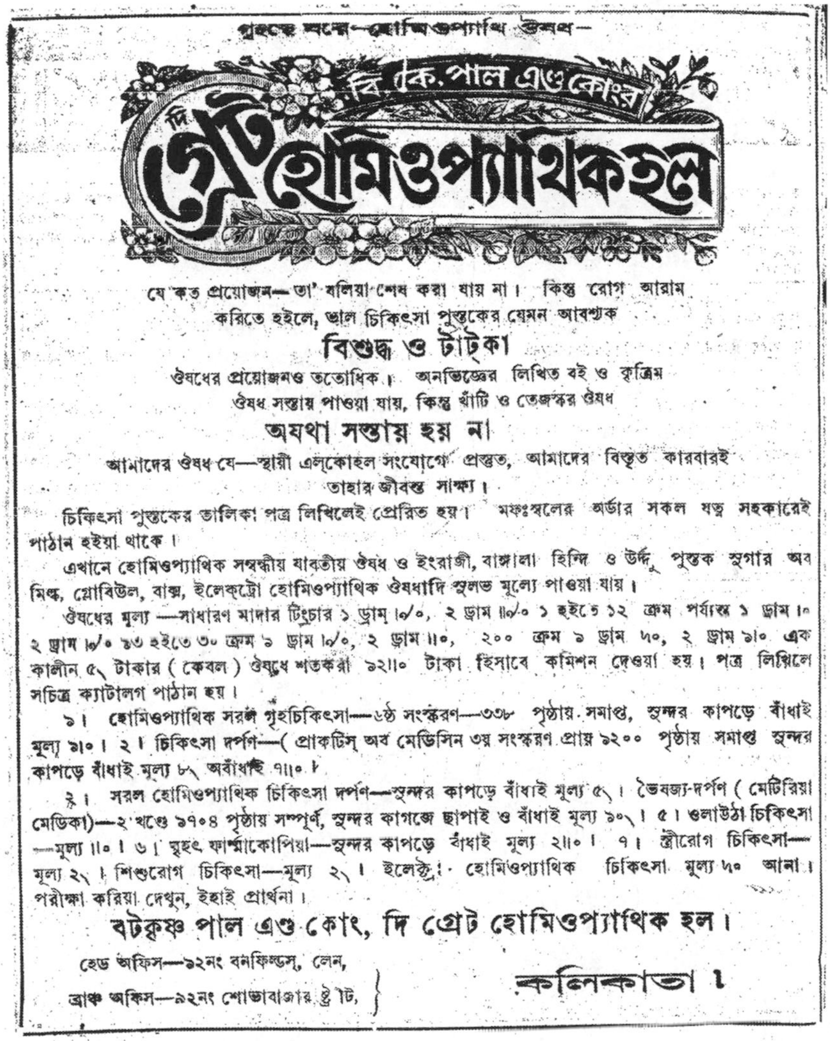

Fig. 1.6 Advertisement of B. K. Pal and Co's Great Homoeopathic Hall in the Bengali journal *Grihasthamangal*, 2, 1 (1928), 6. Reproduced from the collection of the Archives of the Centre for Studies in Social Sciences, Calcutta.

around plague at the time.[153] One of deadliest nineteenth-century epidemic diseases, it was widely held that once taken to the hospital, plague victims hardly ever returned home. The biography noted that despite this stigma, Mahesh Bhattacharya himself, in conjunction with Kumud Bhattacharya (his nephew and then manager of M. Bhattacharya and Company), refused to send Atul to a hospital and committed to treating and nursing him personally. It is detailed how Bhattacharya would visit the patient every two to three hours and make the necessary recommendations for his recovery. The biography further claimed that Mahesh Chandra Bhattacharya looked after his employees even in their old age and gave money in the semblance of a pension to most of them.[154]

In these texts, the virtues of loyalty and trust are discussed repeatedly in the context of generating goodwill in any enterprise. Especially for enterprises committed to therapeutic well-being, the factor of mutual trust was highlighted as of supreme importance. Indeed, trust was named the defining aspect of the relationship between the employer and his employees and also that between the manufacturers and their consumers. Writing on the goodwill of the Hahnemann Publishing Company of the Bhars, the editor of their journal *The Hahnemannian Gleanings* observed, 'the patients come to us in a simple faith: trusting health and even life itself in our hands. The physician is trusted more than anyone else in the world'.[155]

Along with physical well-being, the homoeopathic employers were committed to the emotional as well as moral welfare of their employees; keeping an eye, for instance, on whether 'young men, especially those coming from distant villages to work, fell prey to the seductions of city life'.[156] They were concerned that the people working under them should not become extravagant, indulging too much in alcohol or in frequenting brothels.[157] To encourage 'healthy habits' like reading books in their spare time,

[153] The social stigma placed on plague patients at the turn of the twentieth century, and the frequently brutal segregation enforced upon them by the British colonial authorities, have featured in some excellent works on colonial medicine. See David Arnold, 'Touching the Body: Perspectives on the Indian Plague, 1896–1900' in Ranajit Guha (ed.), *Subaltern Studies V* (New Delhi: Oxford University Press, 1988), pp. 55–90.

[154] Srish Chandra Talapatra, *Mahesh Chandra Charitkatha* (*Life of Mahesh Chandra*), 1946, p. 58.

[155] 'Editorial: New Year's Retrospection and Introspection', *The Hahnemannian Gleanings*, 4, 1 (February 1933), 7.

[156] Srish Chandra Talapatra, *Mahesh Chandra Charitkatha* (*Life of Mahesh Chandra*), 1946, pp. 57–9.

[157] Ibid.

Bhattacharya built up a library exclusively for his employees within the immediate premises of their quarters.[158]

The texts frequently invoked the metaphor of father and son while discussing labour management. Mahesh Chandra argued that the relation between the employer and his employees should exactly replicate the 'bond between a father and his son'. He emphasised that it was the responsibility of the employer to 'protect' his employees from all kinds of corrupting influences, to 'control' them as well as to 'reward' them for their efficiency in the same way he would his own son.[159] He stressed the importance of occasional rewards in the form of commissions, increases in salary and gifts.[160] He further advised that on retirement, and particularly in absence of the employer having an efficient son, trusted old employees could be turned into partners in business.[161]

The boundaries between caste, kinship, blood or professional ties seemed undefined in such texts. A diffused, flexible and inclusive notion of family seemed to emanate from the texts published by the homoeopathic entrepreneurs. Familial relations, as described in these writings, appeared as much acquired as ascriptive. Affective relationship and entrepreneurial partnership often appear overlapping. A group of scholars researching South Asian family life have begun examining the predominance, throughout the nineteenth century, of complex households which included a variety of dependants.[162] They urge us to revisit the historiographic relevance of 'affect' in envisioning such households. What could be the potential roles and positions of dependants, servants (and employees) in such formations? Texts written and published by homoeopathic entrepreneurs on the control and management of labour share such historiographic concerns. Together they project a rather fluid and inclusive notion of family, as it developed around these commercial firms which involved trusted employees recruited through older regional ties, caste and kinship networks, distant relatives and sometimes even mere acquaintances. These different categories of actors seemed easily to form an extended family which dwelt in close vicinity of each other. One finds a caricature of this overt reliance of homoeopathic commercial concerns on their employees in the 1915 drama *Trhyasparsha ba Sukhi Paribar*

158 Ibid., p. 59. 159 Ibid., pp. 76–7. 160 Ibid., pp. 80–1. 161 Ibid.

162 See, for instance, Indrani Chatterjee (ed.), *Unfamiliar Relations: Family and History in South Asia* (Delhi: Permanent Black, 2004), p. 17. Complex households have also been studied by historians of law and those working on the political economy of family from legal vantage points. See Malavika Kasturi, *Embattled Identities: Rajput Lineages and the Colonial State in Nineteenth Century North India* (Delhi: Oxford University Press, 2002); and Rachel Sturman, 'Property and Attachments: Defining Autonomy and the Claims of Family in Nineteenth-Century Western India', *Comparative Studies in Society and History*, 47 (3 July 2005), 611–37.

(*Triangular Impact or the Happy Family*), mentioned earlier in this chapter. Referring to the real-life reputed homoeopath Biharilal Dutta, the father-in-law of Pratap Chandra Majumdar, the author mocked how one of Dutta's long-standing employees assumed himself to be a member of Dutta's family, and consequently a homoeopath by default.[163]

To be sure, such paternalistic language of care, concern and welfare almost invariably converged with concerns about profit maximisation. Mahesh Chandra held that the employer stood to gain profitably in treating the employee as his own son. In *Byabshayee* he argued that enterprises functioning on such an explicitly familial model almost never run the risk of facing workers' strikes.[164]

It is worth noting that as they discussed ways of organising business on the model of the family, these texts at times went further, referring to the institution of family as a kind of business. Both Jitendranath Majumdar and Mahesh Chandra Bhattacharya drew an analogy between '*shong-shaar*' or the household and '*byabsha*', meaning business. Jitendranath in his book *Arther Sandhan* (*Pursuit of Wealth*) observed, 'all householders are businessmen in a sense. But in general, by businessmen one understands only the traders'.[165] On different occasions, they compared the institution of family with business. As he elaborated on the skills of managing a company, Mahesh Chandra observed:

> The will to improve one's condition both in the realm of business as in the domain of the household is contingent on being dependent on others. The more one wishes to improve, the more he is dependent – he needs to take others help and also needs to keep them all in good humor.[166]

The preface to the third edition of *Byabshayee (Businessman)* noted that as much as the author wished to, it was beyond him to write another, separate book on managing a successful household.[167] However, since he believed that 'conducting a business was similar in most ways to conducting a household', he included his reflections on running a successful household in his tract *Byabshayee*, meant for teaching the essentials of successful business. Mahesh Chandra cited specific examples to illustrate the analogy that he drew between running a household and managing a business. Virtues such as frugality, economy and cooperation were shown to be equally important in both spheres. Just as every

[163] Dwijendralal Ray, *Trhyasparsha ba Sukhi Paribar* (*The Triangular Impact or Happy Family*), 2nd edition (Calcutta: Surdham, 1915), pp. 3–4.
[164] Mahesh Chandra Bhattacharya, *Byabshayee* (*Businessman*), 1905, p. 75.
[165] Jitendranath Majumdar, *Arther Sandhan* (*Pursuit of Wealth*), 1932, p. 115.
[166] Mahesh Chandra Bhattacharya, *Byabshayee* (*Businessman*), 1905, p. 144.
[167] Mahesh Chandra Bhattacharya, 'Preface to the Third Edition', *Byabshayee* (*Businessman*), Calcutta: M. Bhattacharya and Company, 4th edition, 1921.

businessman was encouraged to keep a reserve fund for emergencies, so too every household was asked to maintain a secret reserve of cash and kind.[168] Even while analysing certain unsuccessful business ventures of his own in his autobiography, Bhattacharya noted that such experiences had left him enriched with lessons that he later found useful within the realm of his household.[169]

Firms, Family and the Homoeopathic Profession

The familial metaphor, so productive for these writings by the protagonists, was further extended to other related contexts as well. Entrepreneur-physicians practising homoeopathy at the turn of the twentieth century in Calcutta often wrote about their profession itself as if it were one big family. Chapter 2 discusses the production of scientific biographies that projected familial intimacy between the various successful practitioners of homoeopathy. For now, it is sufficient to note that these life stories related to an informal, intimate network of pedagogy involving homoeopathy. Not only were formal institutions teaching homoeopathy absent in the nineteenth century, the foremost advocates of the practice like Mahendralal Sircar and Mahesh Bhattacharya were positively opposed to the idea of a formal pedagogic institution.[170] I already noted in the previous section that entrepreneurs such as Bhattacharya did not think highly of the ability of educational institutes to impart knowledge concerning enterprise. Bhattacharya felt that 'the recruits should first act as apprentices and be put under regular observation until they learnt the fundamentals of their work'.[171] Likewise, for the dissemination of homoeopathic knowledge, these physicians relied more on an informal pupillage network, which they most often referred to in familial idioms.

The Calcutta Homoeopathic College established by the Majumdars in the early 1880s as a very small unit was the only exception to this opinion against institutionalised homoeopathic education. All the noteworthy first-generation homoeopaths in the late nineteenth century were trained as regular doctors at the government-run Calcutta Medical College. Almost all of them learnt homoeopathy informally through reading and

[168] Ibid., p. 23.
[169] Srish Chandra Talapatra, *Mahesh Chandra Charitkatha* (*Life of Mahesh Chandra*), 1946, p. 64.
[170] Mahendralal Sircar's reservation against promoting formal, classroom education to disseminate science and medicine in India is discussed in Pratik Chakrabarti's review of John Lourdusamy's book *Science and National Consciousness in Bengal, 1870–1930*. See Pratik Chakrabarti, *Medical History*, 50, 3 (2006), 403–4.
[171] Mahesh Chandra Bhattacharya, *Byabshayee* (*Businessman*), 1905, p. 64.

interactions with other, similarly inclined physicians. Their life stories record numerous instances of close, near-familial bonds between physicians, nurtured by a shared quest for homoeopathic knowledge. Homoeopathy was widely projected as a science that could be acquired primarily through individual acts of meticulous reading and experimentation. A few like Jitendranath Majumdar were graduates of homoeopathic colleges in America. However, the informal network of pupillage and pedagogy was highlighted as the primary mode of dissemination for homoeopathic knowledge in Bengal. The rhetoric of family was invoked with remarkable frequency to describe the interpersonal relations between the leading physicians since the late nineteenth century.

An example of such relationships, couched in familial terms, was that between Rajendralal Dutta and Mahendralal Sircar. Publications relating to both physicians dramatically emphasised the way Rajendralal inducted Mahendralal into the principles of homoeopathy and taught him the fundamentals, and how Mahendralal forever remained grateful to Rajendralal Dutta and acknowledged him as his mentor.[172] In a letter following the death of Rajendralal, Mahendralal was said to have proclaimed,

> he used to call me his 'father and son' and subscribe himself in all the letters he wrote to me as 'your son and father'. The love that he bore me was not a whit less than that of a father to his son. His faith in me as you know was unbounded. His reverence for me was that of a son. Could I be undutiful to such a man? My personal loss in his death is more than that of any other man.[173]

Mahendralal's friendship with Biharilal Bhaduri, the father-in-law of Pratap Chandra Majumdar, was likewise often highlighted in the context of the pedagogic pupillage network. Pratap Chandra's biography, by his son Jitendranath Majumdar, elaborated how the famous nineteenth-century social reformer Vidyasagar inspired both the leading homoeopaths, Mahendralal and Biharilal, to take up homoeopathy.[174] Vidyasagar, an ardent admirer of homoeopathy, had developed a personal interest in the subject and was said to have built a huge collection of books imported from England and America. Studying at Vidyasagar's library, Mahendralal and Biharilal were known to have developed a fraternal camaraderie that

[172] See Sarat Chandra Ghosh, 'Bharatbarshe Homoeopathic Chikitshar Sorboprothom Pothoprodorshok o Pracharak Dr. Rajendralal Dutta' (The Pioneer Physician and Perpetrator of Homoeopathy in India'), *Hahnemann*, 22, 1 (1939), 14–16.

[173] Sarat Chandra Ghose, 'Homoeopathy and Its First Missionary in India', *The Hahnemannian Gleanings*, 3 (November 1932), pp. 449–50.

[174] Jitendranath Majumdar, 'Dr. Pratapchandra Majumdar', *Hahnemann*, 22, 5 (1939), 260–7.

strengthened over time.[175] Highlighting their role in the dissemination of homoeopathy, Jitendranath claimed that it was only when the two physicians started practising in tandem that 'the people of Calcutta began to realise the tremendous potential of this form of treatment'.[176]

Another instructive example one might cite is the biography of physician Pratap Chandra Majumdar, written by his son Jitendranath. The biography detailed Pratap Chandra's initial interest in homoeopathy, subsequent to his L. M. S degree from the Calcutta Medical College.[177] This interest was primarily stoked by physician Lokenath Maitra, a former student of Rajendralal Dutta. The biography also harked back to the lifelong affection that the two physicians shared since those early days. So deep was the attachment of love and respect that Lokenath always referred to Pratap Chandra as his 'grandson'.[178]

The literature on homoeopathy extensively deployed a host of appellations for familial relations, like 'elder brother', 'son', 'father' or 'grandson', as common tropes to describe the depth of intimacy between physicians. Such a projection of intimate relationships reinforced the inclusive and flexible understanding of family that can be distilled from the texts published by the homoeopathic entrepreneurs. In such an understanding, intimate familial relations were identities that were not always and necessarily inherited through birth but could be acquired in the course of one's life. The fluid, commodious and diffused vision of family represented in such texts were shown to fulfil the purposes both of profit maximisation and knowledge acquisition.

Inherited Family

Such apparently inclusive, accommodative understandings concerning the 'family' were also, however, contradicted within the pages of the very same texts. As the discussions moved away from themes of labour recruitment, management and maintenance towards norms of ownership, inheritance and profit-making, one notices a simultaneous, if paradoxical, celebration of the exclusive, the private and the filial. Simultaneously with the paternal affection due to one's employees, ownership of property and its efficient management were treated as concerns of great importance. The ideal family structure suitable for owning a business was discussed in this context. In the fourth edition of *Byabshayee*, Mahesh Chandra Bhattacharya elaborated on the logistics

175 Ibid., pp. 263–5. 176 Ibid., p. 267. 177 Ibid., pp. 259–60.
178 Sarat Chandra Ghose, 'Daktar Lokenath Maitra', *Hahenmann*, 22, 12 (1939), 309.

of such family structure.[179] While discussing the advantages associated with an extended joint family system, he concurrently drew his readers' attention to its potential pitfalls. His writings powerfully foregrounded a logic of property and material assets in discussions of the relevance of the joint family system. Social histories of the dissolution of the joint family have tended to focus more on its incompatibility with the newer kinds of conjugalities enabled by colonial modernity. The reformed husband and the new conjugality have until recently been at the forefront of the scholarly analysis of changing colonial familial structure.[180] Texts such as *Byabshayee* enable us to think more centrally about the material rationale informing the changing perceptions of the institution of joint family. Pointing out that 'there is hardly any certainty about the profit and loss incurred in any business', Mahesh Chandra recommended that if extended families became involved in the same business, there ought to be clear understandings on the share of each member, preferably through registered deeds.[181] As the focus of discussion shifted towards owning and inheriting enterprise, the rhetoric of a flexible, extended household seemed to fade away slowly.

Keeping aside issues of affect and emotion, the texts sometimes dwelt upon the relative advantages and disadvantages of the joint family system solely from economic points of view. They demonstrated a concern that the joint family setup, if it involved a large number of people, bred laziness and many tended to live off others' income.[182] On the other hand, in joint families the costs of socialisation and the expenses on servants were divided among many. Though the texts emphasised certain benefits associated with the joint family system, smaller families were projected as financially more practicable from a commercial point of view. In *Byabshayee* Mahesh Chandra even contemplated a new kind of family structure for the future, which he termed '*joutha paribar*' or 'cooperative family', where the extended family would live together but share only certain costs between themselves.[183] The second volume of Batakrishna Pal's biography included a whole chapter entitled 'Sukhi Paribar' or 'The Content Family', detailing his thoughts on the subject.[184] Such writings focused great attention on the importance of relationships, such as with one's wife and sons, in

[179] Mahesh Chandra Bhattacharya, *Byabshayee (Businessman)*, 1921, pp. 173–5.
[180] For instance, see Pradip Bose, 'Sons of the Nation: Child Rearing in the New Family', in Partha Chatterjee (ed.), *Texts of Power: Emerging Discipline in Colonial Bengal* (Minneapolis: University of Minnesota Press, 1995), pp. 118–44.
[181] Mahesh Chandra Bhattacharya, *Byabshayee (Businessman)*, 1921, pp. 173–4.
[182] Ibid., p. 174. [183] Ibid.
[184] Gopal Chandra Mukhopadhyay, *Sadhu Batakrishna Pal (The Saintly Batakrishna Pal)*, Vol II, 1919, pp. 176–81.

achieving happiness. A nucleated family structure comprising only parents and children was celebrated as the most convenient one for those involved in commercial enterprise.[185]

Hence, from the perspective of owning a business, these texts seemed to operate within an idiom of restricted, inflexible family defined exclusively by ties of blood. Marriage was considered critical. Positioning himself as a Hindu Aryan, Batakrishna Pal advocated marriage as essential, for it had been prescribed by the Aryan ancestors.[186] Marriage was considered necessary not only for the mere satisfaction of sexual needs, but also the deeper objectives of ensuring balanced conduct of the material and religious practices of life.[187] Both Mahesh Chandra Bhattacharya and Batakrishna Pal discussed the importance of good '*bangsha*', meaning genealogy or familial line of descent. Mahesh Chandra defined a good '*bangsha*' as one that had the reputation of producing knowledgeable, educated and religious men in the past as well as in the present.[188] Criticising the futile hankering for physical beauty, Batakrishna insisted that it was important to follow the rules for marriage prescribed by the ancient lawmakers, as they ensured the well-being not only of each household, but of society at large.[189]

Other than the marital bond, these texts elevated the relationship with male progeny as the most significant one within a family. Such idealisation of a patrilineal family needs to be juxtaposed with the contemporary colonial legal interventions, which defined the Hindu joint family around norms of inheritance by the male child. Batakrishna invoked the teachings of the Vedas to argue that producing a son was one of the main pillars on which rested the Aryan conception of the permanence of the soul.[190] His biography is dotted with his thoughts on the philosophy of immortality of soul, and the importance of male progeny. As Hindu customs required the son to perform all the death rites, the importance of the son within the sphere of the family was supreme.[191] Having referred to such spiritual perspectives, the biography drew an analogy between Batakrishna's own sons and precious gems. Each one of them was eulogised, not only for inheriting his father's professional genius, but for being capable of considerably enhancing his inherited fortunes.[192] Thus, material considerations appeared interwoven with discussions of the spiritual necessity for a family. Mahesh Chandra Bhattacharya maintained that since familial property could be a cause

[185] Ibid., p. 180. [186] Ibid., p. 144. [187] Ibid.
[188] Mahesh Chandra Bhattacharya, *Byabshayee (Businessmann)*, 1921, p. 175.
[189] Gopal Chandra Mukhopadhyay, *Sadhu Batakrishna Pal (The Saintly Batakrishna Pal)*, Vol II, 1919, 1946, p. 150.
[190] Ibid., p. 155. [191] Ibid., pp. 155–7. [192] Ibid., p. 160.

for conflict among sons, having fewer sons helped one avoid confusion over issues of entrepreneurial inheritance.[193]

Hence, exigencies relating to the inheritance of businesses and property resulted in the protagonists, in their writings, celebrating a distinctly patrilineal and nucleated notion of family. One notices a swing in emphasis in these texts from notions of extended household to a more defined kinship identity, as far as business ownership was concerned. Under the section titled 'Pratap Chandra's Family' in the biography of the physician, his son Jitendranath recorded details of his three sons as well as nine daughters.[194] The occupation and identity of his sons-in-law also formed an important part of the description of his family. Jitendranath considered Pratap Chandra fortunate in being able to leave behind him the legacy of a successful and happy family unit. In a particularly narcissistic mode, Jitendranath noted that 'it is not very usual for successful fathers to have sons professionally as flourishing as himself. In Pratap Chandra's case, this has been proven wrong. He is fortunate enough in leaving behind sons who will perpetuate his name when he will be no more'.[195] A parallel understanding of family as the domain of the private and intimate animated the writings. A biography of Rajendralal Dutta in the *Hahnemannian Gleanings* observed,

> Great as Rajendra Dutt undoubtedly was in the arena of public life, he was greater by far in all the sacred relations of private life. Whether as a son, as a father, as a husband . . . he had scarcely any equal and a better, or greater, a noble model my countrymen could not have had.[196]

Index of Success: Family Business

Celebration of the patrilineal family was an essential part of the narrative of the success of these homoeopathic enterprises. One cannot help but note the pompous tone associated with narrating the commercial success of their own enterprises. Such success was invariably ascribed to the intergenerational, patrilineal, familial engagement of the protagonists with homoeopathy. It was considered an important formula for success to incorporate one's own son, or similarly intimate family relations into the overall management and ownership of the firm. The biography of Batakrishna Pal, for instance, discussed how he insisted on having his

193 Srish Chandra Talapatra, *Mahesh Chandra Charitkatha (Life of Mahesh Chandra)*, 1946, p. 26.
194 J. N. Majumdar, 'Dr. Pratapchandra Majumdar', *Hahnemann*, 23, 8 (1940), pp. 454–5.
195 Ibid., p. 455.
196 S. C. Ghose, 'Homoeopathy and Its First Missionary in India', *The Hahnemannian Gleanings*, 3, 8 (September 1932), p. 340.

eldest son Bhootnath Pal assist him in his enterprise.[197] He terminated Bhootnath's education when the latter was only sixteen, and took it upon himself to teach his son the fundamentals of the business. The biographer commented that 'the implication of this wonderful collaboration was soon apparent to relatives, friends, fellow shop-owners and especially to the consumers as the name of B. K. Pal and company spread far and wide'.[198]

Batakrishna had incorporated his two other sons (Harishankar Pal and Harimohan Pal) as well as his nephew Haridas Daw, by appointing them to crucial posts in his enterprise. The third son Harishankar Pal, who was a particularly brilliant student, was also made to give up his education to join his father in the business.[199] Harishankar Pal was put in charge of the homoeopathic department of his father's sprawling drug business, which also involved the import of allopathic drugs. He looked after the pharmacy, The Great Homoeopathic Hall and the extensive homoeopathic publications of the firm.[200] The biographer regarded Harishankar's insights as having 'injected new blood into the veins of the office'.[201] The biography also mentioned the wonderful collaboration between the brothers, referring to Harishankar Pal acting as the 'right hand' of his elder brother.[202] The biography of Batakrishna Pal noted that the firm's profits multiplied as it started investing in innovative practices, such as attractive advertisements under the able leadership of the sons.[203] Indeed, the initiative to advertise proved most rewarding, and advertisements for the business were soon flooding the leading newspapers and journals, as well as the almanacs used extensively by the Hindus.[204] The onus of ownership in most other homoeopathic concerns, including the very successful (and still thriving) Hahnemann Publishing Company, also passed from the father to the sons. Thus, the founder of HAPCO, Prafulla Chandra Bhar, was assisted and later succeeded by his eldest son Gauri Shankar Bhar in the management and ownership of the concern.[205]

197 Gopal Chandra Mukhopadhyay, *Sadhu Batakrishna Pal* (*The Saintly Batakrishna Pal*), Vol I, 1919, pp. 50–1.
198 Ibid., p. 51. 199 Ibid., p. 67.
200 For an extensive list of the publications of the store, see 'Advertisement of the Great Homoeopathic Hall' in *Grihasthamangal*, 3, 1 (1929), 16.
201 Gopal Chandra Mukhopadhyay, *Sadhu Batakrishna Pal* (*The Saintly Batakrishna Pal*), Vol I, 1919, p. 68.
202 Ibid., p. 69. 203 Ibid., p 52. 204 Ibid., p. 52.
205 As narrated by Dr Durga Shankar Bhar, the son of late Gauri Shankar Bhar and current Managing Director of the Hahnemann Publishing Company, in an interview in August 2009.

It was only in the absence of sons that next-of-kin relatives were considered valuable in business ownership and management. The biography of Mahesh Chandra Bhattacharya records the tragic loss of his nineteen-year-old son Manmatha in the year 1908.[206] Narratives of his life, including his autobiography, mentioned his reliance on his nephews Jagadbandhu and Kumud Bhattacharya in the organisation of his work. In his later years, he recognised his adopted son Heramba as a great support. Mahesh Chandra gratefully recounted the crucial role played by his staff, and especially his nephews, in the expansion of his business.[207] Their contribution was felt most when he temporarily retired from active life following his son's untimely death. In his autobiography, he acknowledged that in the four years he was away, his business expanded in the hands of these trusted deputies.[208] The depth of his dependence on his nephews can be sensed from such reminiscences.

The life stories of the physicians Pratap Chandra Majumdar and Mahendralal Sircar similarly illustrate their dependence on their respective sons, Jitendranath Majumdar and Amritalal Sircar. From the 1880s onwards, Pratap Chandra and Jitendranath published and coedited the second oldest homoeopathic journal, *The Indian Homoeopathic Review*, which lasted well into the twentieth century. Advertisements for their firm regularly represented the father–son duo as in charge of the Majumdar's Homoeopathic Pharmacy, which was located at Cornwallis Street with branches at Corporation Street.[209] Jitendranath authored a lengthy biography of his father, serialised in the journal *Hahnemann*, in which he began by detailing the exploits of his grandfather, the famous homoeopath Biharilal Bhaduri, thus keeping in the foreground his family's intergenerational involvement in homoeopathic commerce.[210] This biography publicised Pratap Chandra as the founder of the first homoeopathic school in India. The Calcutta Homoeopathic College established in early 1880s, was later augmented into the Calcutta Homoeopathic Hospital, and was known to be managed jointly by the father and the son.[211]

[206] Srish Chandra Talapatra, *Mahesh Chandra Charitkatha* (*Life of Mahesh Chandra)*, 1946, p. 151.
[207] Mahesh Chandra Bhattacharya, *Atmacharit (My Life)*, 4th edition (Calcutta: Economic Press, 1957), pp. 69–70.
[208] Ibid.
[209] See 'Advertisement of Majumdars Homoeopathic Pharmacy', *Indian Homoeopathic Review*, 19, 6 (June 1910), page number not cited.
[210] J. N. Majumdar, 'Dr. Pratap Chandra Majumdar MD', *Hahnemann*, 23, 5 (1940), 261–7.
[211] J. N. Majumdar, 'Dr. Pratap Chandra Majumdar MD', *Hahnemann*, 23, 6 (1940), 324–5. Involvement of the son is mentioned in a sequel article in *Hahnemann*, 23, 7 (1940), 453.

The second Doctor of Medicine (MD) to qualify from the Calcutta Medical College, Mahendralal Sircar was easily the most reputed physician to have taken up the homoeopathic cause in the nineteenth century.[212] Sircar, however, did not fit into the typical pattern of families involved in homoeopathic enterprise, as neither he nor his son Amritalal formally established any commercial firm. Nevertheless, Mahendralal remained one of the central figures among these intergenerational homoeopathic families in Bengal. From the late 1860s on, he collaborated with his son Amritalal on various publication projects involving homoeopathy. *The Calcutta Journal of Medicine*, which he launched in 1867, boasted of being the first ever homoeopathic journal in the non-western world.[213] Edited as well as published by Mahendralal, the mantle of the journal was taken over by his son following Sircar's death in 1904.[214] Mahendralal Sircar published extensively on homoeopathic remedies from his Anglo-Sanskrit Press at Sankharitollah while his son Amritalal Sircar reworked and republished many of the later editions of his books – for instance, one on treatment of the plague.[215] Together they maintained 'daily written diaries that were preserved in the family' and much of what he had written there 'pertained to their homoeopathic practice and patients'.[216] They also ran a widely known homoeopathic dispensary at their residence.[217] Mahendralal wrote about the popularity of the home dispensary in his journal, mentioning the high numbers of patients attending.[218] The average number of patients treated daily was so staggeringly high – more than a hundred – that it drew him into controversies with fellow physicians like Dr Salzer, who would not believe his numbers.[219]

[212] Chapter 2, which deals with homoeopathic biographies, further discusses the iconic status achieved by Mahendralal Sircar in nineteenth-century Bengali society. Besides highlighting Mahendralal Sircar's other achievements in the field of science, it details the many lives of Sircar that were written comparing him with homoeopathy's German founder, Hahnemann.

[213] 'Editorial: Our Creed', *Calcutta Journal of Medicine*, 1, 1 (1868), 190–1.

[214] See, for instance, Amritalal Sircar, 'Published Monthly: Calcutta Journal of Medicine', *Calcutta Journal of Medicine*, 32, 8 (July 1913), back cover page.

[215] For instance, see Amritalal Sircar, *Therapeutics of Plague*, 4th edition (Calcutta: Anglo-Sanskrit Press, 1913).

[216] See Arun Kumar Biswas (ed.), *Gleanings of the Past and the Science Movement: In the Diaries of Drs. Mahendralal and Amritalal Sircar* (Kolkata: Asiatic Society, 2000), pp. 5–7.

[217] Amritalal Sircar, 'The Late Dr. Mahendralal Sircar, CIE, MD, DL', *Calcutta Journal of Medicine*, 23, 2 (February 1904), 45–66. Also see, Amritalal Sircar, *Obituary Notice of Dr. Mahendralal Sircar* (Calcutta: Anglo-Sanskrit Press, 1905), pp. 37–9.

[218] Mahendralal Sircar, 'Outdoor Homoeopathic Dispensary', *Calcutta Journal of Medicine*, 7, 1 and 2 (1874), 47–52.

[219] Mahendralal Sircar, 'Further Considerations on the Necessity for a Homoeopathic Hospital and Dispensary in Calcutta', *Calcutta Journal of Medicine*, 8, 2 (1876), 57–62.

Mahendralal wrote a follow-up article in his journal justifying his position and reiterating the enormous traffic of patients at his home dispensary.[220]

As much as the entrepreneurs themselves asserted their familial links, such links were perceived and written about by others too. Such familial entanglements were lauded as a marker of the dedication and commitment of these families to the homoeopathic cause. Pratap Chandra Majumdar's obituary notice in the Bengali journal *Hahnemann* explicitly discussed his familial involvement in homoeopathy. Elaborating on Pratap Majumdar's contributions, the obituary referred to his close ties with his father-in-law Biharilal Bhaduri, describing the latter as 'a very competent homoeopathic physician'.[221] The author of the obituary expressed a hope that Pratap Chandra's efficient son Jitendranath Majumdar would soon take up his place as one of the leading practitioners in Calcutta.[222] The fact that the renowned homoeopath N. M. Chowdhury (MD) was his son-in-law was also noted.[223]

Likewise, the familial connection between the legendary Mahendralal and Amritalal Sircar was often written about, notably, in the dedications of several popular tracts. For instance, dedicating his well-received book on homoeopathic therapeutics to Mahendralal Sircar, author C. S. Kali also referred to the presence of his illustrious son in the profession.[224] A collection of the great physician's obituaries, compiled by his son Amritalal himself, is replete with similar references. Navin Kali Devi's poem 'Sunya Bharat' or 'Empty India', while lamenting the death of the departed physician was careful to name his worthy son as the only person competent to fill his shoes.[225]

However, not all such references to the great homoeopathic practices and business enterprises as families were eulogistic in tone. Later in the twentieth century, as these families slowly engaged themselves also in building formal institutions like colleges and hospitals, there was criticism of their mode of functioning, involving (as it did) accumulation of familial capital. The institutions built by the Majumdars, for instance, were often looked down upon as private, family-run affairs. An editorial in the journal *The Hahnemannian Gleanings* wrote about the Pratap Chandra Memorial Hospital, 'the Pratap Chandra Memorial College and Hospital cannot be called

220 Ibid.
221 Anonymous, 'Shok- Sangbad' ('Sad News'), *Hahnemann*, 5, 7 (1922), 383.
222 Ibid. 223 Ibid.
224 C. S. Kali, 'Dedication page', *Homoeopathic Chikitsha Bidhan (Principles of Homoeopathic Treatment)*, Vol II, 13th edition (Calcutta: S. Kyle and Company, 1928).
225 Quoted from Arun Kumar Biswas, 'Preface', *Gleanings of the Past and the Science Movement in the Diaries of Drs. Mahendralal and Amritalal Sircar* (Kolkata: Asiatic Society, 2000), p. VIII.

a public institution proper as the properties have not been transferred into the hands of the committee which the College does not possess (*sic*)'.[226] In their journal *Homoeopathy Paricharak*, a contemporary rival organisation called the Homoeopathy Serving Society accused Hahnemann Publishing Company of attempting to establish '*ekchetiya byabsha*' or 'monopoly business' in homoeopathy.[227]

Conclusion

I have been tracing the reception and reconstitution of ideas around German homoeopathy, since the mid-nineteenth century, in three dispersed colonial sites. By the turn of the twentieth century, a literary readership in Bengal routinely encountered the figure of the homoeopath as a quotidian, valued, if caricatured aspect of their social world. Around the same time, governmental disquiet propelled attempts to control non-state, irregular medicine, which were preoccupied not only with traditional practices like ayurveda and unani, but also with European heterodoxies such as homoeopathy. Allegedly, homoeopathy's 'scientific sounding name' confused consumers into participating in quack practice. Along with the administrative and literary perceptions of the proliferation of homoeopathic practice, I have interrogated the processes of production and investments around homoeopathic knowledge. Homoeopathy's distinct organisation was achieved through a network of Bengali family firms imbued with particular notions of scientific advancement as well as material recompense. Indeed, family emerged not just as the projected consumer but as the crucial generator of this colonial heterodoxy. Unlike the modernising, pedagogic, institution-building initiatives undertaken by the ayurveda and unani revivalists, the homoeopathic entrepreneur-publicists thrived on their crucial interface with the fundamental and intimate institution of the family.[228] Exploring an archive of sociomedical commentaries helped me understand the nineteenth-century visions of an extended joint family system underpinned with values of enterprise, commerce and profit. Histories of heterodox practices such as homoeopathy, much like the recent histories of law, throw new light on the

[226] 'Editorial Notes and Comments', *The Hahnemannian Gleanings*, 3, 6 (June 1932), 236.
[227] 'Editorial: 'Homoeopathy r Dheki' ('Problems of Homoeopathy'), *Homoeopathy Pracharak*, 3, 9 (December 1929), 316–21.
[228] Indeed, existing literature demonstrates that ayurveda was trying to break free of the perception that it was a family and caste-based practice. For an account of the modernising and professionalising initiatives relating to ayurveda since the late nineteenth century through schools, colleges and associations, see Kavita Sivaramakrishnan, *Old Potions, New Bottles: Recasting Indigenous Medicine in Colonial Punjab, 1850–1945* (Hyderabad: Orient Longman, 2006), pp. 53–86.

multiple and often conflicting imaginings of the colonial family, shaped by intersecting discourses of emotion and interest. The following chapters will further trace the role of the family firms in institutionalising homoeopathy as a discrete genre of non-state medicine in myriad other sites; through practices of biographising, processes of translations, as well as quotidian domestic health managements. I will, however, return to explore the governmental reactions towards such unique familial institutionalisation, in order to study the interface between the colonial state and the homoeopathic families in defining what constituted 'scientific' homoeopathy.

2 A Family of Biographies

Colonial Lives of a Western Heterodoxy

'. . . some of the greatest men of India have had the shortest biographies. Many great men have been enwrapped in the folds of oblivion.'[1]

'. . . there is very strong evidence that Bengal does not know its great men.'[2]

'As India entered the colonial era, the earlier hagiographical tradition was beginning to be supplemented, and to some extent supplanted, by a new form of biography, in which greater attention was given to complexity of character and personal motivation, to specific places and events, and to their role in shaping and explaining individual lives.'[3]

In Ghose's three-part serialised biography of homoeopathic physician Rajendralal Dutta, published in the monthly periodical *The Hahnemannian Gleanings* and quoted above, the author repeatedly lamented Bengal's lack of appropriate engagement with the lives of its great men, as compared to the standards set by the West. This lament by the biographer, in conjunction with subsequent observations by historians studying 'life writing practices' in colonial India, hints at a culture of biographising lives, which was proliferating through the nineteenth century.[4]

1 S. C. Ghose, 'Homoeopathy and Its First Missionary in India', *The Hahnemannian Gleanings*, 3, 7 (August 1932), 289.

2 S. C. Ghose, 'Homoeopathy and Its First Missionary in India', *The Hahnemannian Gleanings*, 3, 10 (November 1932), 450.

3 David Arnold and Stuart Blackburn (eds.), *Telling Lives in India: Biography, Autobiography and Life History* (Bloomington: Indiana University Press, 2004), pp. 8–9.

4 This is to collectively indicate the scholarship on writings of life including autobiography, memoir, biography, travelogue and so on. Despite differences among scholars, it is generally agreed that the term 'life story' is preferable to 'life history' as the scope of the former is considered more comprehensive, with no explicit truth claim attached to it. See James Peacock and Dorothy Holland, 'The Narrated Self: Life Stories in Process', *Ethos*, 21, 4 (1993), 367–8. See also David Arnold and Stuart Blackburn (eds.), *Telling Lives in India*, pp. 9–11.

Exploring the depths of popular medical print culture in Bengal, one is astonished at how regularly biographies of homoeopathic practitioners were published, from the latter half of the nineteenth century onwards. These ranged from eulogising accounts of the life of Hahnemann, the eighteenth-century German founder of the doctrine, to the careers of those who were applauded as 'extraordinarily successful and efficient' practitioners of homoeopathy, to the lives of entrepreneurs (mostly also physicians) invested in the production of homoeopathic drugs, print and knowledge – in Chapter 1, most members of this last category were introduced as 'protagonists'. Besides appearing as cheap pamphlets or as heavier tomes, the lives of practitioners were often published serially in the foremost homoeopathic journals such as the *Indian Homoeopathic Review*, *Hahnemann*, *Calcutta Journal of Medicine* and *The Hahnemannian Gleanings*. While occasional autobiographies and memoirs of practitioners were published, biographies remained the quintessential mode of homoeopathic assertion. This distinct archive of Bengali biographies has escaped historical scrutiny so far.

It is important to locate these biographic trends within the larger corpus produced by the colonial Bengali print industry. In their analysis of the burgeoning print market in Bengal, arguably one of the most thriving colonial examples of its kind, Anindita Ghosh and Tapti Roy suggest that although biographies were a fairly peripheral genre until the 1850s, there was a visible shift in the latter half of the nineteenth century.[5] Indeed, following the nineteenth-century enumerations of Reverend James Long, Jatindramohan Bhattacharya and others, it is possible to trace the growing prominence of biography as a genre in the vernacular print market. Despite possible criticisms of such nineteenth-century enumerations, men like Rev. Long had statistically established that since the 1850s the 'tide turned in favour of more useful works' which, among other categories, also included 'biographies of eminent men'.[6]

Over the last decade and a half, histories of colonial book, print and publishing have come to represent an essential strand in analyses of South Asian modernity. These works, as well as those variously reflecting upon the advent of colonial modern subjectivities, have identified biography, along with autobiography, the novel, travel

[5] See Anindita Ghosh, *Power in Print: Popular Publishing and the Politics of Language and Culture in a Colonial Society* (Delhi: Oxford University Press, 2006), pp. 131–3; and Tapti Roy, 'Disciplining the Printed Text: Colonial and Nationalist Surveillance of Bengali Literature' in Partha Chatterjee (ed.), *Texts of Power: Emerging Disciplines in Colonial Bengal* (Minneapolis: University of Minnesota Press, 1995), pp. 38–41.

[6] Ibid., p. 38.

writing, diary and history as significant genres for the expression of an emerging modern self.[7] Yet, of the myriad forms of writing lives, biography seems to have received relatively little attention from South Asian scholars. By contrast, the value of autobiographies and memoirs in recovering the voices of women and other minorities has been recognised, and consequently these genres have received more systematic historical scrutiny.[8] Scholars have only rarely engaged with biographies on their own terms. Biographies typically have been instrumentalised as sources for other kinds of histories; or historians particularly have been more inclined to the critical historical-biographic recreation of renowned lives, most evidently the prominent leaders of our imperial and colonial pasts.[9] Since the 1990s, a growing distrust for metanarratives has further resulted in a fascinating new kind of individual-oriented work that has focused on bringing to life lesser-known figures from more humble backgrounds.[10] Some of these very interesting histories have been

7 See Dipesh Chakrabarty, *Provincialising Europe: Postcolonial Thought and Historical Difference* (Princeton, NJ: Princeton University Press, 2000), pp. 34–5; and Javed Majeed, *Autobiography, Travel and Postnational Identity: Gandhi, Nehru and Iqbal* (Basingstoke: Palgrave Macmillan, 2007). Also see Bhaskar Mukhopadhyay, 'Writing Home, Writing Travel: Poetics and Politics of Dwelling', *Comparative Studies in Society and History*, 44, 2 (2002), 298. Apart from biography, history and novel, Mukhopadhyay includes 'diary writing' as well as 'travel writing' as other modes of modern self-expression.

8 For some representative examples of the use of autobiography or memoir as an analytic tool in understanding gender and patriarchy and/or caste, see Tanika Sarkar, 'A Book of Her Own, A Life of Her Own: Autobiography of a Nineteenth Century Woman', *History Workshop*, 36 (1995), 35–65; Partha Chatterjee, 'Women and the Nation', *The Nation and Its Fragments: Colonial and Postcolonial Histories* (Princeton, NJ: Princeton University Press, 1993), pp. 135–57; Sharmila Rege, *Writing Caste, Writing Gender: Reading Dalit Women's Testimonios* (Delhi: Zuban, 1996); and Meenakshi Mukherjee, 'The Unperceived Self: A Study of Five Nineteenth Century Autobiographies' in Karuna Chanana (ed.), *Socialisation, Education and Women: Explorations in Gender Identity* (Delhi: Orient Longman, 1988).

9 There is a long-established scholarly tradition of political biographies by historians of imperialism. For an earlier representative example, see Percival Spear, *Master of Bengal: Clive and His India* (London: Thames and Hudson, 1975). For more recent critical historical explorations of the lives and thoughts of major nationalist figures, see Judith M. Brown, *Jawaharlal Nehru: A Political Life* (New Haven: Yale University Press, 2003); Benjamin Zachariah, *Nehru* (London, New York: Routledge, 2004); and Sugata Bose, *His Majesty's Opponents: Subhas Chandra Bose and India's Struggle Against Empire* (Cambridge: Harvard University Press, 2011).

10 For some recent explorations, see Richard Eaton, *Social History of Deccan, 1300–1761: Eight Indian Lives* (Cambridge: Cambridge University Press, 2005); Gloria Goodwin Raheja, *Listen to the Heron's Words: Reimagining Gender and Kinship in North India* (Berkeley: University of California Press, 1994); Gautam Bhadra, 'Four Rebels of Eighteen Fifty-Seven' in Ranajit Guha and Gayatri Spivak (eds.), *Selected Subaltern Studies* (Delhi: Oxford University Press, 1988), pp. 129–78; and Clare Anderson, *Subaltern Lives: Biographies of Colonialism in the Indian Ocean World, 1790–1920* (Cambridge: Cambridge University Press, 2012).

informed by the microhistorical approach.[11] Indulging in a strictly person-centred narrative, these scholars have frequently demonstrated how the archival fragments of individual lives can provide an extraordinary window onto the larger social milieu that their subjects inhabited.[12]

Fascinating and significant as these approaches are, what has remained relatively underexplored within this body of scholarship is biography itself as a specific form of historical document. Likewise, the function and relevance of a biography beyond the narration of a single life, as well as the politics of its production, have been neglected. In a recent anthology on life writing practices, the editors usefully raise the point that historians in South Asia have seldom 'paused to consider them (life histories) as *genres* worthy of systemic analysis'. This is indeed truer of biography than of any other genre. To redress this gap in the scholarship, I look into the commercial as well as moral impulses behind the sustained publication of biographies by the adherents of a specific medical ideology. Narration of religious lives, often in the form of hagiographies, are increasingly of interest to scholars studying the manoeuvres of sacred communities.[13] Likewise, here I study the content and function of the plethora of physicians' biographies with relation to the incipient science of homoeopathy in forging medico-scientific communities in Bengal. This essentially interrogates the power of pharmaceutical and print capital in shaping and sustaining heterodox, apparently marginal practices, not directly endorsed by the state.

Yet, this approach is not to stoke any romantic illusion of an uncontaminated 'outside' beyond the regimes of the state, with relation to these nonofficial practices. Even when castigated by the state and the mainstream British scientific authorities in India, these

[11] For an account of the relation between microhistory and biography, see Jill Lepore, 'Historians Who Love Too Much: Reflections on Microhistory and Biography', *Journal of American History*, 88, 1 (2001), 129–44.

[12] For a recent exploration of the current relation between biography and history, see AHR Roundtable Special Issues, 'Historians and Biography', *American Historical Review*, 114, 3 (June 2009). Also see the special issue 'Biography and History: Inextricably Interwoven', *Journal of Interdisciplinary History*, 40, 3 (Winter 2010); and Vijaya Ramaswamy and Yogesh Sharma (eds.), *Biography as History: Indian Perspectives* (Hyderabad: Orient Blackswan, 2009).

[13] See Tony K. Stewart, 'One Text from Many: Caitanya Caritamrita as "Classic and Commentary"' in Wianad Callewaert and Rupert Snell (eds.), *According to Tradition: Hagiographical Writing in India* (Wiesbaden: Harrasowitz Verlag, 1994), pp. 231–48; and Udaya Kumar, 'Writing the Life of the Guru, Chattampi Swamikal, Sree Narayan Guru and modes of Biographical construction' in Vijaya Ramaswamy and Yogesh Sharma (eds.), *Biography as History: Indian Perspectives*, 2009, pp. 53–87.

practices were nonetheless sustained by institutions and processes shaped by colonial modernity, if not the colonial state. In the case of homoeopathy in Bengal, these institutions were the reformed colonial family and more importantly, the modern print culture.[14] I particularly explore the role of the intergenerational family firms, the print culture they promoted, and indeed the role of biography as an exclusive genre of print, in crystallising homoeopathy. This study of the entangled histories of biography, family and homoeopathy in Bengal seeks to broaden our understandings of the modalities through which heterodox sciences were consolidated in dispersed colonial societies such as Tibet, Japan, Transvaal and Egypt.[15] It further illustrates that acculturation of European medicine necessarily drew upon and reinforced local constellations of class, religion, kinship and other networks of familiarities, and unveils the nature of scientific modernity in South Asia.

A 'Biography Industry'

Over the last few years, the historiography of science and medicine has come to focus more and more on what has been characterised as the new 'geographies of nineteenth century science', encompassing sites and experiences beyond the laboratories, clinics or other conventional spaces associated with science.[16] Along with museums, public lectures, galleries

[14] A recent spate of research on the institutions of South Asian family and law explores the ways in which the family as an institution was deeply controlled by the colonial state. Of particular relevance is Ritu Birla's work on colonial legislations and the Marwari family firm, since commerce in homoeopathy was significantly reliant on the family firm model. See Ritu Birla, *Stages of Capital: Law, Culture and Market Governance in Late Colonial India* (Durham: Duke University Press, 2009). Likewise, mechanisms of surveillance of the print market by the state have been pointed out by several south Asian scholars, including Tapti Roy, 'Disciplining the Printed Text: Colonial and Nationalist Surveillance of Bengali Literature', pp. 30–61; and Farina Mir, *Social Space of Language: Vernacular Culture in British Colonial Punjab*.

[15] A range of works has initiated interesting conversations about marginal, often state-censored medico-scientific practices with various forms of print networks. See Vincenne Adams, 'The Sacred in the Scientific: Ambiguous Practices of Science in Tibetan Medicine', *Cultural Anthropology*, 16, 1 (2001), 542–75; Akiko Ito, 'How Electricity Energizes the Body: Electrotherapeutics and Its Analogy of Life in Japanese Medical Context' in Dhruv Raina and Feza Gunergun (eds.), *Science between Europe and Asia, Historical Studies on the Transmission, Adoption and Adaptation of Knowledge* (Netherlands: Springer, 2011), pp. 245–58; Joel Cabrita, 'People of Adam: Divine Healing and Racial Cosmopolitanism in the Early Twentieth Century Transvaal', *Comparative Studies in Society and History*, 57, 2 (2015), 1–36; and Marwa Elshakry, *Reading Darwin in Arabic, 1860–1950* (Chicago: University of Chicago Press, 2013).

[16] David Livingstone and Charles Withers (eds.), *Geographies of Nineteenth Century Science* (Chicago: University of Chicago Press, 2011).

of practical science, panoramic shows and exhibitions, the role of the print market, especially the popular market around print, science, social and individual health has been explored in its various facets, especially in the context of Victorian Britain.[17] The practices challenged by the state and other established authorities related to it were crucially reliant on an increasingly global print network, as illustrated by James Bradley's work on British hydrotherapy and John Kucich's exploration of American spiritualism.[18]

The power of print, along with these other sites, in 'staging (colonial) science' is gradually being acknowledged in histories of South Asian science and medicine. Especially in the case of medicine, the paradigm of 'medical markets' has emerged as an important analytical tool to understand the cultural life of colonial medicine, where the 'marketplace of print' is of increasing importance as a concept.[19] Indeed, a recent spate of fresh research on traditional health and physical cultures in colonial Hyderabad, Punjab, United Province and other parts of north India and Bengal, has opened up conversations about the rapidly growing popular print productions, which owed their development to fast-changing technologies and to the widening horizon of the nineteenth-century reading and consuming public.[20] These works, focusing on facets of traditional knowledge, note that the negotiation with modern print impacted customary practices with changing notions of authority, pupillage and consumption.

[17] See Jonathan Topham, 'Publishing "Popular Science" in Early Nineteenth-Century Britain' in Aileen Fyfe and Bernard Lightman (eds.), *Science in the Marketplace: Nineteenth Century Sites and Experiences* (Chicago: Chicago University Press, 2007), pp. 135–68; and Jonathan Topham, *Scientific Publishing and the Reading of Science in Nineteenth-century Britain: A Historiographical Survey and Guide to Sources, Studies in History and Philosophy of Science*, Part A, 31, 4 (2000), 559–612.

[18] James Bradley, 'Medicine on the Margins: Hydropathy and Orthodoxy in Britain, 1840–1860' in Waltraud Ernst (ed.), *Plural Medicine, Tradition and Modernity, 1800–2000* (London and New York: Routledge, 2002), p. 34; and John Kucich, *Ghostly Communion: Cross-cultural Spiritualism in the Nineteenth Century* (New Hampshire: UPNE, 2004). See the chapter 'Public Spirits: Spiritualism in American Periodicals', pp. 36–58.

[19] See Mark Jenner and Patrick Wallis (eds.), *Medicine and the Market in England and Its Colonies, 1450–1850* (Basingstoke: Palgrave Macmillan, 2007).

[20] Guy Attewell, *Refiguring Unani Tibb: Plural Healing in Late Colonial India* (New Delhi: Orient Longman, 2007), pp. 238–70; Kavita Sivaramakrishnan, *Old Potions, New Bottles: Recasting Indigenous Medicine in Colonial Punjab, 1850–1945* (Hyderabad: Orient Longman, 2006), pp. 104–157; Rachel Berger, *Ayurveda Made Modern: Political Histories of Indigenous Medicine in North India, 1900–1955* (Basingstoke: Palgrave Macmillan, 2013), pp. 75–105; Charu Gupta, *Sexuality, Obscenity, and Community: Women, Muslims and the Hindu Public in Colonial India* (Delhi: Permanent Black, 2001), pp. 30–65; and Projit Bihari Mukharji, *Nationalizing the Body: The Medical Market, Print and Daktari Medicine* (London, New York, Delhi: Anthem Press, 2009), pp. 75–110.

It is perhaps incumbent on new scholarship to go beyond the idea of a monolithic print market, and to explore the various genres and formats of medico-scientific print. Scholars have pointed out that studying the specific formats and genre conventions in the print market is highly instructive of the ideas they seek to convey.[21] While there has been some sporadic work on the function of science text books[22] as also the didactic manuals on health,[23] periodicals have received the most sustained attention from historians of science in South Asia and beyond, who have recognised their role as a significant tool for forging knowledge and opinion in the nineteenth century. Focusing on various aspects, such as 'periodicity'[24] or the formation of a 'common (national) intellectual context',[25] the role of periodicals has been identified as fundamental.[26] While more recent South Asian works are branching out towards deciphering medical advertisements,[27] myriad other areas remain to be explored, not least the world of commercially printed science visuals, which is increasingly being highlighted as yet another important site for the study of science and medicine.[28]

Furthering these historical trends, I focus on the writing and publication of medical biographies. While acknowledging biography to be an important mode in narrating science, especially since the 1960s,

[21] For a couple of authoritative studies, see Robert Darnton, *The Business of Enlightenment: A Publishing History of the Encyclopaedia, 1775–1800*, Cambridge: Harvard University Press, 1987; and William St Claire, *The Reading Nation in the Romantic Period* (Cambridge: Cambridge University Press, 2004).

[22] Dhruv Raina and S. Irfan Habib, 'Ramchandra's Treatise through the "Haze of the Golden Sunset": An Aborted Pedagogy', *Social Studies of Science*, 20, 3 (1990), 455–72.

[23] See Rohan Deb Roy, 'Debility, Diet, Desire: Food in Nineteenth and Early Twentieth Century Bengali Manuals' in Supriya Chaudhari and Rimi B. Chatterjee (eds.), *The Writer's Feast: Food and the Cultures of Representation* (Hyderabad: Orient Blackswan, 2011), pp. 179–205.

[24] James Wald, 'Periodicals and Periodicity' in Simon Eliot and Jonathan Rose (eds.), *A companion to the History of Book* (Oxford: Wiley Blackwell, 2009), pp. 421–32.

[25] Geoffrey Cantor et al. (eds.), *Science in the Nineteenth-Century Periodical: Reading the Magazine of Nature* (Cambridge: Cambridge University Press, 2004).

[26] For explorations in studying the importance of periodicals in the Indian context, see Amit Ranjan Basu, 'Emergence of a Marginal Science in a Colonial City: Reading Psychiatry in Bengali Periodicals', *Indian Economic and Social History Review*, 41, 2 (2004), 103–41. Also see Projit Bihari Mukhari, *Nationalizing the Body*, pp. 92–100. For a recent study of literary periodicals and their readership in Bengal, see Samarpita Mitra, 'Periodical Readership in Early Twentieth Century Bengal: Ramananda Chattopadhyay's Prabasi', *Modern Asian Studies*, 47, 1 (2013), 204–49.

[27] Madhuri Sharma, 'Creating a Consumer: Exploring Medical Advertisements in Colonial India' in Mark Harrison and Biswamoy Pati (eds.), *The Social History of Health and Healing in Colonial India* (New York: Routledge, 2009), pp. 213–28.

[28] See for instance, James Secord, 'Scrapbook Science: Composite Caricatures in Late Georgian England' in A. Shteir and B. Lightman (eds.), *Figuring It Out: Science, Gender, and Visual Culture* (Hanover, New Hampshire: Dartmouth College Press, 2006), pp. 164–91.

historians of science have debated its usefulness as a means of recording the history of science; most agree that 'biography, however useful, exerts a powerfully distorting image of how most science gets done'.[29] Yet, few works other than the important collection of essays by Michael Shortland and Richard Yeo actually delve into the writing, circulation and impact of nineteenth-century medico-scientific biographies.[30] This chapter does precisely that. As noted in the Introduction, popular medical print culture in Bengal is replete with biographies of Hahnemann and of other homoeopathic practitioners, published from the latter half of the nineteenth century.

Biographies narrating individual lives varied in size from slender, cheap, vernacular pamphlets or monographs costing a few *anna* (one-sixteenth of a rupee) to heavier, more expensive English volumes. In addition, lives of practitioners were published serially in the prominent English language journals published, edited and printed by the leading Calcutta–based homoeopathic family firms. Some of these were the *Indian Homoeopathic Review* (published by the Majumdar's Pharmacy), *Homoeopathic Herald* and *Homoeopathy Chikitsha* (published by M. Bhattacharya and Company), *Hahnemann* and *The Hahnemannian Gleanings* (published by Hahnemann Publishing Company), and most importantly *The Calcutta Journal of Medicine*, edited and published by Mahendralal Sircar and his son Amritalal Sircar, uninterruptedly from 1867 to at least 1913. In its heyday under Mahendralal, limited copies were sent for sale in London.[31] Indeed, while most journals boasted a readership beyond the urban centres and extending into the *mofussil*, a few others recurrently drew attention in their editorials to their 'numerous subscribers – clients and readers, within and outside India'.[32] Admittedly, shortages of funds and problems of arrears in running the journals were also occasionally reported.[33]

Yet, the serialised journal articles or stand-alone books hardly exhaust the formats through which the lives of Bengali homoeopaths were made available to the readers. True to the current characterisation of biography as a 'hybrid, unstable genre with many forms', life stories of physicians and of Hahnemann appeared in myriad formats and on remarkably different

[29] Mott Greene, 'Writing Scientific Biography', *Journal of the History of Biology*, 40, 4 (2007), 727–8. Also see Mary Terrell, 'Biography as a Cultural History of Science', *Isis*, 97, 2 (2006), 306–13.

[30] Richard Yeo and Michael Shortland (eds.), *Telling Lives in Science: Essays in Scientific Biography* (Cambridge: Cambridge University Press, 1996).

[31] Arun Kumar Biswas (ed.), *Gleanings of the Past and the Science Movement: In the Diaries of Drs. Mahendralal and Amritalal Sircar* (Kolkata: Asiatic Society, 2000), p. 16.

[32] 'Editorial', Indian Homoeopathic Review, 15, 1 (January 1906), p. 1.

[33] See, for instance, Arun Kumar Biswas (ed.), *Gleanings of the Past*, p. 16.

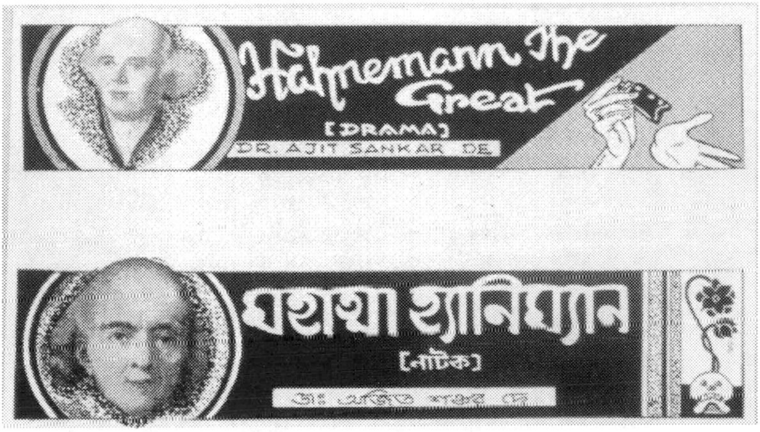

Fig. 2.1 Cover photo of the drama *Hahnemann the Great*, published serially in the journal *Hahnemann*. Reproduced from the collection of the Archives of the Centre for Studies in Social Sciences, Calcutta.

pretexts.[34] Sometimes such lives were narrated as part of published conference papers read out to international homoeopathic congresses. Besides, prefaces, forewords and even dedication pages of books on homoeopathic therapeutics, articles and published lectures in journals, advertisements, journal editorials, obituaries, poems, even plays (see Fig. 2.1) served as platforms for narrating either fragmented or comprehensive lives of Hahnemann and of the various 'key figures instrumental in the spread of homoeopathy in Bengal'. Here I draw upon around fifty such life stories.

Indeed, spanning the last quarter of the nineteenth and the first half of the twentieth century, there seems to have flourished around homoeopathy what in other contexts has come to be described variously as a 'biography industry'[35] or a 'biographical mania'.[36] These characterisations, which refer primarily to the demand, production and readership of such biographies, as well as to the agency and interest of the biographers, can be usefully invoked to understand the nature of the homoeopathic biographic productions in Bengal. An enduring interest in these lives can be assessed from the large

[34] Julie Codell, *The Victorian Artist: Artists' Lifewriting in Britain c. 1870–1910* (Cambridge: Cambridge University Press, 2003), p. 2.

[35] Allen Hibbard, 'Biographer and Subject: A Tale of Two Narratives', *South Central Review*, 23, 3 (2006), p. 31

[36] Julie Codell, 'Constructing the Victorian Artist: National Identity, the Political Economy of Art and Biographical Mania in the Periodical Press', *Victorian Periodicals Review*, 33, 3 (2000), 283–316.

number of biographical works undertaken, as also from the myriad remarks, queries and letters in response, sent to the editors following the publication of these lives. Such readership was often not restricted to the particular journal which originally published the biography. Rivalry between journals was often exposed in the context of the information conveyed in the life stories. An editorial of the journal *Hahnemann*, for example, engaged in a protracted polemic with a rival journal *Homoeopathic Samachar* over the details of Rajendralal Datta's life, which they had published a few months back.[37] The narrators too seemed to be aware of the extensive demand and wide-ranging circulation of their work. Writing in 1909, a biographer of Mahendralal Sircar expressed his confidence regarding the sale of his book: '[a]s many educated Indians like Homoeopathy now-a-days, there is every likelihood of my book being sent to or purchased by them in most educated households'.[38] Such confidence was reaffirmed by the proliferation of many published biographies into multiple editions. The preface to the fourth edition of Mahesh Chandra Bhattacharya's life, published by his own family firm, pompously remarked that the account was inspired by wide-ranging interest in Bhattacharya's life among a Bengali reading public.[39]

Inevitably, this multiplicity of biographies focused not only on communicating the events in the lives of these personalities, but more significantly on what those lives meant. The life stories seemed to fulfil a function as cheaper, popular and more accessible extensions to the proclaimed medical literature. Written in lucid prose for a mass audience, they complemented the more explicitly medical treatise in establishing homoeopathy's genealogy as well as its fundamental principles, in the way artists' biographies in Britain have been shown to operate as complementary texts to actual museum visits and obtuse art criticism.[40] In their meticulous recounting of the founding moment of the sect – the German physician Hahnemann's discovery of the so-called 'law of similars'– the

[37] 'Editorial: Daktar Rajendralal Dutta Sambandhe Homoeopathic Samachar er Uktir Uttor' ('Reply to the Remark on Dr. Rajendralal Dutta by Homoeopathic Samachar'), *Hahnemann*, 22, 3 (1939), 181–3.

[38] Sarat Chandra Ghose, *Life of Dr. Mahendralal Sircar*, 1st edition (Calcutta: Oriental Publishing Home, 1909), p. 55.

[39] Mahesh Chandra Bhattacharya, 'Preface', *Atmakatha* (*My Life*), 4th edition (Calcutta: Economic Press, 1957), page number not cited. Likewise, the monograph *Life of Dr. Mahendralal Sircar*, first published in 1909, was republished in 1935 by Hahnemann Publishing Company on grounds of 'increasing popular demand'.

[40] Julie Codell, *The Victorian Artist*, pp. 6–7.

many lives of Bengali homoeopaths emphasised at once the uniqueness and antiquity and by extension, the superiority of the doctrine.[41] For instance, a typical biography of Hahnemann titled *Homoeopathy Abishkorta Samuel Hahnemann er Jiboni (Biography of Samuel Hahnemann, the Discoverer of Homoeopathy)*, written in 1881, devoted its initial chapters to discussing the discovery that led to enunciation of the homoeopathic theories of healing, based on the 'law of similars', along with Hahnemann's notion of bodily vital force and its derangements as the cause of disease, and also the homoeopathic rationale for minute doses for drugs.[42] Together these life stories seemed to proffer themselves as a contextual literature to understand the central homoeopathic text, namely the *Organon*, much as religious biographies were often conceived as preparatory texts for their relevant scriptures.[43]

Besides, these biographies deployed recurrent typologies of physicians' characters to tease out the specificity of the homoeopathic doctrine in Bengal. For one, they meticulously performed the crucial task of identifying key figures responsible for enunciating the 'homoeopathic reform' in the province. In recurrent biographic tropes, for instance, the life of Hahnemann, the eighteenth-century German founder of homoeopathy, was shown to be analogous to and in dialogue with that of the Bengali physician Mahendralal Sircar, the second MD to qualify from the Calcutta Medical College, was an important personality of nineteenth-century Bengal for more reasons than one.[44] Not least, he was also one of the entrepreneur-physicians discussed in Chapter 1. The biographies enumerated Mahendralal's various involvements with and achievements in the broad field of science, including the establishment of the first native science organisation, the Indian Association for the Cultivation of Science.[45] They especially

[41] The Latin phrase '*Similia Similibus Curatur*', meaning 'like cures like', popularly referred to as the 'law of similars', was widely written about as the core principle of homoeopathy as enunciated by Hahnemann.

[42] Mahendranath Ray, *Homoeopathy Abishkorta Samuel Hahnemann er Jiboni* (*Biography of Samuel Hahnemann, the Discoverer of Homoeopathy*) (Taligunj: Kasi Kharda Press, 1881), pp. 3–17.

[43] See Wianad Callewaert and Rupert Snell (eds.), *According to Tradition: Hagiographical Writing in India*, 1994, pp. 12–13.

[44] Existing historiography has dealt with Mahendralal Sircar's myriad projects concerning science with wider nationalist implications. See, for instance, Pratik Chakraborty, 'Science, Morality, and Nationalism: The Multifaceted Project of Mahendra Lal Sircar', *Studies in History*, 17, 2 (2001), 245–74.

[45] For instance, see Anilchandra Ghosh, 'Daktar Mahendralal Sircar', *Bigyane Bangali* (*Science and the Bengalis*) (Calcutta: Presidency Library, 1931), pp. 19–26.

emphasised the various government recognitions that Sircar received for his pioneering initiative in the 'science movement'.[46] Such scientific attainments were highlighted as conclusive testimony of the undeniable scientific claims of homoeopathy, in which Sircar was equally invested. The biography of Dinabandhu Mukhopadhyay, for instance, candidly argued that 'in Bengal there is an indisputable connection between homoeopathy and the practice of science. This is evident from the fact that Mahendralal Sircar dedicated his whole life to the pursuit and establishment of both in the country'.[47]

The biographies underlined Sircar's distinguished status by narrating his life story with repeated reference to that of Hahnemann. Events in their lives, separated by more than a century, were shown to have remarkable similarities and thus Mahendralal Sircar was presented almost as a modern Bengali reincarnation of Hahnemann. Sircar's life seemed to be the re-enactment of that of the original founder in a different imperial theatre. A slightly later biography of Hahnemann titled 'Asia r Hahnemann: Dr. Mahendralal Sircar' ('Mahendralal, the Hahnemann of Asia') captures precisely this tendency of these biographies – of merging one life into another.[48] The distant and the immediate were locked in constant dialogue with one another in these texts.

The biographies depicted Hahnemann's discovery of the homoeopathic 'law of similars' as the most defining moment in homoeopathy's history. The authors noted Hahnemann's deep unease and disgust with the 'fallacies and uncertainties' of prevalent medicine. The act of discovery, as an answer to such extant fallacies, received substantial importance in the biographies. The sequence of thoughts and events around that one incident received significant attention from the biographers. For instance, Mahendranath Ray, in his biography of Hahnemann, gave a comprehensive review of many contemporary authors who had ventured to write about the event of the discovery.[49] The event of Mahendralal Sircar's 'conversion' to homoeopathy was compared in significance with Hahnemann's 'discovery' of the homoeopathic law. At the fourth annual meeting of the Bengal branch of the British Medical Association in February 1867, of which Sircar was the vice president, he declared his

[46] Saratchandra Ghosh, 'Daktar Mahendralal Sircar er Jibon-katha', *Hahnemann*, 22, 2 (1939), 67, 77–9.

[47] Rashbehari Mukhopadhyay, 'Shworgiyo Raysaheb Dinabandhu Mukhopadhyay er Jiboni' ('Life of Late Honourable Dinabandhu Mukhopadhyay'), *Hahnemann*, 4, 8 (1921), 276.

[48] Satyendranath Ray, *Asia r Hahnemann: Dr. Mahendralal Sircar* (*Mahendralal Sircar: The Hahnemann of Asia*) (Calcutta: Institute of History of Homoeopathy, year not cited).

[49] Mahendranath Ray, *Homoeopathy Abishkorta Samuel Hahnemann er Jiboni* (*Biography of Samuel Hahnemann, the Discoverer of Homoeopathy*), 1881, pp. 23–5.

so-called shift to believing in homoeopathy. Without exception, all his biographies highlighted this incident, and treated it as the single most important factor, like 'Hahnemann's original discovery', behind the propagation of homoeopathy in Bengal. Comparing the role of Mahendralal in popularising homoeopathy with that of Hahnemann himself, one biographer, for instance, noted, '[a]t the time of his (Mahendralal's) conversion, the name of Hahnemann was almost unknown to the nobility, the gentry and the mob of his country', while Sircar's conversion made them aware of the great man's century-old discovery.[50] The biographies regularly contrasted the two events and highlighted the significance of both in the annals of homoeopathy. Even by Mahendralal's own admission, the two events were analogous as they were equally effective in altering ideas around medicine in their respective times. Reflecting on his own career in the pages of his journal *Calcutta Journal of Medicine* in 1902, Mahendralal described his conversion as an act of medical reform, comparable only with the original act of 'discovery' initiated by Hahnemann.[51]

The analogy between the two lives seemed most conspicuous in the context of the aftermath of the events described here. The biographies recorded a startling overlap in the way both Hahnemann and Mahendralal faced stiff professional opposition once they expressed public conviction in homoeopathy. Words like 'professional enmity', 'persecution', 'outcaste', 'struggle' and so on were repeatedly deployed in describing these incidents in the lives of both men. The agonies associated with scientific discovery, and the hardship of initiating a radical change of idea in any context, were shown to bear similarities. Sarat Chandra Ghose argued in a paper read out at an International Homoeopathic Congress, '[l]ike all discoveries, like Harvey's circulation of the blood, like Paracelsus' antimony and like Jenner's vaccination, Hahnemann's homoeopathy was for some time, persecuted with the most remorseless rancour'.[52] In an identical fashion, articles reviewing the conversion of Mahendralal Sircar to homoeopathy referred to the hindrance faced by every innovator in trying to bring about 'progress or reform'.[53]

[50] Sarat Chandra Ghose, *Life of Dr. Mahendralal Sircar*, 1st edition (Calcutta: Oriental Publishing Home, 1909), p. 129.

[51] Mahendralal Sircar, 'The Story of Dr. Sircar's Conversion to Homoeopathy', *Calcutta Journal of Medicine*, 21 (1902), 276.

[52] S. C. Ghose, 'Homoeopathy and Its First Missionary in India', *The Hahnemannian Gleanings*, 3, 7 (August 1932), 289.

[53] 'Review of Indian Daily News', in Mahendralal Sircar, *On the Supposed Uncertainty in Medical Science and on the Relation between Diseases and Their Remedial Agents* (Calcutta: Anglo-Sanskrit Press, 1903), p. 62.

Mahendralal, the author contended, was a victim of such prejudice, as was Hahnemann himself.[54]

Hindu Way of Life

Apart from canonicity, and the projection of personality cults, claims of homoeopathic superiority hinged crucially on the evocative depiction of distinct typology for the physicians' characters. The biographies were careful in highlighting the deep moral integrity of the physicians' personalities, and their righteous commitment to curing social ills. Beyond the mere materiality of drugs, homoeopathy was portrayed as a biomoral regimen for disciplining lives. The practice of homoeopathy was presented as a way to cultivate an ethical, holistic vision, capable of engendering national good. In discussing these virtues, this section explores the discreetly Hinduised idioms through which lives of prominent homoeopathic physicians and entreprebeurs were narrated.

Acquisition and dispensation of wealth remained the two fundamental tropes around which narration of the lives were organised. At one level, homoeopathy's superiority and efficacy was emphasised through careful depiction of its growing popularity across Indian society. Rajendralal Datta's biography described how 'a crowd of eager patients assembled in his house every morning with the punctuality that marks the rising of the sun in the east and as cure followed cure, the crowds grew'.[55] The fact of being summoned by eminent, even princely clients was carefully recorded as an obvious marker of the doctrine's efficacy. Thus, the life history of D. N. Ray noted among his patients Dadabhai Naoraji, the founder of the Indian National Congress, and Byaramjee Malabari, the famous Parsi reformer and editor of the newspaper *Spectator*,[56] while the biographies of other physicians narrated their reputation among the rulers of the princely states of India, such as the Nawab of Bhopal.[57] Apart from the native elites, the names of Englishmen who regularly consulted Bengali homoeopaths featured in these narratives. Rajendralal Datta's life recorded Lord Ripon, Sir Henry Cotton, Sir Peacock, Sir Risley, Sir Harrison, Sir Lambert, Mr

[54] Ibid.

[55] S. C. Ghose, 'Homoeopathy and Its First Missionary in India', *The Hahnemannian Gleanings*, 3, 10 (November 1932), 451.

[56] D. N. Ray, *Daktar D. N. Ray er Atmakatha* (*Autobiography of Dr D. N. Ray*) (publisher not cited, 1929), p. 273.

[57] Sarat Chandra Ghosh, 'Dr. L. Salzer M. D', *Hahnemann*, 22, 6 (1939), 326–7.

Robert Night (editor of the newspaper *Statesman*) and Father Lafont, among his regular patients.[58]

In a related vein, the wealth acquired by these physicians was held up as a palpable measure both of their own repute and of homoeopathy's worth. Wealth was often assessed in terms of the property they managed to acquire and the fortunes they left behind.[59] The life stories were dotted with minutiae of the palatial residences the protagonists had built.[60] The fact that Mahendralal Sircar was one of the highest paid medical practitioners in contemporary Calcutta, and charged a fee of 32 rupees per patient, were adequately highlighted in his biography.[61] It was also carefully mentioned that he had declared a 'prohibitive fee' of rupees 100 per patient once he had formally retired. The elites reportedly were prepared to pay staggering amounts like 2,000 rupees as a consultancy fee after his retirement. The biography noted at the same time that his patients named him 'Dhanwantari' after the legendary Indian healer of the mythical past.[62]

It is, however, significant that in comparison to the physicians' acquisitions, an even greater emphasis was given to the willingness to give up acquired wealth. Narrations of these lives delineated an ethic that prescribed codes for the dispensation of wealth, which was intimately related with Hindu scriptural notions of '*seba*' or 'service', '*kalyan*' or 'well-being', and '*tyag*' or 'sacrifice'.[63] Recent works have dwelt on the centrality of these concepts in the Hindu nationalist lexicon that was emerging from the late nineteenth century onwards.[64] Biographies, in this context, discussed the

58 Saratchandra Ghosh, 'Bharatbarshe Homoeopathy Chikitshar Sorbo pratham Pathopradarshak o Pracharak Dr. Rajendralal Datta' ('The Pioneer Physician and Perpetrator of Homoeopathy in India'), *Hahnemann*, 22, 1 (1939), 19.

59 Biographies and autobiographies of most physicians including Batakrishna Pal, Pratap Chandra Majumdar, Lokenath Maitra, D. N. Ray and so on included elaborate descriptions of the property they acquired through homoeopathic enterprise. For instance, see Jitendranath Majumdar, 'Dr. Pratap Chandra Majumdar M. D', *Hahnemann*, 23, 8 (1940), 452–3.

60 For instance, see Sarat Chandra Ghosh, 'Dr. Brajendranath Bandopadhyay M. D', *Hahnemann*, 23, 3 (1940), 133. Also see Gopal Chandra Mukhopadhyay, *Sadhu Batakrishna Pal* (*The Saintly Batakrishna Pal*), Vol II (Calcutta: Batakrishna Pal, 1919), pp. 168–9.

61 Saratchandra Ghosh, 'Daktar Mahendralal Sircar er Jibon-katha' ('Life of Dr Mahendralal Sircar'), *Hahnemann*, 22, 3 (1939), 137.

62 Ibid., pp. 143.

63 See, for instance, Rashbehari Mukhopadhyay, 'Shworgiyo Raysaheb Dinabandhu Mukhopadhyay er Jiboni' ('Life of Late Honourable Rashbehari Mukhopadhyay'), *Hahnemann*, 4, 8 (1921), 293.

64 See, for instance, R. Srivastan, 'Concept of "Seva" and the "Sevak" in the Freedom Movement', *Economic and Political Weekly*, 41, 5 (2006), 427–38. Also see Raminder Kaur, *Performative Politics and the Cultures of Hinduism: Public Uses of Religion in Western India* (London: Anthem Press, 2005), p. 157.

idea of a 'Mahapurush' or 'Great Man', drawing references from Hindu *shastras*.[65] The biography of Batakrishna Pal, for instance, argued that the attribute of being a millionaire did not necessarily qualify anyone as a 'Mahapurush' nor did such a person inevitably deserve a biography.[66] Only when one possessed the heart to give up hard-earned wealth for the well-being of the people of one's nation and race, could one earn the epithet of a 'Mahapurush' – and claim to have lived life respectfully.[67]

It is important to note that '*seba*' or service to the poor and the distressed was considered the most ethical means of dispensing wealth. Homoeopathy was held up as a powerful ideology which empowered its protagonists to achieve that desired end, as evidenced by a range of biographies detailing their protagonists' commitments towards 'distributing medicines and food free of cost among the sick poor and to minister to their comforts in every imaginable way'.[68] Lives of Mahendralal Sircar, Mahesh Chandra Bhattacharya, Brajendranath Bandopadhyay, Akshay Kumar Dutta and Batakrishna Pal recounted innumerable instances of their selfless help and empathy for the poor, in the form of free treatment and free distribution of drugs.[69] On the death of Akshay Kumar Dutta, the destitute were recorded to have lamented that 'the rich people of the country have many renowned doctors to look after them. But he was like a parent to the poor and the hapless, who had no one else to turn to'.[70] Mahesh Chandra's role in reducing the price of homoeopathic drugs in his Economic Pharmacy provided an exemplary instance of his service to the people.[71] The biographies claimed that such services had a bearing on the welfare of the nation as a whole.[72]

Related to the discourse of 'service' around homoeopathy was the emphasis on charity. Charity or '*daan*' was glorified as the noblest way of utilising the wealth acquired through homoeopathic practice. Whether devoting a whole chapter titled 'Daan Brata' ('Codes of Charity') in

[65] Gopal Chandra Mukhopadhyay, *Sadhu Batakrishna Pal* (*The Saintly Batakrishna Pal*), Vol 1 (Calcutta: Batakrishna Pal, 1919), pp. 6–7.
[66] Ibid., pp. 6–7. [67] Ibid., pp. 6, 174–5.
[68] S. C. Ghose, 'Homoeopathy and Its First Missionary in India', *The Hahnemannian Gleanings*, 3, 8 (September 1932), pp. 338–9.
[69] For instance, see Rashbehari Mukhopadhyay, 'Shworgiyo Raysaheb Dinabandhu Mukhopadhyay er Jiboni' ('Life of Late Honourable Rashbehari Mukhopadhyay'), *Hahnemann*, 4, 7 (1921), 147.
[70] Sarat Chandra Ghosh, 'Dr. Akshay Kumar Datta L. M. S', *Hahnemann*, 23, 4 (1940), 199.
[71] Srish Chandra Talapatra, *Maheshchandra Charitkatha* (*Life of Mahesh Chandra*) (Calcutta: Economic Press, 1946), pp. 31–2.
[72] Ibid., also see, Rashbehari Mukhopadhyay, 'Shworgiyo Raysaheb Dinabandhu Mukhopadhyay er Jiboni' ('Life of Late Honourable Dinabandhu Mukhopadhyay'), *Hahnemann*, 4, 7 (1921), 147.

Batakrishna Pal's biography, or discussing Mahesh Chandra as the author of texts like *Daanbidhi* (*Rules of Charity*), most biographies presented their protagonists as engaged in selfless acts of (often anonymous) charity for the good of society. Discussions on ethical utilisation of wealth further encompassed descriptions of the extraordinarily simple, everyday lifestyle of the protagonists as demonstrated in their diet, clothing and other quotidian habits. Of Mahendralal Sircar's personal lifestyle it was noted that the physician 'always wore Taltollah slippers; whether visiting patients or attending public meetings. The Calcutta public does not remember having seen him in boots or shoes ... He more resembled an old poor Brahmin in these respects than a successful medical practitioner of the town'.[73]

Likewise, Batakrishna Pal's biography recorded the fact that his spectacular changes in fortune had not altered his appearance over the years.[74] The biographer mentioned having seen him in the same simple attire for over fifty years. Men such as Mahesh Bhattacharya categorically condemned extravagance of any kind as sin, especially in a poor, subjugated economy like India's.[75] He held that the cunning colonial powers dominated other nations by luring them into a luxurious lifestyle that played havoc with their social norms.

The biographies of these physicians further represented the physicians as having a deep attachment to their roots, by suggestively referring to their native villages as '*janmabhumi*' or places of birth, and '*desh*' or nation. Evidently, in the context of late nineteenth- to early twentieth-century Bengal, these terms had acquired wide nationalist resonances. Mahesh Chandra Bhattacharya's biography explicitly imparted a nationalistic charge to his life. Describing Mahesh Chandra as a patriot, his biographies explain that the idea of nation in his patriotic imagination was quite narrow in scope.[76] Serving the nation, he believed, necessarily began with one's immediate place of birth. It could then be endlessly extended to include society and the country as a whole.[77] Homoeopathic knowledge was projected as a useful tool to serve the 'interiors' and villages. The biography of Bamacharan Das describes how he abandoned his practice in the city to establish a flourishing practice at his native

[73] Shivnath Shastri, 'Men I Have Seen', *Atmacharit* (*My Life*) (Calcutta: Prabasi Karjalay), 1918 (Reprint Dey's 2003), pp. 503–4.
[74] Gopal Chandra Mukhopadhyay, *Sadhu Batakrishna Pal* (*The Saintly Batakrishna Pal*), Vol II, 1919, pp. 205–7.
[75] Srish Chandra Talapatra, *Maheshchandra Charitkatha* (*Life of Mahesh Chandra*), 1946, pp. 77–8.
[76] Ibid., pp. 8–9. [77] Ibid.

village of Shantipur.[78] This was highlighted as a commendable gesture of self-sacrifice in the larger cause of serving ones '*desh*'.[79]

Indeed, nearly every life story narrated a life shaped by the motif of returning to the protagonist's roots. At some point in the course of their medical or entrepreneurial career in Calcutta, or after retirement, there was a compulsive return to their roots, a 'backward' travel into the 'interiors' of the province. A deep attachment appears in these texts, interchangeably to the 'rural', the 'indigenous', the 'interior' and the '*mofussil*'. Thus, while Rajendralal Dutta's biography depicted his love for indigenous arts and crafts of various kinds,[80] Baridbaran Mukhopadhyay's life recorded his affective ties to his place of birth, Chandannagar.[81] He was 'fluent with its history and felt delighted whenever he heard of that place'.[82] An abiding sense of nostalgia for a rural origin can be sensed as well from D. N. Ray's description of his own childhood.[83] His autobiography records protracted ramblings about his village, its natural beauty, the rural household, food, festivities, sports and other memories of childhood experiences.[84] For these protagonists, working for one's '*desh*' involved service through homoeopathy. The village emerged in these life histories as the nerve centre from where work for the nation ought to begin. Along with other kinds of welfare activities, assisting the penetration of western medical knowledge in the interior was depicted as an important way of accomplishing such work.[85] In these elements of the typical life narrative, one finds clear resonances of the contemporary (Hindu) nationalist agenda of rural reconstruction and improvement.[86]

[78] Sarat Chandra Ghosh, 'Dr. Bamacharan Das L. M. S', *Hahnemann*, 23, 10 (1940), pp. 580–1.
[79] Ibid., pp. 581.
[80] Saratchandra Ghosh, 'Bharatbarshe Homoeopathy Chikitshar Sorbo prothom Pothoprodorshok o Pracharak Dr. Rajendralal Datta' ('The Pioneer Physician and Perpetrator of Homoeopathy in India'), *Hahnemann*, 22, 1 (1939), 23.
[81] Anonymous, 'Paralok e Dr. Baridbaran Mukhopadhyay' ('Late Dr. Baridbaran Mukhopadhyay'), *Hahnemann*, 23, 7 (1940), 428.
[82] Ibid., p. 428.
[83] D. N. Ray, *Daktar D. N. Ray er Atmakatha* (*Autobiography of Dr D N Ray*), 1929, pp. 20–91.
[84] Ibid.
[85] Srish Chandra Talapatra, *Maheshchandra Charitkatha* (*Life of Mahesh Chandra*), 1946, p. 80.
[86] On rural reconstruction as a part of the Hindu nationalist agenda, see Ajay Skaria, 'Gandhi's Politics and the Question of Ashram' in Saurabh Dube (ed.), *Enchantments of Modernity: Empire, Nation, Globalisation* (Delhi and London: Routledge, 2009), pp. 199–233. Also see Surinder S. Jodhka, 'Nation and Village: Images of Rural India in Gandhi, Nehru and Ambedkar', *Economic and Political Weekly*, 37, 32 (2002), 3343–53.

The agency of biographies in shaping cultural memory has been acknowledged in recent scholarship.[87] The recurrent typologies deployed in the narration of the homoeopaths' lives equated the moral propensities of physicians with the inherent value of their doctrine. The virtues of the individual lives were presented as inseparably linked with the craft they practised. The underlying assumption animating the narration of these lives was to sensitise the readers towards an ethically committed, personalised care regimen, which was promised exclusively by a heterodoxy like homoeopathy, distinct from the strictly institutional, depersonalised structures of state medicine. Underlining the impact of these individual lives on the larger society, the biographies constructed the image of a knowledgeable, compassionate, hardworking, selfless and austere physician as the ideal type for an emerging nation.

Of Science and Spiritualism: Vernacular Hahnemann

Although they chimed in with (Hindu) nationalism in describing homoeopathy's features, the biographies hardly ever ceased from emphasising its western roots. The life stories, in fact, simultaneously celebrated homoeopathy as a western marvel, and also a faith-based Indian spiritual practice, embedded in indigenous tradition. Poised within such a contrarian framework, these texts carved out a liminal status for both the heterodox doctrine and its eighteenth-century German pioneer Hahnemann, as radically western yet deeply resonant with Hindu spiritual values. The case of homoeopathy's consolidation and popularisation in Bengal through the market for biographies underlines the centrality of local factors and interest groups, as well as the contingencies of the vernacular print market, in giving medicine a national character. While Chapter 3 looks at the self-proclaimed efforts at 'translating' western homoeopathy for an Indian audience, the biographies also grappled with such issues, particularly as they pertained to the presentation of the German physician as an ideal type for the Bengali audience.

A common feature of most biographies was the glorification of homoeopathy as a significant constituent of the progressive, modernising West. It was projected as an innovative and cutting-edge European science that critiqued the deep-seated orthodoxy of the mainstream of western medicine. Representative biographies of Hahnemann frequently referred to homoeopathy's advent as the

[87] Richard Holmes, 'A Proper Study?' in William St Claire (ed.), *Mapping Lives: The Uses of Biography* (Oxford: Oxford University Press, 2002), p. 12.

'most glorious and beneficent reform'[88] that would 'overturn the whole of the present practice of medicine'.[89] Echoing a common language of radicalism, unorthodoxy, western rationalism and reform, homoeopathy was, to a certain extent, mapped onto extant western-inspired, religious reformist discourses like that of Brahmoism, that had set out to modernise Hinduism as a rational religion in the light of western Unitarianism.[90] Indeed, in highlighting Brahmoism as a 'rational, scientific reformist agenda against orthodoxy and irrationality', the biographies pointed to an affinity between the visions of homoeopathy and Brahmoism. At one level, men like Mahendralal Sircar were reported as champions to the cause of Brahmo reform. It was noted that

> Dr Sircar hated from the bottom of his heart all retrogressive movements. He publicly taunted those educated men who advocated progress in science, literature and politics but propounded retrogressive views in matters of social life. His sympathy for the great reformer Raja Rammohan Roy, were due to the fact of his having inaugurated religious and social reforms.[91]

An obituary volume for Mahendralal Sircar explicitly stated his appreciation of the Brahmo cause, including his donations to the foundation of the Bharatbarshiyo Brahmo Mandir.[92] Nor was Mahendralal alone in this: the biographies of many renowned homoeopaths included appreciative discussions of Brahmo activities, which were praised as 'rational'. Some practitioners, like Pratap Chandra Majumdar and his associates, including M. M. Basu and Akshay Kumar Dutta, were introduced as practising Brahmos. At the same time, the biographies also described contemporary Brahmo leaders as taking profound interest in the German doctrine. Biographies of Pratap Chandra Majumdar, in particular, detailed the abiding faith of the Tagore family, leaders within the Brahmo community, in homoeopathic cure as an acceptable import from the West.[93] Biographies of the physician described how after an instance of quick recovery from serious illness, Debendranath Tagore

[88] Mahendralal Sircar, 'Hahnemann and His Work', *Calcutta Journal of Medicine*, 12, 10 (May 1887), 391–416.
[89] F. C. Skipwith, 'Homoeopathy and Its Introduction into India', *Calcutta Review*, 17 (1852), 19.
[90] For a standard study of Brahmoism as a western-inspired reform agenda in search of a modern, rational religion, see David Kopf, *The Brahmo Samaj and the Shaping of the Modern Indian Mind* (Princeton, NJ: Princeton University Press, 1979).
[91] Quoted in Sivanath Shastri, 'Men I Have Seen' in *Atmacharit* (*My Life*), 1918, pp. 506–7.
[92] Amritalal Sircar, *Obituary Notice of Mahendralal Sircar CIE, MD, DL* (Calcutta: Anglo Sanskrit Press, 1905), pp. 30–3. See especially 'Dr Sircar and Hindu Orthodoxy', p. 49.
[93] J. N. Majumdar, 'Dr. Pratap Chandra Majumdar M. D', *Hahnemann*, 23, 6 (1940), 322–4.

declared his unbounded faith in the homoeopathic ideology, as opposed to allopathy which engaged in 'mere patchwork' of the body. Homoeopathy, for him, represented a more rational, holistic therapeutic.[94] Rabindranath himself, it has been suggested, marvelled at the doctrine. Biographies of Pratap Chandra Majumdar sketched Rabindranath's efforts towards establishing a charitable dispensary in his *zamindari* estate of Silaidaha to promote the free distribution of homoeopathic drugs.[95] The western, unorthodox aspect of homoeopathy was repeatedly played up through similar discussions. Thus Vidyasagar, another pre-eminent reformist and promoter of homoeopathy, was recorded as having built up an enviable private collection of imported books from Europe.[96] Accounts described how the progressive, emancipating doctrine quickly gained a foothold across the colonial world. It was noted that, 'wherever ships go, there is spreading the knowledge of this doctrine and practice. From Rio Janeiro comes proof of its extension, from Labuan and the Spice Isles, from India, New Zealand and Australia, from the steppes of Tartary and from the coast of Africa'.[97]

Yet, as already shown in the previous section, while they highlighted the western, rational, radical and reformist core of the doctrine, the biographies were equally meticulous in discussing its inherent reverberation with India's age-old traditional spirituality.[98] The ascription of a distinct religio-spiritual identity to homoeopathy itself is evident from the frequency with which the biographies resort to literary idioms with underlying Hindu resonance, like 'high priest', 'Guru' or preceptor, '*sheeshya*' or disciple, '*deekha*' or initiation, '*bhakti*' or faith, 'conversion' in depicting the lives of homoeopaths. Though they were evidently propelled by the interests of medical commerce around a professedly western science and catered to the demands of a growing print market, many of the biographies were nonetheless titled 'Charitkatha'.[99] It is difficult to overlook this allusion to an

[94] Ibid., pp. 323–4. [95] Ibid., p. 323.

[96] Jitendranath Majumdar, 'Dr. Pratap Chandra Majumdar M. D', *Hahnemann*, 23, 5, 1940, pp. 261–2.

[97] F. C. Skipwith, 'Homoeopathy and Its Introduction into India', p. 43.

[98] There is an apparent contradiction in the concurrent homoeopathic self-articulations through the rhetoric of Brahmoism on the one hand and Hinduism on the other. However, the contradiction is more a reflection of such articulations being the trend among many Brahmo leaders themselves, especially since the schism of 1866. One needs to remember the varying degrees to which many Brahmo leaders of the later nineteenth century empathised with Hinduism – including Keshab Chandra Sen, Rajnarain Basu and even Rabindranath Tagore, among others. See David Kopf, *The Brahmo Samaj and the Shaping of the Modern Indian Mind*, 1979, pp. 129–48. Especially relevant is the concept of Hindu Brahmoism discussed with relation to Rabindranath Tagore, pp. 287–312.

[99] For instance, see Srish Chandra Talapatra, *Mahesh Chandra Charitkatha* (*Life of Mahesh Chandra*) (Calcutta: Economic Press, 1946).

entire body of Hindu 'Charita' literature of the medieval and early modern times, which was primarily religious and hagiographic in orientation. A profusion of titles as 'Sadhu Batakrishna Pal', 'Prabhu Hahnemann er Proti', 'Maharshi Hahnemann' and 'Mahesh Chandra Charitkatha' reinforces the interpretation that trade in the popular print market was very often 'led by, rather than leading the popular taste', their presentation often slanted towards appealing to a mass readership.[100] I have already explored how the depiction of individual lives of physicians was woven around recurrent typologies of piety, service, temperance, sacrifice and charity – ideas that had begun acquiring a significant position in the Hindu nationalist lexicon from the late nineteenth century. Often expressed through English language texts, such processes of vernacularisation illustrate that the 'vernacular' is more about the 'style and sensibility they stood for', rather than any particular language.

Indeed, the fractured, hybrid, ambiguous identity of homoeopathy is captured most convincingly in the many lives of Friedrich Christian Samuel Hahnemann circulating in Bengali print from the 1860s onwards. Biographies of Hahnemann collectively appropriated the distant figure of a German physician as the central, 'original' figure around which Bengali homoeopaths came together as a distinct community. On the one hand, the vernacular lives of Hahnemann echoed the late nineteenth- to early twentieth-century western, heterodox discourse around the advanced nature of homoeopathic knowledge. Hahnemann, accordingly, was held up as a rational scientist and a critical scholar. Widely read and knowledgeable, he was described as 'a thinker – and a very original one'[101] His logical bent of mind and his aptitude for questioning the established order of things were put forward as marks of a great intellect.[102] Depicted as the quintessential scientist engaged in laborious research, it was argued that 'his discovery was not the mere theory of a chamber philosopher indulging in idle reveries, but a plain induction from facts and experiments ... after a series of trials covering many years of his life'.[103] He was credited with anticipating future directions in scientific research, his biographers concluding that 'the Chemistry of our day is more and more approaching Hahnemann ... the infinitely little is becoming infinitely potent and the bulk and energy of particles are seen to be in inverse ratio'.[104]

[100] Anindita Ghosh, *Power in Print*, 2006, pp. 24–5.
[101] James C. Wood, 'Value and Limitations of Homoeopathy', *The Hahnemannian Gleanings*, 3 (December 1932), p. 501.
[102] Mahendranath Ray, *Homoeopathy Abishkorta Samuel Hahnemann er Jiboni* (*Life of Samuel Hahnemann the Inventor of Homoeopathy*), 1881, pp. 23–4.
[103] F. C. Skipwith, 'Homoeopathy and Its Introduction into India', pp. 22–3.
[104] Himangshushekhar Ghosh, 'Hahnemann O Adhunik Bigyan' ('Hahnemann and Modern Science'), *Hahnemann*, 23, 1 (1940), 22–3.

On the other hand, an impressive array of biographies approached Hahnemann through the prism of spirituality and faith. He was portrayed as a sacred, mystic persona in possession of divine powers. Quoting the Hindu text *The Bhagavad Gita*, these biographies drew analogies between Hahnemann and the scriptural divine power that was reborn periodically to restore religion on earth.[105] Depicting him as a 'chosen messiah',[106] it was argued that Hahnemann was sent with the preordained mission to cure millions of ailing people with his talent, sacrifice and compassion.[107] He was addressed with epithets like '*Sadhu*' or the hermit, '*Guru*', '*Maharshi*' and '*Prabhu*', terms which loosely stood for 'spiritual head'. The journal *Hahnemann* published a series of poems on Hahnemann the practitioner in its different issues across 1925, which were titled variously, 'Prabhu Hahnemann er Proti', 'Guru Hahnemann er Proti', 'Maharshi Hahnemann er Proti' and the like (see Fig. 2.2).[108]

In addition to such subtle references, there were more explicit instances of comparisons between Hahnemann and major deities. A poem titled '*Deboddeshe*' ('*To the Divine*'), published in the journal *Hahnemann*, for instance, compared Hahnemann with both Siva and Buddha.[109] Hinting at Hahnemann's experimentation on himself with different drugs, the poet drew an analogy between the German physician and Lord Siva who, according to Hindu mythology, had consumed poison in order to save the gods. His determination to overcome disease and human distress was analogised with Buddha's spiritual quest towards defeating death. Analysing the dramatic effect of Hahnemann on the Bengalis, the biographies asserted that 'he has shown the path to salvation from diseases, has liberated them from fear ... has transformed drugs into sweets'.[110] Comparing his discovery to a holy blessing, a poem titled *Hahnemann* described the rising popularity of the doctrine in every household.[111] Faith in homoeopathy was coupled with a deep devotion towards Hahnemann in such households. An instance of the heightened

105 Ibid., p. 20.
106 Bhupendranath Bandopadhyay, 'Smriti Sabha' ('Memorial Meeting'), *Hahnemann*, 9, 1 (1926), 34.
107 Himangshushekhar Ghosh, 'Hahnemann O Adhunik Bigyan' ('Hahnemann and Modern Science'), *Hahnemann*, 23, 1 (1940), 20.
108 For another representative example, see Kalikumar Bhattacharya, 'Prabhu Hahnemann er Proti' (To Hahnemann the Divine'), *Hahnemann*, 8, 5 (1925), 1.
109 Radharaman Biswas, 'Deboddeshe' (To the Almighty), *Hahnemann*, 23, 1 (1940), 190.
110 Anonymous, 'Presidential Address at the Annual Meeting of the Midnapore Hahnemann Association', *Hahnemann*, 10, 2 (1927), 65–6.
111 Saratchandra Ghosh, 'Hahnemann', *Hahnemann*, 22, 1 (1939), 1.

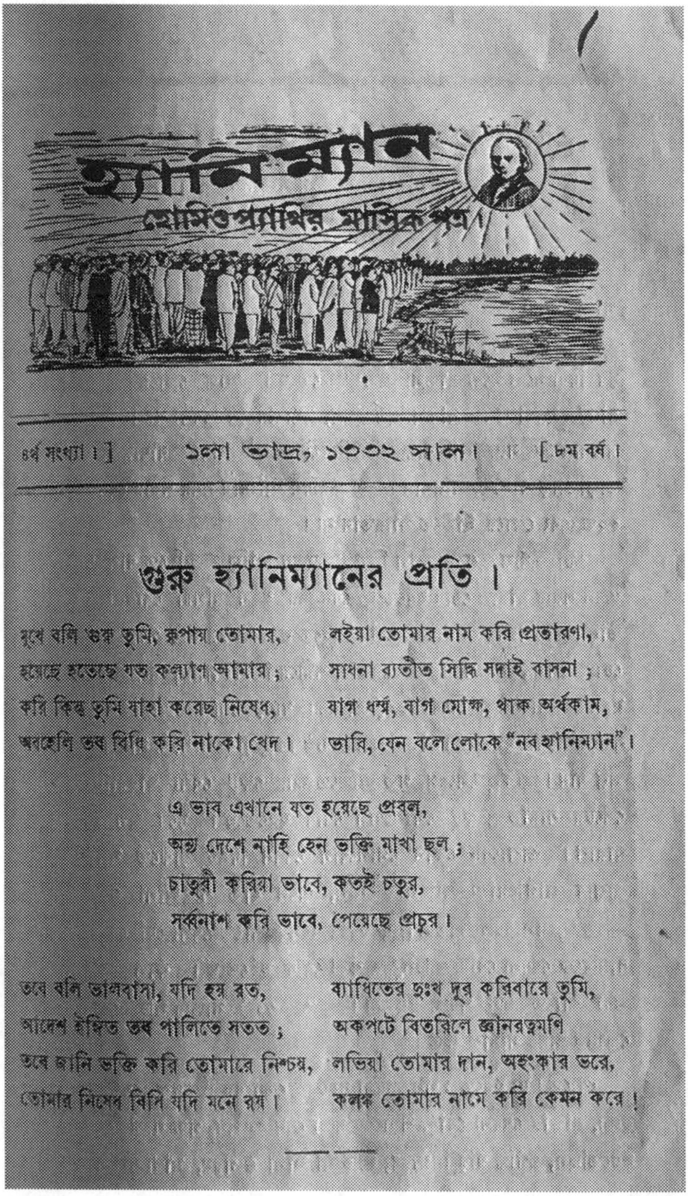

হ্যানিম্যান

হোমিওপ্যাথির মাসিক পত্র।

৪র্থ সংখ্যা।] ১লা ভাদ্র, ১৩৩২ সাল। [৮ম বর্ষ।

গুরু হ্যানিম্যানের প্রতি।

মুখে বলি গুরু তুমি, কৃপায় তোমার,
হয়েছে হতেছে যত কল্যাণ আমার ;
করি কিন্তু তুমি যাহা করেছ নিষেধ,
অবহেলি তব বিধি করি নাকো খেদ।

লইয়া তোমার নাম করি প্রতারণা,
সাধনা ব্যতীত সিদ্ধি সদাই বাসনা ;
যাগ ধর্ম্ম, যাগ মোক্ষ, থাক অর্থকাম,
ভাবি, যেন বলে লোকে "নব হ্যানিম্যান"।

এ ভাব এখানে যত হয়েছে প্রবল,
অন্য দেশে নাহি হেন ভক্তি মাখা ছল ;
চাতুরী করিয়া ভাবে, কতই চতুর,
সর্ব্বনাশ করি ভাবে, পেয়েছে প্রচুর।

তবে বলি ভালবাসা, যদি হয় রত,
আদেশ ইঙ্গিত তব পালিতে সতত ;
তবে জানি ভক্তি করি তোমারে নিশ্চয়,
তোমার নিষেধ বিধি যদি মনে রয়।

ব্যাধিতের দুঃখ দূর করিবারে তুমি,
অকপটে বিতরিলে জ্ঞানরত্নমণি
লভিয়া তোমার দান, অহংকার ভরে,
কলঙ্ক তোমার নামে করি কেমন করে !

Fig. 2.2 Poem Titled 'Guru Hahnemann er Proti' ('To Hahnemann, the Spiritual Guru'), in *Hahnemann*, 8, 1 (1925), 1. Credit: Hahnemann Publishing Company Private Limited, Kolkata.

literary exposition of such emotions can be found in the drama 'Shantir Sandhan' ('In Search of Peace') published in the journal *Homoeopathy Paricharak*.[112] It captured a scene where the hero, a homoeopathic physician, literally worshipped the image of Hahnemann with appropriate Hindu rituals. When confronted by his wife, the physician justified his act by describing the spiritually transformative influence on his being as being caused by an exposure to Hahnemann's principles.

Biography, History and a Familiar Science

Such remarkably expedient representation of homoeopathy through the life stories of its practitioners, as well as the life story of its founder, I argue was often facilitated by the practitioners' considerable agency in the biographic market. In her insightful work on artists' biographies in nineteenth-century Britain, Julie Codell demonstrates that through the nineteenth century, Victorian artists increasingly 'came to control their public image . . . became their own agents for the circulation and reproduction of their identities as well as of their works'.[113] She elaborates on the intimate friendships with critics, journalists and art dealers through which artists indirectly ended up shaping their public image. Likewise, relations of 'intimacy' and 'familiarity' were, in fact, crucial determinants in shaping homoeopathy as it appears through life writings.

As I have already noted, at the heart of the homoeopathic discourse in colonial public culture was a range of intergenerational family firms. The biography industry focusing on homoeopathy was fundamentally held together by these commercial firms, as they assumed multiple overlapping roles in relation to the printed lives. The entrepreneur-physicians and their firms were primarily the patrons and publishers of these life stories, but also frequently their authors and almost invariably their subjects. Apart from explicit blood relations, the biographies also repeatedly highlighted near-familial relationships of friendship, alliance and intimacy between the protagonists and eminent physicians related to these firms. Exceptional professional camaraderie between the entrepreneur-physicians was projected as a hallmark of homoeopathic commerce based on the family-firm structure: the mouthpiece journals of these firms recurrently emphasised that 'harmony should be the basic principle upon which true friendship and good business can last and

[112] Ajit Shankar De, 'Shantir Shandhan' (In Search of Peace), *Homoeopathy Pracharak*, 2, 1 (April 1928), 42–5.
[113] Julie Codell, *The Victorian Artist*, pp. 8–9.

flourish'.[114] Further, as Chapter 1 noted, publications by these homoeopathic family firms, especially in the form of biographies, also represented the entrepreneur-physicians, their descendants, students and associates sharing cordial interpersonal relations in an informal network of pedagogy and pupillage. An illustrative example is the relationship of Rajendralal Dutta and Mahendralal Sircar. All the printed lives of both physicians dramatically highlight the way Rajendralal inducted Mahendralal to the principles of homoeopathy, inspiring him to 'convert' from the orthodox state medicine he had studied at the Calcutta Medical College. They also relate that Mahendralal remained grateful to the Rajendralal, acknowledging him as his mentor.[115]

Because fathers and sons, uncles and nephews, teachers and students, mentors and disciples often ended up sharing relations in print as authors, publishers and subjects of homoeopathic biographies, it is important to situate such life writings within the complex processes of their publications. More striking than the rhetoric and reality of 'family' relations, perhaps, is the fact that such relationships of intimacy were invoked variously and recurrently in print. The persistent proclamations of familial, affective relationships between those who propagated homoeopathy had the effect of constructing it as an overwhelmingly family-oriented science. Not meant only for consumption by colonial domesticities, homoeopathy was projected as a science that was even produced within the realm of the colonial family. In this respect, its history resonates with those of other non-state, traditional practices like ayurveda and unani. The historiography has fleetingly hinted at the links between such traditional bodies of knowledge and indigenous, intergenerational practising families.[116] Further, these narrative approaches publicised Bengali homoeopathy as an emotive, informal, personalised and familial domain populated by men committed to a shared mission of popularising a heterodox, European science for the good of the nation.

[114] 'Editorial: New Year's Retrospection and Introspection', *The Hahnemannian Gleanings*, 4, 1 (February 1933), 10–11.

[115] For instance, see Sarat Chandra Ghosh, 'Bharatbarshe Homoeopathic Chikitshar Sorboprothom Pothoprodorshok o Pracharak Dr. Rajendralal Dutta' (The Pioneer Perpetrator of Homoeopathic Treatment in India Dr Rajendralal Dutta), *Hahnemann*, 22, 1 (1939), 14–16.

[116] For a discussion of elite Muslim families like the Azizi family, and their role in the modernisation of traditional unani, see Seema Alavi, *Islam and Healing: Loss and Recovery of an Indo-Muslim Healing Tradition 1600–1900* (Basingstoke: Palgrave Macmillan, 2008), pp. 14–16. On the comparably powerful presence of 'hereditary' practising families like that of Bhai Mohan Singh Vaid or Hakim Ajmal Khan, and their ties with commercial print and pharmaceuticals, see Kavita Sivaramakrishnan, *Old Potions, New Bottles: Recasting Indigenous Medicine in Colonial Punjab (1950–1945)*, 2005, pp. 106–8.

Such tropes of representing the protagonists in an informal, familiar, intimate network had serious ramifications for the proclaimed purpose of the biographies. Beyond the immediate and narrow agenda of chronicling individual lives, the vernacular biographies, almost without exception, shared wider convictions of a loftier purpose for writing history. In these texts, the authors frequently paused to reflect on the importance of biography as an academic genre and included their thoughts on the very acts of writing and recording the lives, as they did. They referred to an entrenched Victorian culture of writing and memorialising lives of eminent personalities. They expressed regret that Indians compared dismally with the English in celebrating and recording prominent lives for posterity. Referring to Rajendralal Dutta's entrepreneurial skills, one biography lamented, 'had he been born among more appreciative people, they would certainly have recognised in him the stuff of which the Howards and the Hampdens are made'.[117]

Biography was contended to be a significant means of recording the past. Indeed, through biographies, most authors claimed to have been engaged in the writing of history. While the relationship between biography and history has been a matter of much unresolved concern for the historians of our times, it is somewhat unusual for late nineteenth- to early twentieth-century writing that many homoeopaths' biographies proclaimed their own function as chronicling the history of their time. They emphasised an integral relation between individual lives and the history of the times they were lived in. Such texts argued that the 'personal element plays so important a part in the history of every moment that no one can afford to ignore it or to treat it with indifference'.[118] To these biographers, narrating a life dedicated to the cause was the most effective way of recounting and recording homoeopathy's history. A monograph on the life of Mahendralal Sircar, for instance, declared at the outset,

> The life of Dr. Sircar was connected in such imperishable links with the *history* of Homoeopathy in India that any attempt to write a *biography* of this great man necessitates a fair exposition of the Rise and Development of Homoeopathy in India and any biography bereft of it will not be found to be interesting and withal it will prove the incompleteness of the book.[119]

Thus, narrating histories of medicine and writing biographies of significant physicians were considered analogous and equivalent processes.

[117] S. C. Ghose, 'Homoeopathy and Its First Missionary in India', *The Hahnemannian Gleanings*, 3, 8 (September 1932), 339.

[118] S. C. Ghose, 'Homoeopathy and Its First Missionary in India', *The Hahnemannian Gleanings*, 3, 7 (August 1932), 294.

[119] Sarat Chandra Ghose, *Life of Dr. Mahendralal Sircar*, 2nd edition (Calcutta: Hahnemann Publishing Company, 1935), p. 27.

A number of journals such as *The Hahnemannian Gleanings* launched serial publications featuring biographic sketches of important personalities to give their readers 'a taste of the history of homoeopathy in India'.[120] It is noteworthy that the late nineteenth- to early twentieth-century biographer-physicians felt compelled to speak in the language of 'history'. The historiography tracing the emergence of a nationalist consciousness has elaborated on the crucial importance attached to the writing of pasts of the nation.[121] They have shown how such writings in Bengal since the mid-nineteenth century were increasingly imbued with post-Enlightenment thinking, which regarded the western rationalist-positivist notion of 'History' as the most desirable mode of knowing the past of a people.[122] In late nineteenth-century Bengal, the strong intertwining of the struggle for a national identity with historical writing resulted in a proliferating culture of public engagement with history.[123] The compulsion of these homoeopathic physicians to identify their biographic endeavours as history is consonant with this early twentieth-century proclivity towards what has been described as an 'enormous public enthusiasm for history'.[124]

In their eagerness to write histories through biography, the authors of homoeopaths' life stories were often drawn into the early twentieth-century concerns over the writing of credible histories. Indeed, what constituted history was a contentious topic in late colonial India. Dipesh Chakrabarty has shown the growing ascendancy of the notion of professional, 'scientific' history in India since the late nineteenth century, informed by an entrenched faith in the Rankean rationalist-positivist understanding of objective, unbiased historical truth.[125] However, others have attempted to demonstrate the limits to such notions of 'scientific' history among sections of the Indian

[120] 'Editorial Notes and News: Reminiscences of Old Torch-bearers of Homoeopathy in India', *The Hahnemannian Gleanings*, 9 (June 1939), 266–7.

[121] Partha Chatterjee, 'Nation and Its Pasts', *The Nation and Its Fragments: Colonial and Postcolonial Histories* (Princeton, NJ: Princeton University Press, 1993), pp. 88–94. Also see Daud Ali (ed.), *Invoking the Past: The Uses of History in South Asia* (Delhi: Oxford University Press, 2002).

[122] Partha Chatterjee, *Nation and Its Fragments*, pp. 88–92. [123] Ibid., pp. 109–15.

[124] Dipesh Chakrabarty, 'Public Life of History: An Argument Out of India', *Public Culture*, 20, 1 (2008), p. 145. Also see Kumkum Chatterjee, 'The King of Controversy: History and Nation Making in Late Colonial India', *American Historical Review*, 110, 5 (2005), 1454–5.

[125] Dipesh Chakrabarty, 'Public Life of History', pp. 145–6; and 'Bourgeois Categories Made Global: Utopian and Actual Lives of Historical Documents in India', *Economic and Political Weekly*, 44, 25 (June 2009), 68. Also see Dipesh Chakrabarty, 'The Birth of Academic Historical Writing in India' in Stuart Macintyre et al. (eds.), *The Oxford History of Historical Writing, Vol 4: 1800–1945* (Oxford: Oxford University Press, 2011), pp. 528–9.

intelligentsia.[126] In her analysis of the early twentieth-century controversies surrounding the status of 'Kulagranthas' (a specific kind of genealogical literature), Kumkum Chatterjee shows that parallel notions of history persisted among various sections of Bengali society. She designates these notions as popular/romantic history, identifying them as valuing emotion, memory or community over any idealised notion of objectivity or rationality promoted by scientific history.[127]

Operating within this intellectual milieu, the physician-biographers too, I argue, came to represent another faction of the Bengali intelligentsia, who registered their differences with the plausibility of the mandate of scientific history. From a pragmatic standpoint, they ended up critiquing the notion of 'objectivity' and privileged the virtue of 'familiarity' and 'intimacy' as more fundamental in writing biographies. Biography as a genre, these authors argued, thrived essentially on intimate, familial, private and informal sources of information.

Engaging with contemporary notions of 'objectivity' and 'rationality', these texts, nonetheless, hinted at their limits when it came to writing credible biographies. Thus, at one level, in a lecture published on Hahnemann's birth anniversary in 1887, Mahendralal Sircar alerted his readers to the importance of writing objective, critical biographies, which did not degenerate into hero worship of their subjects.[128] Mahendralal warned that such exercises made 'men and events acquire a magnitude and an importance which they do not intrinsically possess'.[129] Before narrating a biography of Hahnemann himself, he reflected upon the importance of a critical biography to 'judge of him (Hahnemann) as a man, and of his place in the history of science and medicine'.[130] Such analytic distance was often measured in terms of temporality. Thus, in his introduction to the *Life of Dr. Mahendralal Sircar*, the author gave vent to his anxiety over the timing of his act of writing. He was aware that,

> He [Mahendralal] lived so long and lived so manfully and nobly and was so warmly cherished in the affection of numerous readers that it still seems *too soon* to venture on a critical estimate of his labours and works in the world.[131]

Yet, the authors were equally concerned with the other crucial requirement of scientific history, viz., collection of verifiable facts. To them, access to reliable sources and information was far more fundamental to

[126] See Partha Chatterjee and Raziuddin Aquil (eds.), *History in the Vernacular* (Delhi: Permanent Black, 2008), pp. 1–22.
[127] See Kumkum Chatterjee, 'The King of Controversy', pp. 1464–75.
[128] Mahendralal Sircar, 'Hahnemann and His Work', pp. 391–416. [129] Ibid.
[130] Ibid.
[131] S. C. Ghose, Preface, *Life of Dr. Mahendralal Sircar*, 1st edition (Calcutta: Oriental Publishing Company, 1909), p. i.

the writing of biographies. They pointed out that accessing sources and verifiable facts were necessarily related to the familiarity and intimacy one shared with one's biographic subject. They unequivocally confessed that the virtues of 'intimacy', 'affective attachment' and 'familiarity' with sources had been, for them, indispensable in writing biographies. Accordingly, the biographies routinely highlighted the closeness and intimacy between their authors and the subjects.

Indeed, these texts show the reliability and verifiability of the information they furnish as being inherently predicated on such intimacies. The truth claim of biographies was presented as resting on the perceived intimacies between the author and the subject. Most biographies identified the author by their relationship to the subject, ranging from sons, brothers-in-law and sons-in-law, to close family friends or professional associates. The biographer of Mahesh Bhattacharya informed the readers, on the very first page, of his fifty years of association with the family, just as biographer Jitendranath Majumdar made no effort to conceal his deepest reverence for his father and subject, physician Pratap Majumdar.[132] The personal, affective elements of the author–subject relation were played up to the extent that the biographer of Batakrishna Pal, his friend and fellow homoeopath, expressed his sense of loss and helplessness at Batakrishna's death.[133] In instances where familial and other intimate friendships were not asserted, the texts still exuded a sense of an exceptional professional camaraderie. Sarat Chandra Ghosh, himself a homoeopathic practitioner, editor of the widely circulating *The Hahnemannian Gleanings* and author of many serialised biographies in journals, expressed his excellent relationship with all his subjects. In his biographies he quoted personal conversations and letters, described private meetings and the like. His biography of Mahendralal Sircar in the journal *Hahnemann*, for instance, included an entire section elaborating the 'extremely amicable relation' between them.[134] Such shared closeness with the subject rendered his portrayal of Mahendralal's life as 'most reliable', compared to other biographies of the physician.[135] At the same time, the biographer of Mahesh Bhattacharya revealed his anxiety in being too intimate 'with not only Bhattacharya, but his entire

[132] Srish Chandra Talapatra, *Maheshchandra Charitkatha* (*Life of Mahesh Chandra*), 1946, p. 3. Also see J. N. Majumdar, 'Dr. Pratap Chandra Majumdar MD', *Hahnemann*, 23, 5 (1940), 261–7.

[133] Gopal Chandra Mukhopadhyay, *Sadhu Batakrishna Pal* (*The Saintly Batakrishna Pal*), Vol II, 1919, pp. 191, 292.

[134] Saratchandra Ghosh, 'Daktar Mahendralal Sircar er Jibon-katha' ('Life of Dr. Mahendralal Sircar'), *Hahnemann*, 22, 3 (1939), 137–41.

[135] Saratchandra Ghosh, 'Daktar Mahendralal Sircar er Jibon-katha' ('Life of Dr. Mahendralal Sircar'), *Hahnemann*, 22, 2 (1939), 67–71.

family'.[136] In a self-critical mode, he mused on the possible hindrances to objective analysis engendered by such long-term familiarity.[137]

Thus, in establishing the relation between biography and history, the physician-biographers spoke also on the methodological dilemma between cultivating historical objectivity, and the procurement of sources through personal relations. Biography was projected as a kind of history which essentially privileged the virtues of 'intimacy' over any idealised notions of objectivity. In their pragmatic rejection of objectivity, the homoeopathic biographies constitute an important counterpoint to the emerging academic project of writing 'scientific' history. Their quandary between objectivity and intimacy hinted towards the larger issues of politics of archiving and the problem of sourcing related to the craft of writing history. In his recent work, Dipesh Chakrabarty reveals the problematic nature of public archives in early twentieth-century India, showing how 'facts' or 'sources' were often caught up within various kinds of 'privileged communities'.[138] Access to such networks or communities was often determined through private relations of friendship and enmity. With specific examples from Bengal and Maharashtra, he demonstrates how the process of accessing 'original' historical sources for public consumption was often fraught with hidden stories of enmity, rivalry, friendship, inheritance and alliance.[139]

More general scholarship on knowledge formation in the nineteenth century also argues for the centrality of networks of friendship, alliance and intimacy as crucial, latent determinants of knowledge and history.[140] Uncovering the processes by which homoeopathy was consolidated through public assertions of intimacy contributes to this scholarship. Further, in privileging 'intimacy' and 'familiarity' over objectivity, the homoeopaths, as practitioners of a family-oriented, informal, intimate science, claimed a special status for themselves, as indeed for other sectarian groups caught up in family, caste, kinship or sacred networks, as producers of authoritative biographies.

[136] Srish Chandra Talapatra, *Maheshchandra Charitkatha* (*Life of Mahesh Chandra*), pp. 3–4.

[137] Ibid. [138] Dipesh Chakrabarty, 'Bourgeois Categories Made Global', pp. 67–8.

[139] Ibid., pp. 71–4.

[140] William Lubenow, 'Intimacy, Imagination, and the Inner Dialectics of Knowledge Communities: The Synthetic Society, 1896–1908' in Martin Daunton (ed.), *The Organisation of Knowledge in Victorian Britain* (Oxford: Oxford University Press, 2005), pp. 357–70.

Conclusion

While exploring the writing and publication of an extensive repertoire of biographies around physicians practising homoeopathy in Bengal, I have refrained from attempting a biographical exploration of any individual life. Instead, I have analysed the relevance of the *genre* of biography with relation to the colonial trajectories of homoeopathy. Even as the historiography studying the 'new geographies of nineteenth-century science and medicine' is expanding to explore various facets of the profusion of print culture around science, popular medico-scientific biographies have barely been explored as a site, especially in South Asia.[141] Exploration of the myriad kinds of colonial medical lives reiterate biography's contribution to a significant democratisation of science and medicine. Posing as contextual, even complementary text to actual works of science or medicine, these biographies upheld a certain egalitarian promise of a 'republic of science' reaching out even to the functionally literate.

The larger point that this chapter has driven home is the relationship between the life stories and practices marginalised by the state or scientific authorities. In the absence of any substantial state records in British India, the chapter identifies the systematic publication of biographies as a significant arena of assertion for a heterodox, family-based practice like homoeopathy. By recurrently recounting the life of the founding figure Hahnemann (also the author of the central text of homoeopathy the *Organon*), the lives of physicians dedicated to homoeopathy, the significance of their activities, and the socioreligious sensibilities that informed such activity, these life stories elevate homoeopathy to a creed professed by a distinct collective of men inspired by a vision of ethical living. In so doing, they offer a glimpse into the complex relationship between texts, society and the practices actively censured by the state, which are often caught up within family, caste, kinship or sacred networks. Following Arjun Appadurai, this chapter has noted that the very survival and availability of these texts, mostly in their now-obscure-yet-still-continuing entrepreneurial concerns, signify the power of such alternative archives as the 'material site of a collective will to remember'.[142]

Such traces of the resilience of unorthodox, marginalised practices also caution us to resist the temptation to draw any conclusions that lead to

[141] In a recent anthology on new sites to study science, Bernard Lightman urges a more serious engagement with science biographies. See Bernard Lightman and Aileen Fyfe (eds.), *Science in the Marketplace: Nineteenth Century Sites and Experiences*, 2007, p. 14.

[142] Arjun Appadurai, 'Archive and Aspiration' in Joke Brouwer and Arjen Mulder (eds.), *Information is Alive* (Rotterdam: V2_Publishing/NAI Publishers, 2003), pp. 16–17.

a straightforward narrative of victimhood around these practices. Their imbrication in the 'domains of politics and profiteering' can be assessed from role of the homoeopathic family firms with relation to the biographies. In contending that biographies are as much the story of the biographers and publishers as of their subjects, I have traced the intertwined trajectories of commerce, print capital, nationalist ideology and medical knowledge with relation to a western heterodox sect in Bengal.

The case of homoeopathy's popularisation through the biographic market underlines the importance of local factors and interest groups, as well as the contingencies of the vernacular print market in rendering medicine national. It contends that the acculturation of European medicine and print capitalism necessarily drew upon and reinforced networks of familiarities, including those of religions, class, kinship and family. Hence, while here I have discussed the role of biographies in rendering Hahnemann as a Hindu icon, the following chapter looks into the self-proclaimed efforts at 'translating' western homoeopathy for an Indian audience.

The importance of local factors and interest groups becomes manifest even in the particular favouring of biography over other kinds of print platform. The biographer-physicians reflected on the status of biography vis-à-vis history. Though they were active participants in the 'enormous public enthusiasm for history', nonetheless, these physician-biographers also posed a critique to the emerging western notion of 'scientific' history. Asserting biography-writing and history-writing as analogous processes, these authors, nonetheless, insisted on the importance of 'familiarity' as a virtue in narrating authentic biographies. As practitioners of a science heavily invested in familial ethos and networks, the homoeopaths claimed for themselves, and indeed other sectarian groups, a special status as producers of authoritative biographies.

3 A Science in Translation

Medicine, Language, Identity

'Our vernacular friends do not know the principles of Homoeopathic law of cure and many other things collateral to science like the above one. They therefore are very anxious to know them and requested us to translate our great master's *Organon of the Art of Healing* into our own vernacular.'[1]

'Homoeopathic science is their science, to be able to use it in India, we need to adapt it to our situation and make it our own.'[2]

In the third volume of the popular homoeopathic journal *Hahnemann*, physician Sripati Chandra Boral wrote a long letter to the editors titled 'Protibaad' or 'Protest', in response to an article previously published in the journal.[3] The article had used the phrase '*paap byadhi*' in place of the unique Hahnemannian term 'psora', understood to be a underlying disease causing a certain bodily condition.[4] Sripati Chandra Boral expressed himself as being very disappointed with the use of '*paap byadhi*', which literally means 'sin disease', as the 'vernacular synonym' for 'psora'. His letter led to a protracted correspondence on the topic, involving different physicians as well as the editors of the journal, which spanned several volumes of *Hahnemann*. In an article titled 'Homoeopathic Philosophy' for instance, author S. C. Thakur, in reference to Boral's letter,

[1] Nilambar Hui, 'Our Letter to the Publisher' in *Sadrisa Bigyan Sutra* (*Principles for the Science of Similars*) (Calcutta: Sanyal and Company, 1896), page number not cited.

[2] K. Chatterjee, 'Bharate Kromo Somosya' ('The Problem of Potency in India'), *Hahnemann*, 8, 5 (1925), 406.

[3] Sripati Chandra Boral, 'Protibaad' ('Protest'), *Hahnemann*, 3, 4 (1920), 169–73.

[4] 'Psora', like 'vital force', was a unique concept enunciated by Hahnemann, which recurs in most discussions of homoeopathic principles. Simply put, according to Hahnemann diseases were of two kinds, *acute* and *chronic*. Chronic diseases were considered more deep-seated and difficult to cure. According to homoeopathic discussions, 'psora' was the most fundamental of the three miasmas causing chronic diseases in humans. The theory of miasma originates in Hahnemann's book *The Chronic Diseases*, which was published in 1828. Here he declared that this theory was the result of twelve years of the most painstaking work on difficult cases of a chronic character, combined with his own historical research into the diseases of man.

proposed '*adi* disease' meaning 'fundamental malady' as the synonym for 'psora'.[5] These discussions on the correct vernacular rendering of this particular scientific term opened up several significant issues. Medical biographies, as we read in Chapter 2, contributed towards a construction of the image of homoeopathy as a western doctrine infused with indigenous values. Simultaneously, however, there were more specific and concerted efforts at 'translating' European homoeopathy 'into our own vernaculars'. Authors like Sripati Chandra Boral were convinced of the urgency of translation as a means to disseminate useful knowledge from the West. Boral held that 'it is for the purpose of national development that one needs to enrich one's mother tongue with several [scientific] jargons. It is the best way to educate our people'.[6] He highlighted the role of journals like *Hahnemann* in explaining western sciences in Bengali.[7]

The authors participating in such debates over translation were, evidently, concerned with the modalities, constraints and implications of such translations, as they engaged in extensive discussions of the best way to interpret 'scientific terms'. Some argued against innovating new words in Bengali, saying 'it is unwise to create a new word in any language without investing deep thoughts on the subject'.[8] Others, like Boral, contended for direct incorporation of English and German words into the Bengali language. They reasoned that, 'if there is a term whose idea is not prevalent in our country, and it is difficult to get a Bengali synonym, we should incorporate that foreign word as it is. As examples, we can refer to English words like chair, bench, hospital and so on which have been incorporated as such into Bengali'.[9] Further, discussions on the translation of 'psora' involved contentions over the 'correct reading' of original texts like Hahnemann's *Organon*. In a letter to the Bengali journal *Hahnemann*, author Manomohan Dey, for instance, registered his disagreement with other practitioners like Nilmani Ghatak.[10] Emphasising his own reading of *Organon*, Manomohan Dey argued that the phrase 'spiritual sickness' was most appropriate to describe the term 'psora'.[11] In response, Sripati Chandra Boral pointed out that the Bengali synonyms of 'psora' that were being proposed were hardly literal translations and were, in fact, based on certain 'religio-cultural interpretations' of homoeopathic tenets. Dismissive of such culturally informed interpretations, he argued that they pitched discussions around body and health at a level that was analogous to discussions in the 'philosophical texts of our country'.[12] In reply to Boral's letter, the editors of *Hahnemann* strongly

[5] S. C. Thakur, 'Homoeopathic Philosophy', *Hahnemann*, 3, 8 (1919), 284–9.
[6] Sripati Chandra Boral, 'Protibaad' ('Protest'), p. 169. [7] Ibid. [8] Ibid. [9] Ibid.
[10] Manomohan Dey, 'Patra' ('Letter'), *Hahnemann*, 8, 11 (1925), 601–4.
[11] Ibid., p. 604. [12] Sripati Chandra Boral, 'Protibaad' ('Protest'), p. 169.

defended translations relying on cultural interpretations.[13] To them, such interpretations were in fact the hallmark of a work of good translation.

This discussion reveals translation as a complex process involved in the negotiation of meaning not only across languages, but also across cultures. Indeed, as recent work contends, the process of translation should be viewed as a study of both the linguistic as well as the sociocultural strategies by which concepts, terms and even theoretical constructs are made legible across cultural borders and rendered stable over time.[14] These works point towards the creative tension involved in the idea of 'translatability' in negotiation of meaning across languages and locales. Thus, the discussions around the translation of the homoeopathic concept of 'psora' seem representative in opening up two burning issues related to scientific translations. The first was whether translation ought to be literal or culturally nuanced in nature; and the second, whether or not foreign words ought to be engrafted onto vernacular languages. Similar deliberations on language and culture will be encountered here, as authors translated a range of other therapeutic concepts such as 'homoeopathy' itself as '*amiya-patha*', and 'vital force' as '*jiboni shakti*'. Contending that homoeopathy was a science for the attainment of longevity, authors of such translations pointed out that since '*amiya*', i.e. '*amrita*'[15] or the elixir of life leads to immortality, tracts on homoeopathic principles were justifiably titled 'Amiya-Patha', i.e. the path leading to the attainment of immortality or '*amrita*'.[16] These texts supported '*amiya-patha*' as the Sanskrit rendering of homoeopathy.[17]

Though the homoeopathic physicians were significant participants in the translation of European knowledge, they were hardly the only group engaged in acts of translation. On the contrary, there is a rich literature that has characterised translation as a 'central act of European

[13] Editors, 'Mantabya' ('Comment'), *Hahnemann*, 3, 4 (1920), 173–7.

[14] See Marwa Elshakry, 'Knowledge in Motion: The Cultural Politics of Modern Science Translation in Arabic', *Isis*, 99, 4 (2008), 701–30. Also see Lydia Liu, *Translingual Practice: Literature, National Culture and Translated Modernity: China 1900–1937* (Palo Alto: Stanford University Press, 1995); and, edited by the same author, *Tokens of Exchange: The Problem of Translation in Global Circulations* (Durham: Duke University Press, 2000).

[15] *Amrita* literally means deathless. It is a magic potion that gives eternal life. It also means elixir of life. In Indian mythology, *visha* (poison) and *amrita* emerged during the churning of the sea. Shiva drank the poison and stored it in his Adam's apple.

[16] Chandra Shekhar Kali, *Brihat Olautha Samhita (Enlarged Compendium for Treatment of Cholera)*, 13th edition (Calcutta: C. Kylye and Company, 1926), pp. 1–2.

[17] Ibid., p. 1.

imperialism'.[18] These scholars have studied the keen interest early orientalists took in translating Indian works into English, as well as early nineteenth-century administrative efforts in translating western knowledge into Indian vernaculars.[19] The adoption of translation as a 'pedagogical strategy' by the East India Company has been explored in a recent spate of research. While Michael Dodson's work on the Benares College and the Delhi College delved into the vernacular translations of European science as well as Christianity by colonial educationists,[20] Ishita Pande has looked specifically into the discussions on the dissemination of western medico-scientific ideas through the Translation Committee and Native Medical Institution, under the superintendence of John Tytler in Calcutta in the 1820s and 1830s.[21] Together, these works chart the ways in which the colonial translation discourses equated language with civilisation, creating myriad hierarchies of languages between the East and the West, to constitute colonial India as the somewhat deficient 'other' of the progressive West. Some considered the Indian languages unfit vehicles for the transmission of rational science and religion, while others like James Ballantyne at Benares College committed themselves to the linguistic enhancement of Indian languages through diverse translation techniques.

What still remains to be explored, however, is how these issues played out in the domain of the popular print market around science. Indeed, the project of importing modern science in the colonies through a process of translation has too often been seen to work in collusion with the state. Hence, it has been suggested that in colonial India 'science was not encumbered with the task of constructing hegemony', as the state remained more of an 'externality' to the social fabric.[22] Yet, as an instance of a western science that the colonial state did not actively perpetrate, the popular practices of translation around homoeopathy provide a distinct

[18] Michael Dodson makes the point drawing upon Eric Cheyfitz's *Poetics of Imperialism: Translation and Colonisation from the Tempest to the Tarzan*. See Michael Dodson, *Orientalism, Empire, National Culture, India 1770–1880* (Basingstoke: Palgrave Macmillan, 2007), p. 118.

[19] See Tejaswini Niranjana, *Siting Translation: History, Post-Structuralism and the Colonial Context* (Berkeley: University of California Press, 1992); Kate Teltscher, *India Inscribed: European and British Writing on India* (Delhi: Oxford University Press, 1995); Bernard Cohn, 'Command of Language and Language of Command' in *Colonialism and Its Forms of Knowledge: The British in India* (Princeton, NJ: Princeton University Press, 1997), pp. 16–56.

[20] Michael Dodson, *Orientalism, Empire, National Culture, India 1770–1880*, 2007.

[21] Ishita Pande, *Medicine, Race and Liberalism in British Bengal: Symptoms of Empire* (New York: Routledge, 2010), pp. 119–38.

[22] Drawing upon Ranajit Guha's idea of 'dominance without hegemony', Gyan Prakash makes this point. See Gyan Prakash, *Another Reason: Science and the Imagination of Modern India* (Princeton, NJ: Princeton University Press, 1999), pp. 9–10.

narrative of science's popular reception. I trace the efforts of the Calcutta-based family firms to translate homoeopathy for a vernacular audience, that at once reified the power of western science and language (chiefly English), while offering the promise of a possible democratisation and even cultural reinterpretation of knowledge.

Existing scholarship on popular science translation has mostly dwelt upon the thoughts of prominent Indian intellectuals, like Rajendralal Mitra in relation to western science and Girindrashekhar Basu in relation to western psychiatry, who insisted that 'Indian interests must govern the translation of western science'.[23] In his well-known monograph, Rajendralal Mitra proposed a scheme whereby commonly used Bengali terms could be retained, depending on specific criteria in different instances. In other cases, new terms could be formed using root words from Sanskrit. For the rest, European terms had to be adopted. Both Gyan Prakash and Partha Chatterjee read Mitra as urging his readers to locate translation as a means by which to become aware of the unequal power relations pertaining to language (and knowledge), as well as to challenge the claim of English as the universal lingua franca for science.[24]

In tracing how these extant official and proto-nationalist discourses on translation were mapped onto a popular culture around homoeopathy, I explore what constituted authentic, effective or useful linguistic translation in the Bengali print culture. The chapter is attentive to discussions on perceived power imbalances and hierarchies between languages. Beyond the realm of language, the homoeopaths' conviction and their sustained translation efforts resisted the official scepticism about the incommensurability of European and Indian knowledge systems. Reflecting upon the troubled acknowledgement of 'modern science's image as free enquiry and its operation as an instrument of colonial domination', Gyan Prakash has theorised a sense of 'alienation' suffered by the colonised in negotiating modern science. Yet, the sheer enthusiasm around homoeopathic translation promoted a profound sense of 'equivalence' rather than alienation. Bolstered with the sense of equivalence, the Bengali authors of homoeopathy went a step further to advocate culturally sensitive, locally embedded translation practices. Echoing the guidelines set by men like Rajendralal Mitra, they denigrated the practices of 'servile, verbatim translation like a Chinese copy,

[23] Amit Ranjan Basu, 'Emergence of a Marginal Science in a Colonial City: Reading Psychiatry in Bengali Periodicals', *Indian Economic and Social History Review*, 41, 2 (2004), 115–17.

[24] Partha Chatterjee, 'The Disciplines of Colonial Bengal' in Partha Chatterjee (ed.), *Texts of Power: Emerging Disciplines in Colonial Bengal* (Minneapolis: University of Minnesota Press, 1995), p. 22. Gyan Prakash, *Another Reason*, pp. 50–1.

with patch and all'.[25] Hence, the homoeopathic scheme of translation produced a vernacular science where homoeopathy could be understood as *amiya-patha*, where the theory of 'vital force' was explained in reference to Indian philosophy and practices of caste system and Hahnemann became analogous to the Hindu deity Siva and Hanumana. While championing a deliberate decision to indigenise the content, the translators were nonetheless conscious of displacements of form. In particular, the format of vernacular discussions of science, as well as displacements beyond the urban enclave of Calcutta, emerged as points of significant deliberation. Taken together, translation with its various facets constructed homoeopathy as a modern western science in harmony with Indian philosophical thoughts. It further helped define homoeopathy's 'other' in the Bengali print culture: the practitioners of state medicine or 'allopathy' on the one hand, and the 'spurious' practitioners of homoeopathy in the *mofussil* on the other.

Translation and Language

The entrepreneur-physicians and their homoeopathic commercial enterprises discussed in the earlier chapters upheld homoeopathy's western origin. Through their myriad publications in the form of advertisements, journals, manuals, medical monographs, as well as biographies and memoirs, these figures projected themselves as entangled with the West through ceaseless transactions of ideas, drugs, people and pharmaceutical expertise. This needs to be contextualised within the general sense of awe-infused enthusiasm for 'science' as a symbol of modernity and progress. In all such transactions, there was a strong sense of excitement in engaging with the very latest in 'modern science'. For instance, in a report of the International Homoeopathic Congress in his journal *Indian Homoeopathic Review*, Jitendranath Majumdar proudly depicted his role in representing India in 'the most representative Congress meeting that was ever held' at London.[26] He noted how he applied himself to learning from these gatherings, with a view to improving homoeopathy in Bengal.[27] The leading homoeopathic journals routinely published articles that gave accounts of the progress of homoeopathy in the Anglophone world. The article 'World Progress in Homoeopathy' in the journal *The Hahnemannian Gleanings*, closely noted the steps that were being

[25] Rajendralal Mitra, *A Scheme for the Rendering of European Scientific Terms in India* (Calcutta: Thacker, Spink and Company, 1877), p. 18.
[26] Jitendranath Majumdar, 'The International Homoeopathy Congress', *The Indian Homoeopathic Review*, 20, 9 (September 1911), 257–63.
[27] Ibid.

taken in the American homoeopathic colleges and schools of Chicago, Illinois, Boston, Massachusetts and elsewhere to popularise the doctrine.[28] Emphasising a rising global popularity of homoeopathic science, it asserted that 'biological works and scientific investigations in various countries from various sources have confirmed the truth enunciated by Hahnemann'.[29]

The flow of knowledge was not always represented as unidirectional from the West to India. Mahendralal Sircar's report, for instance, detailed the impact of his own paper on 'Homoeopathy in the Treatment of Malarious Fevers', which was eventually published in the *Transactions of the British Homoeopathic Congress* in London.[30] Exchange with the West was highlighted in various ways. A 1934 editorial in the journal *The Hahnemannian Gleanings* jubilantly noted the appointment of a foreign contributing editor based in New York, who was attached to the New York Homoeopathic Medical College and Flower Hospital.[31] The editorial looked ahead to the future exchange of ideas with the New York-based Dr Stearns, who was interested in 'obtaining from India as great a number of snakes as possible and snake venoms' for his own research.[32]

Bengali writers primarily emphasised the importance of reading key western texts to the development of homoeopathic knowledge. Hahnemann's *Organon of the Healing Art*, often referred to simply as *Organon* (1810), his *Materia Medica Pura* (six volumes between 1811 and 1827) and *Chronic Disease* (1828) were the main homoeopathic texts under discussion, although texts by authoritative European homoeopaths were of equal importance. Writing in the journal *Hahnemann* published by the Hahnemann Publishing Company, author Gyanendra Mohan Pan proclaimed that 'to acquire proper knowledge on various facets of homoeopathy one needed to read the texts by the homoeopathic giants like Hahnemann, Herring, Kent, Farrington and others'.[33] Reading western texts was publicised as far preferable to attending schools or colleges as far as learning homoeopathy was concerned.

28 George Royal, 'World Progress in Homoeopathy', *The Hahnemannian Gleanings*, 3, 6 (June 1932), 213–18. Also see Julia Minnewa Green, 'Homoeopathy in the United States', *The Hahnemannian Gleanings*, 7, 10 (November 1936), 437–43.

29 'Editorial: New Year's Retrospection and Introspection', *The Hahnemannian Gleanings*, 4, 1 (1933), 3.

30 Mahendralal Sircar, 'British Homoeopathic Congress of 1874, *Calcutta Journal of Medicine*, 7 (June–July 1874), p. 241.

31 'Editorial Notes and Comments', *The Hahnemannian Gleanings*, 5 (March 1934), 91–2.

32 Ibid., p. 92.

33 Gyanendra Mohan Pan, 'Edesh e Homoeopathy Chikitshar Unnotir Ontoray Ki?' ('What are the Hindrances to the Development of Homoeopathy in India'), *Hahnemann*, 21, 10 (1938), 585.

In the preface to his book *Olautha Samhita*, published by C. Kylye and Company, author Chandra Shekhar Kali enumerated in detail the advantages of reading texts for oneself.[34] As the principal of the Calcutta Homoeopathic College run by the abovementioned company, he emphasised that 'it is a matter of less significance to graduate or fail or to be part of any big college. The more important thing is to be able to cure a patient as efficiently as possible. For that, you have to read the texts closely for yourself, judge symptoms and apply drugs'.[35]

At the same time, it was equally acknowledged that such texts were beyond the reach of most Bengali readers, as they were in European languages. Despite recognising the doctrine's German roots, a range of homoeopathic texts pledged to help 'the Bengali readers unfamiliar with English language'.[36] These texts promised, in their introductions or in a separate translator's note, to render homoeopathy 'into Bengali for the benefit of our friends who do not know English and for its further spread'.[37] Letters to the editors of leading journals, requesting translations of important texts, revealed twin concerns over the price of the original texts, as well as their being in English.

Writing in 1938, *mofussil*-based physician Dharmadas Das requested the editor of the Bengali journal *Hahnemann* to translate a specific section of the sixth edition of Hahnemann's *Organon*.[38] His letter noted that he had failed to locate a Bengali version of that particular edition in any reputed Calcutta-based homoeopathic store. He urged the editor that his response would be 'immensely helpful to the English-ignorant homoeopathic physicians as him', further reminding them that 'many are unable to read English or procure English texts for want of money'.[39] Indeed, along with language, the relatively high cost of books was put forward as another significant impetus for the translation of European texts. In a separate 'Translator's note' attached to the first edition of his translation of Hahnemann's *Nature of Chronic Diseases*, author Yaminikanta Gangopadhyay argued,

> The price of the original text is too steep. It is not possible for the general reader to purchase and read it. Therefore, I am translating the original tenets from the English text in simple language, which can be easily followed by everyone.

[34] Chandra Shekhar Kali, 'Preface', *Brihat Olautha Samhita* (*Enlarged Compendium for Treatment of Cholera*), 1926, pp. 1–5.
[35] Ibid., p. 4–5.
[36] Nilambar Hui, 'Translator's Notes', *Sadrisa Bigyan Sutra* (*Principles for the Science of Similars*), 1896, page number not cited.
[37] Ibid. [38] Dharmadas Das, 'Jigashya' ('Question'), *Hahnemann*, 21, 10 (1938), 545.
[39] Ibid., p. 545.

It would be possible for every potential reader to perceive the crux of the book and know enough of chronic diseases to help others.[40]

Moreover, translation into Bengali was considered especially necessary for the production of a standardised Bengali homoeopathic pharmacopoeia. Such translations were considered essential for the preparations of drugs, and hence, in fundamental ways were relevant to the pharmacies and their consumers. Thus, the preface to the first edition of the pharmacopoeia *Bheshaja Bidhan (Pharmaceutical Prescription)*, published by Mahesh Chandra Bhattacharya's M. Bhattacharya and Company in 1892 stated,

The whole supply of medicine for our firm having been obtained from Germany and America, it has occurred to us that in the absence of a reliable Bengali treatise on the manipulation of such drugs, it would be quite impossible for our customers unacquainted with English to prepare their own dilutions.[41]

Although the need for translation was widely perceived, there was hardly any unanimity with regard to the ways of executing it. Accessing Hahnemann's original works was a matter of significance, and most authors insisted on translating the key original texts of Hahnemann himself, including the *Organon, Chronic Diseases* and *Materia Medica Pura*. While beginning his serial translation of *Organon* for the journal *Hahnemann*, author R R Ghosh argued, 'Hahnemann had incorporated all that was to know of homoeopathy in his *Organon*'.[42] Sharing a similar conviction, translator/author Nilambar Hui in his book *Sadrisa Bigyan Sutra* (*Principles for the Science of Similars*) promised to provide a comprehensive translation of *Organon*'s 292 principles along with their scientific explanations, which was meant to 'dispel any darkness in the reader's mind'.[43] As already noted, along with Hahnemann, works by other European homoeopaths of repute were also held in high esteem.

It is important to note, however, that the zeal for popularisation reigned over any essential obsession with a translation's fidelity to the original texts. A number of authors emphasised the futility of translating any particular key text in its entirety. Instead, most texts advertised themselves as compilations and translations of bits and

[40] Yaminikanta Gangopadhyay, 'Translator's Notes', *Hahnemann's Nature of Chronic Diseases* (Dacca: Baikunthanath Press, 1933), page number not cited.
[41] Mahesh Chandra Bhattacharya, 'Preface to the First Edition', *Bheshaja Bidhan (Pharmaceutical Prescription)*, 5th edition (Calcutta: M. Bhattacharya and Company, 1920), page number not cited.
[42] R. R. Ghosh, 'Organon ba Homoeopathy Bigyan' ('Organon or the Science of homoeopathy'), *Hahnemann*, 1, 1 (1918), 11.
[43] Nilambar Hui, 'Translator's Preface', *Sadrisa Bigyan Sutra* (*Principles for the Science of Similars'*), 1896, page number not cited.

pieces of various English texts for the benefit of the readers and students of homoeopathy. Indeed the impulse to popularise, rather than to produce a faithful replica of the original, becomes clearer when one focuses on texts such as the *Diseases of Children and their Homoeopathic Treatment* that explained at the outset which portions had been retained and rejected from the original text.[44] The author justified such acts of selective translation, stating, 'translating the whole text is a time consuming and expensive exercise that is not necessarily more helpful for the readers'. The approach to translation in such texts often decentred Hahnemann as the sole repository of homoeopathic principles, focusing more on reputed western physicians' interpretation of him. Writing in 1921, Mahendranath Bhattacharya in the introduction to the first edition of his *Contributions Towards a Knowledge of the Peculiarities of all Homeopathic Medicines*, advertised the book as a 'Bengali translation of high quality and well-known works on homoeopathic relationship, aggravation, amelioration etc. by reputed American professors Dr. Herring, Gaurency, Kent and Dr. C. Von Bonncinghausen'.[45] Bhattacharya argued that the book, being a translation of the works of reputed scholars, required no further certificate of its merit.[46] The preface to the 1892 edition of *Bheshaja Bidhan* by Mahesh Chandra Bhattacharya similarly mentioned a whole list of 'books consulted in the compilation of this manual ... great pains have been taken to systematise the matter compiled for the work'.[47] Most such translated works even had bilingual titles in Bengali and English. Thus, *Bheshaja Bidhan* was simultaneously titled as *The Pharmaceutists Manual: A Companion to the German and American Homoeopathic Pharmacopoeias*. Many authors recommended reading translations of key texts like *Organon* along with other specialised compilations. Such compilations were often made reader-friendly by incorporating specific instructions for reading the various authors together. Mahendranath Bhattacharya included a short note explaining the meaning of various signs that had been deployed by him to distinguish and communicate the various parts that were

[44] Bipin Bihari Maitra, *Diseases of Children and Its Homoeopathic Treatment* (Calcutta: Maitra and Company, 1887), p. 1.

[45] M. N. Bhattacharjee, 'Advertisement to the First Edition', *Contributions Towards a Knowledge of the Peculiarities of all Homoeopathic Medicines* (Hooghli: Mahendranath Bhattacharya, 1921), p. 1.

[46] Ibid., p. 2.

[47] Mahesh Chandra Bhattacharya, 'Preface', *Bheshaja Bidhan (Pharmaceutical Prescription)*, 1st edition (Calcutta: M. Bhattacharya and Company, 1892), page number not cited.

translations of different western authors.[48] In *Bheshaja Bidhan* Mahesh Chandra Bhattacharya noted,

The preparations of drugs according to the German homeopathic pharmacopoeia and American homoeopathic pharmacopoeia are expressly marked by the words 'American' and 'German' in the manual. Where neither of these words occurs, the preparation is to be understood to be made according to the German homoeopathic pharmacopoeia.[49]

Often the authors published their translated works serially over a period. Such serial and systematic translations of original English texts were considered ideally suited for pedagogic purposes. Most leading journals included serial translations of one or more homoeopathic texts.[50] Translated works were also compiled in the form of series of books. In the preface to his book *Homoeopathic Chikitsha Bigyan* (*Homoeopathic Medical Science*), Biharilal Bhaduri noted that he would 'draw upon various English texts and compile them in his monograph, but would not do it all at a time'.[51] He stated that for the convenience of both the readers and the author, he would publish the book in various volumes, adding that one volume would be published systematically every two months.[52] The *Datta's Homoeopathic Series* published by B. Datta and Company included several contemporary newspaper reviews praising their effort at serialised translations. It quoted *Sulabh Samachar* of 9th Chaitra 1282 (1875), praising the series for its immense benefit to Bengali readers by 'translating all available homoeopathic texts each month volume by volume into pure Bengali language'.[53] By way of explicating how, gradually and systematically, more and more of the homoeopathic *materia medica* was being translated every month, this review added that the 'first issue has already covered discussions on Arnica and Ipecac and some parts of Aconite'.[54]

[48] M. N. Bhattacharjee, *Contributions towards a Knowledge of the Peculiarities of all Homoeopathic Medicines*, 1921, pp. 2–3.

[49] Mahesh Chandra Bhattacharya, *Bheshaja Bidhan (Pharmaceutical Prescription)*, 1st edition (Calcutta: M. Bhattacharya and Company, 1892), p. xi.

[50] All leading journals published a number of serial translations of 'original' texts. Some of the longest running serial translations of homoeopathic principles were: 'Organon ba Homoeopathy Bigyan' ('Organon or the Science of Homoeopathy') in *Hahnemann*, 'Etiology in Homoeopathy' in *The Hahnemannian Gleanings*, 'Shantir Sandhan' ('In Search of Peace'), in *Homoeopathy Paricharak*.

[51] Biharilal Bhaduri, 'Preface', *Homoeopathic Chikitsha Bigyan* (*Homoeopathic Medical Science*) (Calcutta: Saraswat Jantra, 1874–77), page number not cited.

[52] Ibid.

[53] Basanta Kumar Datta (ed.), 'Review of Datta's Homoeopathic Series' in *Datta's Homoeopathic Series in Bengalee*, 3, 3 (March 1876), cover page.

[54] Ibid.

The deployment of language received critical attention from the translating authors. Indeed, easy communication with the readers was considered an important merit of translated works. In the introduction to his *Homoeopathic Bhaishajya Tattva Chikitsha Pradarshika* (*Guide to the Materia Medica of Homoeopathic Treatment*), author Hariprasad Chakrabarti noted that the book retained the exact language which he used in his lectures explaining homoeopathic principles to his students.[55] He explained that 'the presentation may lack a little in organisation but facilitates the understanding of the readers'.[56] A 1927 promotional advertisement for the book *Chikitsha Darpan* (*Mirror of Medicine*), published by Batakrishna Pal and Company, proclaimed that 'although there are numerous other homoeopathic tomes written in the mother tongue, yet we can safely certify that you have not come across a tract written in a more simple and lucid language'.[57] In their efforts to reach out to the largest possible number of readers, books like *Bheshaja Bidhan* deliberately included a column of text in English, side by side with its Bengali translation, for the convenience of the 'educated gentlemen of the N. W. P, Orissa, Madras etc'.[58] Other authors like Hariprasad Chakrabarti, reaching out to all 'including the native doctors and Kavirajes', were careful not to use any 'provincial dialect or term in writing'.[59] Chakrabarti explained that such 'provincial rustic language' was not comprehensible to all and could not be looked up in dictionaries. He further added that since it was easier for the readers to follow Bengali, he had retained the original English names of the drugs and diseases by writing such names in the Bengali script. However, to avoid confusion he also 'inserted the translations of the meaning of those words'.[60] Hence, vernacular translation of homoeopathy did involve considerable negotiations with the English language. In any case, the overall linguistic quality of their writing remained an arena of concern for the authors. In his *Brihat Olautha Samhita* (*Enlarged Compendium for Treatment of Cholera*), Chandra Shekhar Kali was thus particular to highlight a letter from one

[55] Hariprasad Chakrabarti, Preface, *Homoeopathic Bhaishajya Tattva o Chikitsha Pradarshika* (*Guide to the Materia Medica of Homoeopathic Treatment*) (Calcutta: Chikitsha Tattva Jantra, 1902), page number not cited.
[56] Ibid.
[57] 'Advertisement of Chikitsha Darpan' in Anonymous, *Homoeopathic Mowt e Saral Griha Chikitsha* (*Simple Domestic Treatment According to Homoeopathy*), 7th edition (Calcutta: Batakrishna Pal and Company, 1926), page number not cited.
[58] Mahesh Chandra Bhattacharya, 'Preface', *Bheshaja Bidhan* (*Pharmaceutical Prescription*), 1st edition (Calcutta: M. Bhattacharya and Company, 1892), page number not cited.
[59] Hariprasad Chakrabarti, 'Bigyapon or Advertisement', *Bhaishajya Tattwa o Chikitsha Pradarshika* (*Guide to the Materia Medica of Homoeopathic Treatment*) (Calcutta: Chikitsha Tattwa Jontro, 1902), page number not cited.
[60] Ibid.

of his readers who extensively praised the author's works saying, 'such books in one of our Indian vernaculars is a complete surprise'.[61]

The authors garnered legitimacy for their translations through myriad means. The entrepreneur-physicians at the helm of the homoeopathic families, whom we encountered in Chapter 1, were frequently invoked. The author Haricharan Chatterjee, for instance, cited in the preface to his *Practical Materia Medica* a list of western authors whose works have inspired his own. He elaborated on the fact that the late Mahendralal Sircar had taken keen interest in his compilations and was most satisfied with the outcome. He let his readers know that Mahendralal had not only read the whole draft but had also suggested crucial revisions and changes at various places.[62] Indeed Mahendralal Sircar and Rajendralal Dutta were among the most cited names in a range of texts translating western homoeopathic works.[63]

A number of texts included correspondence between the translators and the original publishers or authors to demonstrate the legitimacy of their publications. Correspondence illustrating the consent of the original western publishers or authors was cited as a feature of credible acts of translation. Such correspondence also presented the Bengali translators as part of a global network of science popularisers. The book *Contributions Towards a Knowledge of the Peculiarities of all Homoeopathic Medicines*, for instance, included a '*onumati patra*' or 'permission letter' that contained a message from the English author R. Gibson Miller granting the translator permission to 'translate into Hindustani or any other language you desire'.[64]

In the author-translators' letters seeking such permission, the emphasis was often not as much on the specific language as on the effort to 'vernacularise' homoeopathy. Writing in 1896, author Nilambar Hui included his correspondence with the 'reputed America based firm Boericke and Tafel' in his monograph. He sought permission to translate their particular version of the *Organon of the Art of Healing*.[65] In the letter, Hui repeatedly characterised his effort as one of 'translating it [*Organon*] into our own vernacular' for the benefit of 'our vernacular friends'.[66]

[61] Chandra Shekhar Kali, 'Banga Bhashar Gaurab o Samadar' (Prestige and Appreciation of Bengali Language'), *Brihat Olautha Samhita* (*Enlarged Compendium for Treatment of Cholera*), 1926, page number not cited.

[62] Haricharan Chatterjee, 'Mukhobondho or Preface', *The Practical Materia Medica of Homoeopathic Treatment* (Dacca: Popular Library Patuatoli, 1911), page number not cited.

[63] For dedication to Rajendralal Dutta, see Biharilal Bhaduri, *Homoeopathic Chikitsha Bigyan* (*Science of Homoeopathy*), 1874–77, Dedication page.

[64] M. N. Bhattacharjee, 'Advertisement to the First Edition', *Contributions Towards a Knowledge of the Peculiarities of all Homoeopathic Medicines*, 1921, pp. 2–3.

[65] Nilambar, 'Our Letter', *Sadrisa Bigyan Sutra* (*Principles for the Science of Similars*), 1896, page number not cited.

[66] Ibid.

The 'vernacular' in such writings emerged both as the language as well as the context and the people in which and for whom homoeopathy needed to be translated.

Yet, the issue of language remained central to the efforts to vernacularise homoeopathy. The readers were often reminded of the multiple acts of translation that the texts were undergoing, sometimes from German or French to English before being translated into an Indian language. In his translation of the *Organon*, Nilambar Hui included the letter of permission from the American publisher Boericke and Tafel, who while granting him the right to translate, urged him to 'give due credit to our house as well as Dr. Wesselhoeft the translator of the German (version)'.[67] Indeed, translations from German to English featured frequently. In their promotional advertisements, as shown in Fig. 3.2, the Hahnemann Publishing Company frequently mentioned titles of English books that had been translated from the 'original' German into English under the aegis of their publication department.[68] However, the authors often cautioned the readers against the problems inherent in such acts of multiple translations. The article 'On Translations of Hahnemannian Pathogenesis: With a Plea for a new English Version' in the *Calcutta Journal of Medicine* discussed at length how the earliest English translations from German often failed to capture the specific essence of the German writings.[69] It argued that 'some 5000 of Hahnemann's symptoms are quotations from authors – English, Latin, French, Italian as well as German. It is easy to see what confusion is made when these are retranslated into English from Hahnemann's rendering of them into German'.[70] German and English were not the only European languages invoked in the homoeopathic literature in Bengal. In the 1868–69 volume of the *Calcutta Journal of Medicine*, Mahendralal Sircar reported a series of 'public conferences in homoeopathy' which were 'translated from the French of Dr. Jousset by the editor'.[71] Hence, as Figs. 3.1 and 3.2 reveal, at various moments English itself emerged as the language through which homoeopathy was translated and vernacularised for the Bengali readers.

[67] Nilambar Hui, 'Onumati Patra or Permission Letter', *Sadrisa Bigyan Sutra (Principles for the Science of Similars)*, 1896, page number not cited.

[68] See 'Advertisement of Hahnemann Publishing Company' in *Hahnemann*, 8, 11 (1925), 600.

[69] Richard Hughes, 'On Translations of Hahnemannian Pathogenesis: With a Plea for a New English Version', *Calcutta Journal of Medicine*, 8, 5 and 6 (1876), 311–15.

[70] Ibid.

[71] Mahendralal Sircar, 'Public Conference upon Homoeopathy: On the Reform of Hahnemann as the Basis of Positive Therapeutics', *Calcutta Journal of Medicine*, 1, 1 (January 1868), 14–15.

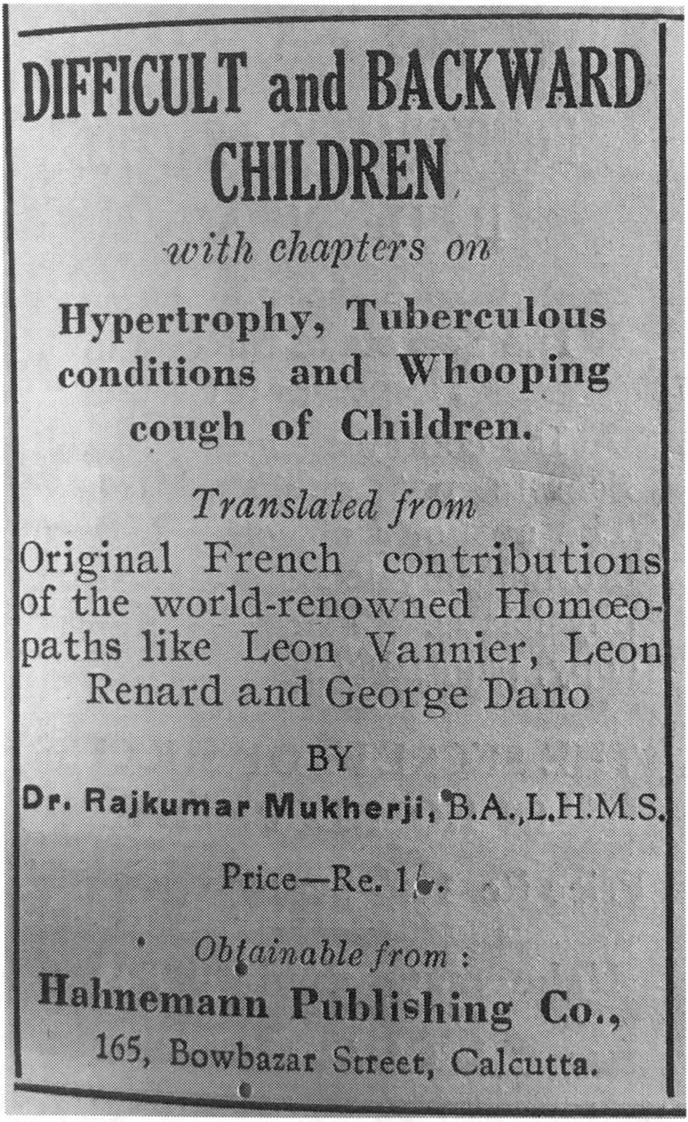

Fig. 3.1 Advertisement for a monograph on children's disease translated from French original, *Hahnemannian Gleanings*, 9 (May 1938), 11. Credit: Hahnemann Publishing Company Private Limited, Kolkata.

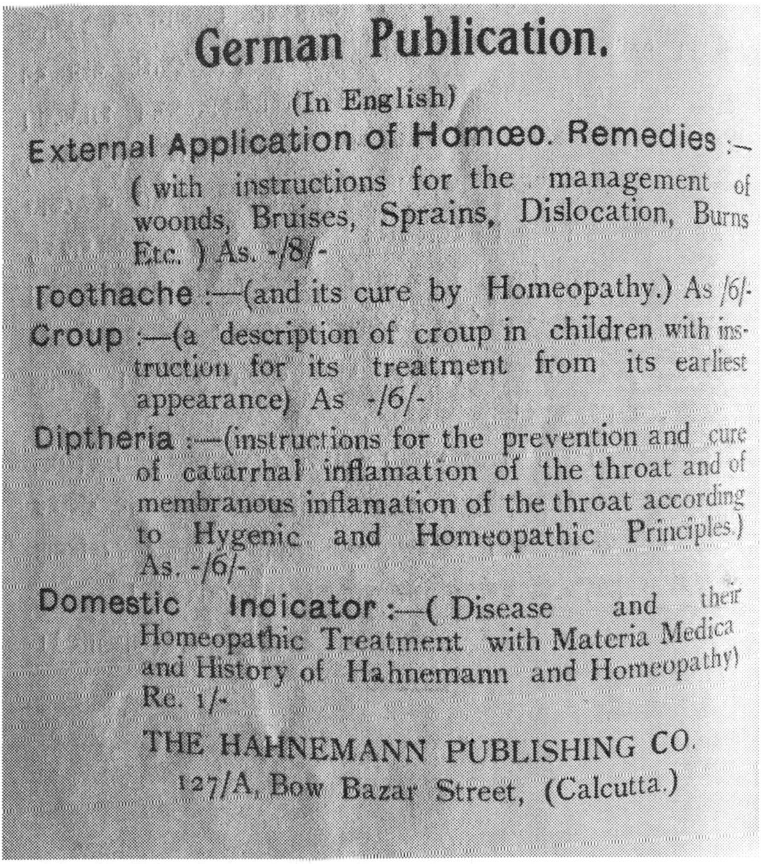

Fig. 3.2 Advertisement for German books in English in the Bengali journal *Hahnemann*, 9, 8 (1925), 404. Credit: Hahnemann Publishing Company Private Limited, Kolkata.

Indeed, in the 'notes on translations' included by authors in their works, Bangla or the Bengali language figured often as a moment in a continuous chain of multiple translations. Thus, in a short note in his book *Olautha Samhita* author Chandra Shekhar Kali described it as 'a matter of great honour for both Bengal and the Bengali language'[72] that the private secretary to Raja H. H. Jahvar of Bombay had sought Dr Kali's

[72] Chandra Shekhar Kali, 'Banga Bhashar Gourab o Samador' ('The Prestige and Recognition of Bengali Language'), *Brihat Olautha Samhita (Enlarged Compendium for Treatment of Cholera)*, 1926, page number not cited.

permission to translate his Bengali books, like *Chikitsha Bidhan*, into Mahratta [Marathi].[73] The importance of the author/publisher's consent may be assessed from Dr Kali's words of caution to the secretary. While granting his wholehearted consent to the translation of his Bengali books into Mahratti, Dr Kali cautioned, 'I beg to ask your goodness to note down, that without my permission you should not allow your translated Mahratta books of mine to be translated into any other Language. And this letter of mine be printed into those translated books of yours'.[74] Taken together, these instances affirm translation as a continuum involving various languages, that constantly remade the original. Under such circumstances, the vernacular revealed itself as a flexible, mutating and relative category.

There was a simultaneous concern with the impact of these works of translation on Bengali as a language. Opinion remained divided on whether scientific translations were beneficial for the healthy advancement of a language. The journal *Hahnemann*, edited by Basanta Kumar Dutta, published a series of articles titled 'Homoeopathic Bangla Sahitya' or 'Homoeopathic Bengali Literature', which reflected upon the proliferation of homoeopathic literature in Bengali.[75] In the first instalment of his article, as early as in 1884, the author pointed out that while literary forms like drama, novel and poetry formed the bulk of Bengali publications in the late nineteenth century, homoeopathic authors too were becoming significant contributors to the language.[76] A review published in the newspaper *Samaj Darpan* on 4th Chaitra 1875, likewise, confirmed that of all the various categories of physicians, homoeopathic authors were the most active in writing Bengali texts.[77] The reviewer opined that such overabundance of writing had a distinctly positive impact on the language as a whole. He argued that extensive translations of scientific texts had a beneficial and enabling impact on Bengali language. This review pointed out, as it was contended in other contexts around the same time, that assimilation of foreign scientific terms led to expansion of a language.[78] Many held that the translated texts ought to be discussed in

[73] Ibid. [74] Ibid.

[75] It should be noted that *Hahnemann* was the name of several journals circulating in Bengal since the late nineteenth century. *Hahnemann*, edited by Basanta Kumar Datta, was different from the *Hahnemann* published by the Hahnemann Publishing Company of the Bhar family.

[76] Basanta Kumar Datta, 'Homoeopathic Bangla Sahitya' ('Homoeopathic Bengali Literature'), *Hahnemann*, 2, 10 (1884), 181.

[77] 'Review by Samaj Darpan' in Basanta Datta (ed.), *Datta's Homoeopathy Series in Bengalee*, 3 (March 1876), promotional advertisement at the end.

[78] The 'politics of neologism' in science translation has been a recurrent theme in the historiography. For a recent discussion, see Marwa Elshakry, 'Knowledge in Motion:

greater detail in scientific journals for the benefit of general readers. They held that such translation efforts would 'nourish the growing limbs of the Bengali language'.[79]

At the same time, publications from the period demonstrate others disputing such convictions. Some authors and publishers were alarmed at the way homoeopathic publications were flooding the print market. To them, the plethora of translated works that were published in Bengali did not have any appreciable impact on the language. They held that widespread and arbitrary translations by authors of dubious competence did more harm to a language than good. The author of the article 'Homoeopathic Bengali Literature', expressed serious reservations against the arbitrary ways in which the bulk of the homoeopathic texts were being translated.[80] Following an extensive survey of the published books, the author identified three broad trends in translations. He noted that in the first kind of translation, all the English terms were retained and the authors only inserted Bengali verbs. The second kind, he complained, was of outright bad quality, what he termed as the '*Battala*' standard. He castigated the publication standard of such tracts, including their print, letters, illustrations full of floral margins and the like. He identified a third trend of translating English words variously, using different vernacular synonyms.[81] He regretted the lack of any coherence and standardisation, pointing out the tremendous confusion such translations caused for the readers.[82] Thus, by many contemporary commentators, such writings were considered deeply injurious to the cause of both homoeopathy as a science and Bengali as a language.[83]

Critical reflections on the ill effects of such unsystematic, extensive translations stoked larger questions about the reception of western science in a colonial context. By the early years of the twentieth century, along with manoeuvres in language, the question of the *context* in which a scientific text was being translated emerged as a significant theme for discussion. Literal translations of western texts, with straightforward transliterations,

The Cultural Politics of Modern Science Translation in Arabic', pp. 713–20. For a South Asia-specific discussion that dwells on the missionary-orientalist policies of translation implicating science as well as religion, see Michael Dodson, 'Translating Science, Translating Empire: The Power of Language in Colonial North India', *Comparative Studies in Society and History*, 47, 4 (2005), 809–35.

[79] 'Review by Sulabh Samachar' in Basanta Datta (ed.), *Datta's Homoeopathy Series in Bengalee*, 3 (March 1876), cover page.

[80] Basanta Kumar Datta, 'Homoeopathic Bangla Sahitya' ('Homoeopathic Bengali Literature'), *Hahnemann*, 2, 12 (1884), 222.

[81] Ibid.

[82] Basanta Kumar Datta, 'Homoeopathic Bangla Sahitya' (*'Homoeopathic Bengali Literature')*, *Hahnemann*, 2, 10 (1884), 183.

[83] Ibid.

were strongly opposed by many. Some even considered such literal translations as acts of political subservience. As the author K. Chatterjee explicitly argued in the journal *Hahnemann*, while translating Anglo-American texts it was not advisable to follow their contents unconditionally and completely.[84] In support of his argument, he elaborated on the differences in climate, food habit, dressing patterns, as well as beliefs and customs between India and the West. Similarly, a range of texts claiming to translate homoeopathy put a premium on the experiences of physicians working in India. For instance, the author of *Berigny and Company's Bengali Homoeopathic Series*, Harikrishna Mallik, was careful to note that his writings, while being translations of western texts, were also adequately contextualised to suit the mental and physical health of the people inhabiting Bengal.[85] In the introduction to the fourth manual in the series, he explained that although 'the tract is mostly a translation from Borjo', he had integrated the knowledge gained from working among the people in Bengal. He elaborated on his method of innovating on the doses, keeping in mind the context and his readers while translating that particular text.[86]

Literal translations that did not take into account the specific context of Bengal – its physical and emotional landscape – were labelled inadequate. It was pointed out that although 'homoeopathic science is *their* science, to be able to use it in India, we need to adapt it to our situation and make it our own'.[87] Evidently chiming in with nationalist sensibilities, in such arguments the process of 'translation' came to acquire a much wider significance with relation to homoeopathy. Arguing for contextualising science, authors like K. Chatterjee held that translations had to be sensitive to factors like '*desh, kal, patra*' or 'time, place and individuals'.[88] Hahnemann's homoeopathy, as we shall see in what follows, was increasingly projected as compatible with and even inherited from 'Indian classics'.

Hindu Homoeopathy

As noted in the introduction, the official-colonial-orientalist efforts in translation resulted in discourses on hierarchies of languages and

[84] K. Chatterjee, 'Bharate Kromo Samasya' ('The Problem of Potency in India'), *Hahnemann*, 8, 8 (1925), 405–7.
[85] Harikrishna Mallik, 'Upokramanika or Preface', *Berigny and Company's Bengali Homoepoathic Series Number IV: Sadrisa Byabastha Chikitsha Dipika (Glossary for Treatment According to the System of Similars)* (Calcutta: Berigny and Company, 1870), pp. 1–2.
[86] Ibid.
[87] K. Chatterjee, 'Bharate Kromo Samasya' ('The Problem of Potency in India'), pp. 405–7.
[88] Ibid.

civilisations. Many like John Tytler of the Native Medical Institution firmly believed in English as a 'language of reason' as opposed to the native languages. To them, translation of European knowledge to Indian vernaculars was a near-impossible mission, given the conceptual non-equivalence of the two knowledge systems. Tytler in fact distinguished between 'ideas of sensation' which to him were the same throughout the world, as opposed to 'ideas of reflection' which were constructed and therefore culturally determined. Proclaiming the distinction in 1834, he argued,

> where nations like those of Europe have similar manner and frequent intercourse, the ideas [of reflection] thus formed will, like those of sensation, be nearly the same, and expressed by parallel words, among nations, on the other hand, whose manners are different, and between whom intercourse is comparatively rare, as those of Europe and Asia, it will in almost all cases, happen that the ideas of reflection are quite different, and that there are few or no parallel words by which those of the one language can be expressed in the other.[89]

Through their sustained efforts at translation spanning the second half of the nineteenth century, the homoeopathic popularisers systematically challenged any such notion of 'non-equivalence'. By the early decades of the twentieth century, these translations moved from a phase of deliberations around literal linguistic translations to more culturally sensitive interpretations. Existing literature on translations of psychiatry shows that men like Girindrashekhar Basu had begun, by the early twentieth century, to avoid literal translation and to promote translations 'that were done at the level of concepts which were then explained in the context of Indian philosophy and culture'.[90] The homoeopaths, too, promoted a sense of symmetry, arguing for a deep embedded harmony between homoeopathic principles and Indian philosophical thought. In a series of articles and monographs, the 'science' of homoeopathy was shown to have deep religio-philosophic resonance, as the authors argued that even though it represented 'scientific medicine of the highest order', one could hardly grasp its tenets by 'only reading the materia medica'.[91] It was

[89] John Tytler, 'On Native Education', the Calcutta literary gazette, Nos 1, 25, p. 382. Quoted in Michael Dodson, *Orientalism, Empire, National Culture, India 1770–1880*, p. 130. For detailed discussion of Tytler's policies of translation at the Native Medical Institution, see Ishita Pande, *Medicine, Race and Liberalism in British Bengal: Symptoms of Empire*, 2010, pp. 77–82.

[90] Amitranjan Basu, 'Emergence of a Marginal Science in a Colonial City: Reading Psychiatry in Bengali Periodicals', pp. 134–7.

[91] Anonymous (Translated from the English of Herbert A. Roberts), 'Jeebani Shakti' ('Vital Force'), *Hahnemann*, 20, 7 (1937), 362. Also see Gyanendra Mohan Pan, 'Edesh e Homoeopathy Chikitshar Unnotir Ontoray Ki?' ('What Are the Hindrances to the Development of Homoeopathy in India'), p. 583.

pointed out that, to perfectly comprehend homoeopathy, it was necessary to perceive its '*darshonik tattwa*' or its 'philosophical basis'.[92] These texts identified the theory of 'vital force' and the 'administration of infinitesimal or minute doses of drugs' as the two fundamental principles preached by Hahnemann. Through discussions in a range of texts, authors contended that both these fundamental features resonated heavily with Hindu philosophical thought as delineated in the Vedas and Upanishads, including the ayurvedic corpus. The article 'Kromo Nirnay ba Matra Bijnan' or 'Science of Determining Doses' in the journal *Hahnemann* asserted that 'the basis of true homoeopathy is spirituality. It is very apparent from the texts of Hahnemann and those of his principal disciple Kent, that there are distinct overlaps between their thoughts and Hindu philosophy'.[93] While exploring the Hindu philosophical affinities, these turn-of the-century texts were also evidently in conversation with the nationalist efforts at reviving and homogenising the scriptural foundations of Hindu philosophy and religion.

In 'Amiya Samhita', a serially published long article in the journal *Hahnemann*, author Nalininath Majumdar emphasised the philosophic underpinnings of homoeopathic thoughts. He argued that 'true medicine' or the science of healing could not be studied without reference to '*dharma*' or religion, which was also essentially related to the body and the world.[94] Justifying the title 'Amiya Samhita', the author interpreted the term 'homoeopathy' as the science to attain long life. Since, according to the Hindu Puranas, '*amiya*', i.e. '*amrita*'[95] (the elixir for life that led to immortality), the tract on homoeopathic principles was justifiably termed 'Amiya [meaning *Amrita*] Samhita'.[96] Indeed, the word '*amiya*' was used time and again as a Bengali variant of the word 'Homoeo' in several texts. In the introduction to his book *Brihat Olautha Samhita*, Chandra Shekhar Kali too invoked 'Amiya-Patha', i.e. the path leading to the attainment of immortality or 'amrita'.[97] He, and some others upheld 'amiya-patha' as the Sanskrit term for homoeopathy.[98]

[92] Anonymous (Translated from the English of Herbert A. Roberts), 'Jeebani Shakti' ('Vital Force'), p. 362

[93] Haricharan Ray, 'Kromo Nirnay ba Matra Bijnan' ('The Science of Potency'), *Hahnemann*, 1, 11 (1918), 322–3.

[94] Nalininath Majumdar, 'Amiya Samhita' ('Collection of Principles Ensuring Immortality'), *Hahnemann*, 8, 4 (1925), 192–3.

[95] See note 15.

[96] Nalininath Majumdar, 'Amiya Samhita' ('Collection of Principles Ensuring Immortality'), *Hahnemann*, 8, 4 (1925), 196.

[97] Chandra Shekhar Kali, 'Preface', *Brihat Olautha Samhita* (*Enlarged Compendium for Treatment of Cholera*), 1926, pp. 1–2.

[98] Ibid., p. 1.

Interestingly, the word '*samhita*', which had a distinct resonance with Hindu classical texts, appeared in the titles of many texts. Discussing the many meanings of the word '*samhita*', C. S. Kali emphasised that it primarily stood for a collection of tenets compiled by the *rishis* or Indian sages. He pointed out that his book *Olautha Samhita* was justifiably named as it was also a collection of tenets compiled by the 'German *rishi*' Hahnemann.[99] Just as '*amiya*' emerged as the vernacular term for *homoeo*, various other Bengali terms, often with Hindu resonances, began circulating in the homoeopathic translations. It was argued that the Sanskrit phrase '*samah samang samayati*' captured the meaning inherent in the Latin '*similia similibus curantur*' used by Hahnemann in delineating the homoeopathic law of similars.[100] Likewise, the most appropriate Bengali translation of the term 'potency' in relation to the strength of homoeopathic drugs was identified as '*shakti*', which had distinct Hindu connotations.[101] Articles like 'Oushadh er Shakti Tattva' or 'Principles Relating to the Potency of Drugs' explicitly reminded the readers of the Hindu iconography of *shakti* and the cult of worship of *shakti* or the mother goddess among the Hindus.[102] Together, such usages demonstrate attempts at going beyond the practices of transliteration or 'engrafting', to innovate what has been recently referred as 'archaising', i.e. using older words and terms, sometimes with religious references.[103]

The theory of 'vital force' as explicated by Hahnemann was regarded as a core doctrine of homoeopathy in the translations. 'Vital force', translated as '*jiboni shakti*', was the staple of a range of articles that pitted the 'theory of vital force' against orthodox medicine's 'germ theory of disease'. As the author of the article 'Jiboni Shakti' in the journal *Hahnemann* elaborated, the homoeopaths considered life itself to be constituted equally of three parts: the body, the mind and spirit, and the vital force which was the 'spirit like force, the dynamis that animates the material body'.[104] Of the three constituent elements of life, the 'simple, invisible, immaterial, spiritual, indivisible and qualitative' vital force was considered the most

[99] Ibid., p. 2.

[100] For instance, see the cover of the journal *Hahnemann* edited by Basanta Kumar Datta. The emblem on the cover describes the Sanskrit phrase as the translation of the Latin phrase.

[101] Chandra Shekhar Kali, 'Preface', *Brihat Olautha Samhita (Enlarged Compendium for Treatment of Cholera)*, 1926, pp. 3–4.

[102] G. Dirghangi, 'Oushadh er Shakti Tattva' ('Theories Relating to the Potency of Drugs'), *Hahnemann*, 3, 8 (1920), 297.

[103] Marwa Elshakry, *Reading Darwin in Arabic, 1860–1950* (Chicago and London: University of Chicago Press, 2013), pp. 17–18.

[104] Anonymous (Translated from the English of Herbert A. Roberts), 'Jeebani Shakti' ('Vital Force'), pp. 362–3.

fundamental.[105] As author C. Roy elaborated in an article in the journal *The Hahnemannian Gleanings*, 'our body is a mere vehicle or abode of the vital force ... and without the animating power of the vital force, the body is a mere mass of matter dead and defunct in every way'.[106] To the Bengali homoeopaths, following the *Hahnemannian* corpus of thought, derangement of this all-important, invisible spirit-like vital force was the primary cause of disease, rather than any emerging notion of germs. Author S. N. Roy reminded the readers in his article 'Rog Kahake Bole?' or 'What Is Disease?' that neither dead bodies nor inanimate objects experience diseases.[107] Diseases, then, were caused by the 'derangement of the body's immaterial vital force' by the 'dynamic influence upon it of a morbific agent inimical to life'.[108] The homoeopaths following Hahnemann further held that the 'morbific force' disturbing the vital force of the body was also invisible and immaterial. Hence, they categorically denied the role of any material agent, i.e. germs or bacteria, in causing diseases. Diseases to them were caused by the impact of invisible, immaterial force on the vital force of the body. The article 'Comparison of Homeopathy with Allopathy and Other Medical Systems' stated, 'the allopaths argue that coma bacilli causes cholera, but they confuse the effect with the cause ... visible germs are not the disease causing entities rather their effects '.[109] The article 'Bacteria r Shohit Rog er Ki Sombondho' ('What is the Relation between Bacteria and Disease?') in the journal *Homoeopathy Paricharak* voiced similar convictions, saying 'germs *seek* diseased tissue rather than being the cause of the diseased tissue'.[110]

These elaborate discussions on the vital force reverberated with and reinforced different Hindu thoughts and practices. G. Dirghangi's article on homoeopathic drugs in the journal *Hahnemann*, for instance, argued how the concept of vital force was

[105] C. Roy, 'The Spiritual Power of Medicine Does Not Accomplish its Object by Means of Quantity but by Potentiality and Quality', *The Hahnemannian Gleanings*, 1, 1 (February 1930), 59.

[106] Ibid., p. 57.

[107] S. N. Roy, 'Rog Kahake Bole' ('What Is Disease'), *Hahnemann*, 6, 12 (1923), 555.

[108] Anonymous (Translated from the English of Herbert A. Roberts), 'Jeebani Shakti' ('Vital Force'), p. 366.

[109] Kamal Krishna Bhattacharya, 'Homoeopathy Bonam Allopathy O Onyanyo Chikitsha Pronali' ('Homoeopathy vs. Allopathy and Other Medical Systems'), *Hahnemann*, 23, 6 (1940), 345.

[110] Kalikumar Bhattacharya, 'Bacteriar Shohit Rog er Ki sombondho' ('What Is the Relation between Bacteria and Disease'), *Homoeopathy Paricharak*, 2, 12 (March 1929), 463–9.

useful in rationalising the caste hierarchies of the Hindus.[111] Following Hahnemann, some argued that vital force could not be the same in any two persons – it always varied with the personality of every individual.[112] Hence, the Hindu distinction between men belonging to the highest Brahmin caste and the lowest Sudra caste could be easily explained by the difference in their vital force.[113] The author of this text asserted that the three different qualities of '*sattwah, tamah and rajah*', as explained in the Vedas as the basis for caste hierarchies, corresponded perfectly to the potential variations of vital force as explicated by Hahnemann.

Similarly, discussions on the homoeopathic concept of vital force invoked elaborations on Hindu philosophical schools. It was argued that the spiritual nature of the 'vital forces' resonated deeply with Indian thought, since most philosophical schools in India were engaged with assessing the nature of spirit or mind, vis-à-vis body. The essential point of contention, as stated by author Kamal Krishna Bhattacharya, was that 'oriental thinking considers spirit to be the cause of matter while occident believes in the primacy of matter'.[114] As C. Roy's article 'Etiology in Homoeopathy' candidly said, the western world, their world-view, thought process, indeed their 'whole metaphysics itself, from Locke's time onwards, has been physical: not a spiritual philosophy, but a material one'.[115] Through invocations of contemporary debates in philosophy, several authors including Kamal Krishna Bhattacharya, Nalininath Majumdar, C. Roy, Umapada Mukhopadhyay, Kali Krishna Bhattacharya and others writing in various journals established that the 'eastern' philosophical tradition, much like the Hahnemannian tradition, celebrated the supremacy of spirit as 'infallible and most logical'.[116] These authors affirmed that an invisible, immaterial force variously termed as '*Brahma*', '*Atma*', '*Purush*', '*Shabda*' or '*Paramanu*' by ancient philosophers and in various traditional texts or 'Shastras', was identified as the centre and the cause of the material world. Nalininath Majumdar in his 'Amiya Samhita' discussed how the Nyaya school of Indian

[111] G. Dirghangi, 'Oushadh er Shakti Tattva' ('Theories Relating to the Potency of Drugs'), pp. 300–1.
[112] Anonymous (Translated from the English of Herbert A. Roberts), 'Jeebani Shakti' ('Vital Force'), pp. 362–7.
[113] G. Dirghangi, 'Oushadh er Shakti Tattva' ('Theories Relating to the Potency of Drugs'), p. 300–1.
[114] Kamal Krishna Bhattacharya, 'Homoeopathy Bonam Allopathy O Onyanyo Chikitsha Pronali' ('Homoeopathy vs. Allopathy and Other Medical Systems'), p. 341.
[115] C. Roy, 'Etiology in Homoeopathy', *The Hahnemannian Gleanings*, 1, 1 (1930), 53–4.
[116] For instance, see Kamal Krishna Bhattacharya, 'Homoeopathy Bonam Allopathy O Onyanyo Chikitsha Pronali' ('Homoeopathy vs. Allopathy and Other Medical Systems'), p. 344.

philosophy, especially scholars like Gautam and Kanad, anticipated modern theories of the 'atom'.[117] Such arguments pointed out strong similarities between the Nyaya conception of the primacy of 'paramanu' and Hahnmenann's notion of the vital force. It was also claimed that the most recent contemporary research by eminent scientists like Jagadish Chandra Bose and Einstein conformed to such ancient Nyaya philosophical ideas as well as Hahnemann's ideas.[118]

Such Indian conceptions of the immaterial spirit, the homoeopathy popularisers argued, were reflected not only in the theory of vital force, but also in the homoeopathic notion of drugs. Indeed, as is widely known, the Hahnemannian idea of prescribing the minutest dose of a drug had been a matter of long-standing controversy among the scientific community in Europe and in India.[119] For the drugs to attain efficacy in such doses, it was contended that they needed to be 'potentised' – a specialised process by which drugs were diluted to such an extent that they were rendered invisible, and yet acquired tremendous strength. Homoeopathic authors claimed that such concepts had parallels in ancient Indian thought.[120] Author Benoytosh Bhattacharya, asserted that 'the qualities and powers residing in the ions of the homoeopathic potentised drugs have already been described in a picturesque manner in the *Taittiriya Upanishad*, one of the immortal philosophical works of India'.[121]

Apart from indicating specific references to ayurveda, homoeopathic translators also went to great lengths in drawing upon eclectic Hindu rituals and practices to establish their common underlying similarity, that is, belief in the power of immaterial, minute substance as propounded by Hahnemann. In his 'Amiya Samhita', Nalininath Majumdar explicated how the power of the minute was most clearly discernible from the Hindu practices like '*shradhha*' or the death rites, as well as from Hindu astrologic practices.[122] He discussed the ways in which ancient Hindu astrology was based on the understanding that the faintest rays of distant planets

[117] Nalininatha Majumdar, 'Amiya Samhita' ('Collection of Principles Ensuring Immortality', *Hahnemann*, 8, 10 (1925), 525.

[118] Kamal Krishna Bhattacharya, 'Homoeopathy Bonam Allopathy O Onyanyo Chikitsha Pronali' ('Homoeopathy vs. Allopathy and Other Medical Systems'), p. 341.

[119] See Robert Jutte, Guenter B. Risse and John Woodward (eds.), *Culture, Knowledge and Healing: Historical Perspective of Homoeopathic Medicine in Europe and North America* (Sheffield: European Association for the History of Medicine and Health Publications, 1998).

[120] See Abhaypada Chattopadhyay, 'Chikitsha Jogote Homoeopathy' ('Homoeopathy in the Medical World'), *Chikitshak*, 4 (1926), 38–9.

[121] Benoytosh Bhattacharya, 'Preface', *The Science of Tridosha* (Calcutta: Firma K. L. Mukhopadhyay, 1975 [1951]), page number not cited.

[122] Nalininath Majumdar, 'Amiya Samhita' ('Collection of Principles Ensuring Immortality'), *Hahnemann*, 9, 1 (1926), 31.

and sun were capable of controlling life cycles on earth.[123] Likewise, Kamal Krishna Bhattacharya pointed out that the eastern philosophy of *atma* or spirit attributed immense potential to the spirit after the death of the material body. Such a conception of the phenomenon of death, he argued, was analogous to the homoeopathic process of dilution or potentisation, where the extinction of the material medicinal substance released latent, infinite power, just as the immensely powerful *atma* was released with the death of the physical body.[124] Nalininath Majumdar also detailed the concept of the emancipated spirit or '*atma*', as well as the notion of '*pinda*' or sacrificial offering to the soul to highlight the affinity between such profound yet subtle philosophies with homoeopathic principles.[125] He expressed regret that some 'modern materialist' Hindus were incapable of appreciating such intricate philosophy and expressed agnosticism both towards these traditional customs, and towards homoeopathic principles.[126] Majumdar was critical of the argumentative nature of many western-educated Indians, who demanded 'scientific' explanations of every truth. He proclaimed that modern science was, in reality, slowly approaching the truths already inherent in ancient Indian philosophy.[127]

It is evident, then, that Bengali discussions of homoeopathic principles were steeped in references to Hindu practices and metaphors. Such interpretations suggested that western homoeopathic science was in perfect harmony with what they simultaneously celebrated as classical Hindu philosophy. By elaborating on the overlap between homoeopathy and Hinduism, these texts contributed towards making 'it our own' by a process of translation which was not merely linguistic. Such Hinduised readings further enabled the recurrent iconisation of Hahnemann.

As we have seen earlier, biographies of Hahnemann frequently compared him to religious icons of indigenous origin, such as Siva and Buddha.[128] Tracts discussing vernacular translations of homoeopathy abound in such religious metaphors. For instance, commenting on the declining influence of the Vedas among contemporary Hindus, Nalininath Majumdar referred to Hahnemann as the *avatar* or

[123] Ibid., pp. 27–31.
[124] Kamal Krishna Bhattacharya, 'Homoeopathy Bonam Allopathy O Onyanyo Chikitsha Pronali' ('Homoeopathy vs. Allopathy and Other Medical Systems'), p. 345.
[125] Nalininatha Majumdar, 'Amiya Samhita' ('Collection of Principles Ensuring Immortality'), *Hahnemann*, 9, 2 (1926), 96–7.
[126] Ibid., p. 97.
[127] Nalininath Majumdar, 'Amiya Samhita', *Hahnemann*, 8, 7 (1925), 349.
[128] See Chapter 2, section titled 'Of Science and Spiritualism: Vernacular Hahnemann'.

incarnation of Siva in the Kaliyug.[129] He represented it as a sheer divine blessing that 'with the declining impact of Vedas in India, Hahnemann was born as an incarnation of Lord Siva to drive home such Vedic ideas under the name of homoeopathy or amrita-path'.[130] Resonances of such vernacular association between Hahnemann and Hindu gods spilled out beyond the colonial period and the Bengali print market. Mishr Harivansh Lal Sundd, a retired army man and an amateur homoeopath in Punjab, composed an encyclopaedic life of the monkey-god Hanumana in the late 1990s. Written in light of Tulsidas's *Ram Charit Manas*, the iconic sixteenth-century epic poem on Rama's life, Sundd's *Sri Sankat Mochan Hanuman Charit Manas* (*Life of Hanumana, Preventer of Crisis*) discussed the myriad facets of Hanumana's personality in great detail. In discussing his great quality as a 'redeemer of health' and his knowledge in surgery and medicine, Sundd explicitly described Hahnemann as a modern reincarnation of the monkey-god.[131]

Even in the colonial era, the inflection of homoeopathy with Hindu connotations was commonplace in disparate forms of literature. Amritalal Basu was a notable figure of Bengali theatre in the late nineteenth century.[132] In his early life, Basu was trained as a homoeopath by the leading Varanasi-based physician Lokenath Maitra, whose biography is discussed in Chapter 2.[133] Published in 1903 and written as a long poem, Amritalal Basu's memoir titled *Amrita Madira* recounted his days with Lokenath Maitra at Kasi.[134] The poem is full of religious allusions in describing homoeopathy and its appeal among the people. It reflected upon the immense popularity of the doctrine in Kasi, a place ascribed

[129] *Avatar* in Hinduism describes a deliberate descent of a deity from heaven to earth, or a descent of the Supreme Being. It is mostly translated into English as 'incarnation', but more accurately as 'appearance' or 'manifestation'. Kali Yuga is the last of the four stages that the world goes through as part of the cycle of 'yugas' or ages supposedly described in the Indian scriptures. Kali Yuga is associated with the apocalyptic demon Kalki, not to be confused with Goddess Kali. For a scholarly deployment of the concepts in understanding nineteenth-century Hindu *bhadralok* sensibility, see Sumit Sarkar, 'Kaliyuga, Chakri, Bhakti: Ramkrishna and His Times', *Writing Social History* (Delhi and New York: Oxford University Press, 1997), pp. 282–357.

[130] Nalininath Majumdar, 'Amiya Samhita' ('Collection of Principles Ensuring Immortality'), *Hahnemann*, 8, 7 (1925), 344–5.

[131] Harvansh Lal Sundd, *Sri Sankat Mochan Hanuman Charit Manas* (*Life of Hanuman, Preventer of Crisis*) (Delhi: Aravali Books International, 1998), pp. 439–40.

[132] Amritalal Basu (1853–1929), dramatist and actor, born in Calcutta, was one of the pioneers of the nineteenth-century public theatre in Bengal. A close associate of the legendary Girish Chandra Ghosh Basu, he was fondly termed 'Rasaraj' or the 'king of wits'. He acted in the historic staging of Nil Darpan (1872), and some of his celebrated productions were Til Tarpan (1881), Sati Ki Kalankini (1874), Model School (1873). He was elected the joint President of the Calcutta Bangiya Sahitya Parishad in 1923.

[133] Saratchandra Ghosh, 'Daktar Lokenath Maitra', *Hahnemann*, 22, 12 (1939), 708–10.

[134] Amritalal Basu, *Amrita Madira* (*The Intoxicating Elixir*) (Calcutta, 1903), pp. 79–84.

with considerable religious significance in Hindu Puranas.[135] It compared homoeopathic drugs with '*amrita*' or 'elixir for life', which assured immortality, and upheld it as the only form of western medicine that the Hindus could happily consume without any fear of losing their faith. The poem insisted that Hindu widows as well as children could benefit from homoeopathy.

Translation as Exclusion: Homoeopathy vs. Allopathy

Evidently, the discussions aimed at translating homoeopathy onto the specific Bengali milieu were entrenched within a growing Hindu nationalistic impulse towards constructing a classical Indian past. These efforts, and the discussions they initiated, had wider ramifications in the realm of the Bengali print market. Discourses around translation were entwined with indigenising homoeopathy in ways that delineated its unique status as opposed to practitioners and authors of other western medical sciences. Indeed, it was argued that the innovative and culturally sensitive translations entrenched homoeopathy as more familiar and ubiquitous to the Bengali readers in comparison to any other doctrine.

These claims were upheld specifically in opposition to the practitioners of state medicine, recurrently referred by the homoeopaths as 'orthodox' or the 'allopaths'. A series of articles published in homoeopathic and other medical journals since the late nineteenth century highlighted the ability of homoeopathic translators to adapt its doctrines within prevailing vernacular contexts. While asserting such abilities, these writings often took the form of allegations against practitioners of 'orthodox' medicine, i.e. the 'allopaths'. In his article in *The Hahnemannian Gleanings*, J. N. Chowdhury for instance noted that 'the allopaths of this country are being trained and patronised by the power that be and its super-masters in that distant island'.[136] It was argued that such 'over-guidance' was rendering the allopaths 'impotent and dependent'.[137] Chowdhury argued that the allopathic practitioners and authors lacked any potential to produce culturally sensitive readings of the western tenets. He stated that they never innovated upon its doctrines or contextualised them sensitively. He complained that the allopaths mindlessly 'simply reproduce what their over-sea masters [*sic*] are pleased to observe

[135] Kasi (or Banaras), housing the famous Vishwanath Temple of Lord Siva, is a highly revered religious site for the Hindus.
[136] J. N. Chowdhury, 'Recognition, a Blessing or a Curse', *The Hahnemannian Gleanings*, 1, 5 (June 1930), 208–9.
[137] Ibid.

and this has entailed no small suffering on the public here'.[138] Such authors lamented the lack of any state support for homoeopathy. In his introduction to the third volume of *Berigny and Company's Bengali Homoeopathic Series*, Harikrishna Mallik described homoeopathy as '*Raj shohay biheen*', i.e. 'without any state support'.[139] As a homoeopathic author, he felt compelled under the circumstances to assert homoeopathy's merits as 'scientific medicine' as opposed to allopathy.

Indeed, the self-proclaimed allopathic and homoeopathic authors in the popular print market were engaged in long contentious tussles over the relative scientific merit of their crafts.[140] The issues involving translation, contextualisation and innovative interpretation were drawn into this ongoing polemic between practitioners of the contesting medical traditions.[141] Literature involving squabbles between allopathic and homoeopathic physicians can be traced in Bengali print culture since the early 1870s, and continued well into the twentieth century. These texts were published mostly in the popular medical journals, which dealt broadly with issues of health and hygiene as well as in specialised journals dedicated exclusively to either homoeopathy or 'orthodox' medicine. Correspondence and discussion among these physicians in the pages of these journals often took the form of unpleasant debates. The thread run by 'allopathic' practitioner Pulin Chandra Sanyal and 'homoeopath' Haranath Ray in *Chikitsha Sammilani* is a typical example. The dialogue and debate between this particular pair of physicians ran into several volumes of *Chikitsha Sammilani*, beginning in the fourth volume of the journal in 1887.[142]

These conversations, debates and correspondence published since the 1870s in Bengali yielded a series of binary oppositions, which fed into the

138 Ibid.

139 Harikrishna Mallik, 'Mukhobondo or Introduction', *Berigny and Company's Bengali Homoeopathic Series Number III: Sadrisa Byabastha Chikitsha Dipika* (*Glossary for Treatment According to the System of Similars*) (Calcutta: Berigny and Company, 1870), pp. 1–2.

140 See Shinjini Das, 'Debating Scientific Medicine: Homoeopathy and Allopathy in late Nineteenth Century Medical Print in Bengal', *Medical History*, 56, 4 (2012), 463–80.

141 Such correspondence between contending, rival physicians has been an integral part of the history of homoeopathy in different contexts. For an in-depth study of the American context, see J. H. Warner, 'Orthodoxy and Otherness: Homoeopathy and Regular Medicine in Nineteenth Century America' in Robert Jutte, Guenter B. Risse and John Woodward (eds.), *Culture, Knowledge and Healing: Historical Perspective of Homoeopathic Medicine in Europe and North America*, 1998, pp. 5–30. Also, see Naomi Rogers, 'American Homoeopathy Confronts Scientific Medicine', pp. 31–65 in the same book.

142 Haranath Ray, 'Homoeopathic Mowt e Jowr Chikitsha' ('Homoeopathic Treatment of Fever'), *Chikitsha Sammilani*, 4 (1887), 122–6. Also see Pulin Chandra Sanyal, 'Ini Abar Ki Bolen' ('What Does He Say'), *Chikitsha Sammilani*, 4 (1887), 304–8.

stereotypical descriptions of allopathy and homoeopathy in the vernacular. The cheapness of homoeopathic drugs as opposed to the expensive allopathic medicine; heroic doses of allopathy in contrast to the minute doses in homoeopathy; homoeopathic reliance on a single 'law of cure' as compared to a thorough allopathic disregard for any particular therapeutic law; gentle, sweet homoeopathic drugs as opposed to the bitter-tasting, pungent-smelling, harsh allopathic remedies; rationalistic deductions in allopathy as distinct from the inductive cure in homoeopathy enabled by experimental drug proving – these were some of the common binary distinctions that characterised this literature.[143] To a great extent, the labels 'allopathy' and 'homoeopathy', and the sets of characteristics respectively associated with them, were being neatly delineated through these polemics to a wider reading public. The exclusive ability of homoeopathic authors and practitioners to innovate upon the tenets received from the West, to integrate their own experiences to read homoeopathy contextually, and provide a culturally sensitive interpretation of a European science, were similarly parts of relevant homoeopathic assertions. It was repeatedly argued that such features set homoeopathy apart from the dominant western medical practice like allopathy in Bengal.

Apart from failing to 'translate' imaginatively and sensitively, it was alleged that the allopaths were further guilty of adopting unacceptable expressions and gestures in their polemical opposition to the homoeopaths in the realm of popular print. Such objectionable language, homoeopathic texts lamented, flouted the exalted norms of respectable scientific debate established in and inherited from the West. While emphasising the need to indigenise and translate, the homoeopathic texts thus appeared also to assert a pristine moral code for conducting and narrating western science in the vernacular. Indeed, the form and expression of scientific writing emerged as an important index as much as the content of science. Existing literature, particularly by Gyan Prakash, explicates how scientific ideas across cultures effected 'inappropriate transformations', and displacements in meanings.[144] In the homoeopathic schema, therefore, respectable acts of scientific writing in Bengali were often required to display a balance between imaginative repackaging

[143] The essential scientific claim of homoeopathy lay in its discovery of a law of medicine. Hahnemann 'discovered' the law '*similia similibus curantur*' meaning 'like cures like' in 1790, as discussed in Chapter 2. Widely known as the 'law of similars', it came to be recognised by the homoeopathic practitioners as the fundamental truth of homoeopathy.

[144] See Gyan Prakash, 'Translation and Power', *Another Reason: Science and the Imagination of Modern India*, 1999, pp. 49–85. Also see Pratik Chakrabarti, *Western Science in Modern India: Metropolitan Methods, Colonial Practices* (Delhi: Permanent Black, 2006).

of western science, as well as uncontaminated Victorian moral uprightness in form and expression. Innovative translation of science in the vernacular, homoeopaths warned, should be delimited by obvious moral guidelines. In so doing, homoeopathic writers upheld their own works as benchmarks of credible, respectable and effective rewriting of science in Bengali. The homoeopathic authors were often extremely careful about what could and could not be included in scientific discussions concerning therapeutics. Certain idealised norms of scientific discussion were central to their writings. In his introduction to the fourth manual in *Berigny and Company's Bengali Homoeopathic Series*, Harikrishna Mallik, for instance, portrayed his hesitancy to introduce a discussion involving venereal diseases. He argued that discussion of those diseases invariably entailed the use of vulgar or '*ashleel*' words and phrases. He considered it inappropriate to use such words in serious scientific discussions on treatment. He feared that discussions involving such unchaste words could be revolting to the 'taste' of the respectable men for whom they were meant.[145] Questions of 'morality' and 'taste', thus, remained integral to acts of scientific translations.

Reflecting upon the hostile literature generated by the conflict between the allopathic and homoeopathic authors, physician Keshablal Dey also invoked the varying 'tastes' of the authors in a letter to the editor of the journal *Hahnemann*.[146] He further underlined that such scientific writings should not be belligerent in their tone.[147] The appropriate style and demeanour for registering disagreements and arguments on scientific issues were topics of frequent discussion. In a text carefully compiled by Mahendralal Sircar, the newspaper *Hindu Patriot*, for instance, was quoted as condemning the aggressive tone in which 'he [Mahendralal Sircar] was denounced as a Homoeopath, the grossest personal attack was allowed to be made on him' by the practitioners of allopathy.[148]

In all these homoeopathic writings, there was a deep sense that allopaths were violating the pristine, immaculate norms of discussing 'western science'. The aggressive and inappropriate tone and style of the allopathic writers were condemned. In his monograph, Mahendralal Sircar complained how the 1867 scientific meeting of the Bengal Medical Association, where the allopaths attacked him for publicly embracing homoeopathy, turned out to be a 'farce' and

[145] Harikrishna Mallik, 'Introduction', *Berigny and Company's Bengali Homeopathic Series No. IV: Sadrisa Byabastha Chikitsha Dipika* (*Glossary for Treatment According to the System of Similars*) (Calcutta: Berigny and Company, 1870), page number not cited.

[146] Keshablal Dey, 'Protibaad' ('Protest'), *Hahnemann*, 5, 10 (1922), 514–15. [147] Ibid.

[148] Mahendralal Sircar, *On the Supposed Uncertainty in Medical Science and on the Relation between Diseases and Their Remedial Agents* (Calcutta: Anglo Sanskrit Press, 1903), p. 67.

a 'comedy' rather than an 'engaged scientific discussion'.[149] These homoeopathic publications repeatedly alleged that the allopathic attacks directed at them were falling short of, and becoming distorted caricatures of, a certain given standard of western scientific discussion. It was pointed out that attempts at '*somalochana*' or 'scientific critique' frequently ended up being mere '*jhagra*' or 'outright quarrel'. An anonymous homoeopathic author in *Chikitsha Sammilani* expressed regret that,

> Informed debates involve a lot of reading and learning. In place of debating uneducated men simply, shout. It is very difficult to critique, very easy to quarrel. It is embarrassing to see educated men quarrel in the name of debating and critiquing.[150]

Discussions about translations and the norms of conducting and narrating western science in the vernacular, therefore, emerged in the homoeopathic discourse as a powerful tool to delineate itself from any other western medical doctrines. It helped the homoeopathic authors define their 'other' in the print market. The homoeopathic publications projected 'translation' as a tool of exclusion that rendered homoeopathy most suited for a vernacular audience. Interestingly, the trope of 'acceptable translation' was often invoked to express scorn against certain groups of homoeopathic practitioners as well, particularly those located beyond the urban enclaves. The following section traces how 'translation' as a concept was also invoked and emphasised by the homoeopathic authors in defining 'authentic homoeopathy'.

Policing 'Mofussil' Practices

I have so far traced two interrelated yet different processes of 'translation' as they recurred in homoeopathic publications of the late nineteenth to early twentieth century. Just as translation, at one level, was a linguistic exercise involving communication between at least two languages, at another, it was related to processes of contextualisation and imaginative articulation of cultural meanings. The two processes often came together, as I illustrated, in targeting the 'allopaths' as practitioners of illegitimate translations. They were also instrumental in delineating a space for pure homoeopathy that reflected the inherent class bias of the translated texts. Although they advocated innovative contextualisation and cultural reinterpretation of western science, a considerable bulk of the homoeopathic

[149] Ibid., pp. 55–6.
[150] Anonymous, 'Letter to the Editor', *Chikitsha Sammilani*, 5 (1888), 98.

publications also asserted a hierarchy of spaces and authorship in relation to what they considered as 'good translation'. Highlighting a 'difference' between the practices of western medicine in the urban centres of Calcutta or Dacca and beyond, these urban publications admonished disparately dispersed *mofussil* or suburban practitioners. Indeed, these publications constructed an active urban-*mofussil* binary, in constituting the *mofussil* as a place where science inevitably turned into its caricature. Unbridled innovations, irrelevant reinterpretations and associated ill-translations of the meaning and purpose of homoeopathy in the *mofussil* were emphatically discouraged. Such trends were condemned even as the village practitioners referred to their specific sociocultural contexts as the impulse behind such innovations. Indeed, *mofussil* efforts in cultural innovation were castigated as serious threats to the sanctity of 'scientific' homoeopathy.

The homoeopathic literature illustrates an entrenched concern at the increasing bulk of vernacular homoeopathic publications. The Calcutta-based authors regularly blamed the *mofussil* readers for such overproduction of cheap printed texts. The journal *Hahnemann* published a series of editorial articles in 1884 titled 'Homoeopathic Bangla Sahitya' or 'Homoeopathic Bengali Literature'. The author expressed his disappointment with the overproduction of Bengali homoeopathic tracts, pointing out their various disadvantages.[151] He registered dismay at the linguistic standard and the arbitrary nature of translation in these publications. As already noted in the first section, these authors regretted the disparaging impact of such publications on the Bengali language as a whole. The editor Basanta Kumar Dutta, owner of the Calcutta-based B. K. Dutta and Company, was convinced that the *mofussil* and village-based ill-educated people of various lower-middle-class professions were primarily responsible for the increasing demand of those cheap translated tracts.[152] He felt that such inefficient, random translations were in wide circulation among the semi-literate village people, who chose to read them in plenty as they considered it to be the easiest route to a respectable profession like medicine. Indeed, Dutta tried to raise the alarm, saying, 'the semi-literate unintelligent people in the villages diligently buy and read these substandard, cheap tracts. Hence, with the swelling of such bad publications there is a simultaneous increase in the ranks of these ill-taught physicians'.[153] The article elaborated on the

[151] Basanta Kumar Datta, 'Homoeopathic Bangla Sahitya' ('Homoeopathic Bengali Literature'), *Hahnemann*, 2, 10 (1884), 181–3.
[152] Basanta Kumar Datta, 'Homoeopathic Bangla Sahitya' ('Homoeopathic Bengali Literature'), *Hahnemann*, 2, 11 (1884), 202.
[153] Basanta Kumar Datta, 'Homoeopathic Bangla Sahitya' ('Homoeopathic Bengali Literature'), *Hahnemann*, 2, 10 (1884), 182.

horrible inefficiency of the village-based physicians who blindly emulated the cheap homoeopathic translations. One can hardly miss the unmistakable ring of scepticism about homoeopathy practised and consumed in the *mofussil*. The author reiterated that 'the standard, good quality texts and physicians are not adequately appreciated beyond the capital (i.e. Calcutta)'.[154]

The history of standardisation of any language is significantly related to broader changes within the social formation in terms of the emergence of new classes and their ideologies.[155] Existing literature maps the changing discursive role of the Bengali *bhadralok* in shaping the Bengali language over the course of the nineteenth century.[156] The attempts of this western-educated upper class at regulating the standards of non-urban publications can be located within this broader story of 'guardianship over language'. Yet, in case of homoeopathy, control over language was entwined also with assessing the scientific merit of the publications.[157] Thus, through the late nineteenth and early twentieth century, related to the issue of language, the use of 'patent drugs' by homoeopathic physicians in the *mofussil* was a topic of typical urban concern.[158] In a letter to the journal *Hahnemann*, Ramcharan Sadhukhan noted that it was a common sight in the villages for the 'homoeopathic practitioners' to possess and prescribe from a repertoire of patent drugs.[159] His letter blasted a particular *mofussil* homoeopath, Amulya Kumar Chandra, who allegedly promoted his own patent '*deshabandhu batika*' in the pages of *Hahnemann*. Sadhukhan complained that the drug concerned was misleadingly advertised as a 'guaranteed cure of all kinds of malarial fevers'.[160] It also promised to cure all patients 'within forty-eight hours'.

[154] Ibid., p. 182.
[155] Drawing upon Renee Balibar's work on the development of French language and transformation of class relationships in France, Tithi Bhattacharya shows developments in the Bengali language in the context of class; see Bhattacharya, *Sentinels of Culture: Class, Education and the Colonial Intellectual in Bengal, 1848–1885* (Delhi: Oxford University Press, 2005), p. 217.
[156] Ibid., pp. 192–219.
[157] In the context of colonial Punjab, Kavita Sivaramakrishnan's work has explored in depth the interrelated trajectories of language and medical reforms. See Kavita Sivaramakrishnan, *Old Potion, New Bottle: Recasting Indigenous Medicine in Colonial Punjab 1850–1940* (Hyderabad: Orient Blackswan, 2006).
[158] *Columbia Encyclopaedia* describes patent medicine as packaged drugs that can be obtained without prescription. It clarifies that the term was formerly used to describe quack remedies sold by peddlers, the sense in which it appears in the homoeopathic literature of this time.
[159] Ramcharan Sadhukhan, 'Patra' ('Letter'), *Hahnemann*, 9, 10 (1926), 435–6.
[160] Ibid., p. 435.

Interestingly, Amulya Kumar Chandra replied in the journal *Hahnemann* with a long letter defending his use of patent drugs. His letter invoked the contingencies of rural situations in justifying his use of the said '*deshabandhu batika*'. He emphasised that 'only physicians practising in the villages would know the widespread havoc caused by malaria with the onset of monsoon every year'.[161] He described the socioeconomic conditions of the hard-pressed farmers for whom the monsoon was a very busy season. Such cultivators were the bulk of the patients in rural Bengal. Amulya Kumar Chandra argued that his prescription of patent medicine was essentially related to the treatment of a large number of patients at a particular time of the year in villages. He wrote that his innovations were imperative on a combination of factors like the incapacity of his patients to visit him every day or pay the fees regularly, their compulsion to be in the field daily, the lack of any possibility of gathering their precise symptoms and so on. The author reminded the readers that 'no one should be misled into believing that I have recommended deshbandhu batika in every case of malaria. It is to be prescribed only in the rural situations described by me where due to the aforementioned constraints, fever cannot be controlled by any other means'.[162]

Indeed, elaborating on their specific contexts, the practitioners based in the *mofussil*, in turn, often highlighted their differences from the city-based big urban pharmacies and authorities. A lengthy advertisement for the 'Electro Homoeopathic Pharmacy' appeared in the manual titled *Homoeopathic Mowt e Manashik Rog Chikitsha* (*Homoeopathic Treatment of Mental Diseases*), published from the village of Khagra in Murshidabad district in 1904.[163] This advertisement stated that the pharmacy had branches at various *mofussil* locations in Saidabad and Berhampore, and a clientele dispersed across districts of Bhagolpur, Munger, Chattagram and Noakhali.[164] At one level, the advertisement noted that their drugs were as good in quality and as well-packaged as those of the 'reputed pharmacies in Calcutta'.[165] However, it also underlined that the *mofussil* pharmacies rendered certain services that could hardly be matched by their urban counterparts. The advertisement presented a list of these services, which included helping the ailing patients who visited Murshidabad for treatment find suitable places to stay.[166]

161 Amulya Kumar Chandra, 'Patra' ('Letter'), *Hahnemann*, 9, 10 (1926), 543–5.
162 Ibid., p. 546.
163 'Advertisement of Electro Homoeopathy Pharmacy' in Bipin Bihari Dasgupta, *Homoeopathy Mowt e Manashik Rog Chikitsha (Treatment of Mental Health According to Homoeopathy)* (Murshidabad: Kanika Press, 1904), page number not cited.
164 Ibid. 165 Ibid. 166 Ibid.

The advertisement of another *mofussil*-based store, National Pharmacy, offered a range of similar services.[167] The pharmacy, it claimed, performed multiple functions beyond those conducted in the urban homoeopathic pharmacies. National Pharmacy, for instance, promised to 'supply special items of Murshidabad including silk cloth, buttons and other trinkets made of ivory ... at reasonable prices'.[168] They even pledged to assist their consumers and others in multifarious other functions including paying taxes, seeking legal advice on specific cases, appointing city-based lawyers and the like.[169] These pharmacies, typically, also listed a number of 'patent drugs' as an important distinguishing feature of the *mofussil* homoeopathic pharmacies (see Fig. 3.3). Advertisements for the National Pharmacy included a long list of drugs including 'Hysteria Cura', 'Firingi Domon', 'Ringworm Ointment', 'Gonorrhea Drop', 'Nervina' and others. The Pharmacy declared itself the 'sole agents of the patent drugs'.[170]

The urban publications condemning the *mofussil* displacements remained unconvinced by such innovations. Highlighting his position against the use of patent drugs, Ramcharan Sadhukhan, for instance, appealed to the editors as well as the larger medical fraternity to curb such practices.[171] He argued that by recommending the 'unscientific' patent drugs, homoeopath Amulya Kumar Chandra only highlighted his personal ignorance in 'homoeopathic science'.[172] He urged that regular publication of advertisements promoting these 'unscientific' practices by journals like *Hahnemann* would cause immense harm to 'real homoeopathy'.[173]

Yet, one also notices a traffic across the urban-*mofussil* divide on these issues of translation and displacement. A shift is detectable around the second quarter of the twentieth century, when big Calcutta-based established pharmacies like M. Bhattacharya and Company, Hahnemann Publishing Company, Batakrishna Pal and Company and others began advertising their own patent drugs (see Fig. 3.4). For instance, a promotional brochure for M. Bhattacharya and Company, published in the journal *Banik* in 1930, advertised a range of patent homoeopathic drugs including the anti-malarial drug malogen.[174] From

[167] 'Advertisement of National Pharmacy' in Bipin Bihari Dasgupta, *Homoeopathy Mowt e Manashik Rog Chikitsha (Treatment of Mental Health According to Homoeopathy)*, 1904, page number not cited.
[168] Ibid. [169] Ibid. [170] Ibid.
[171] Ramcharan Sadhukhan, 'Patra' ('Letter'), *Hahnemann*, 9, 10 (1926), 436.
[172] Ibid., p. 436. [173] Ibid., p. 436.
[174] 'Advertisement of M. Bhattacharya and Company', in *Banik*, Shravan [1337] 1930, pp. 29–36.

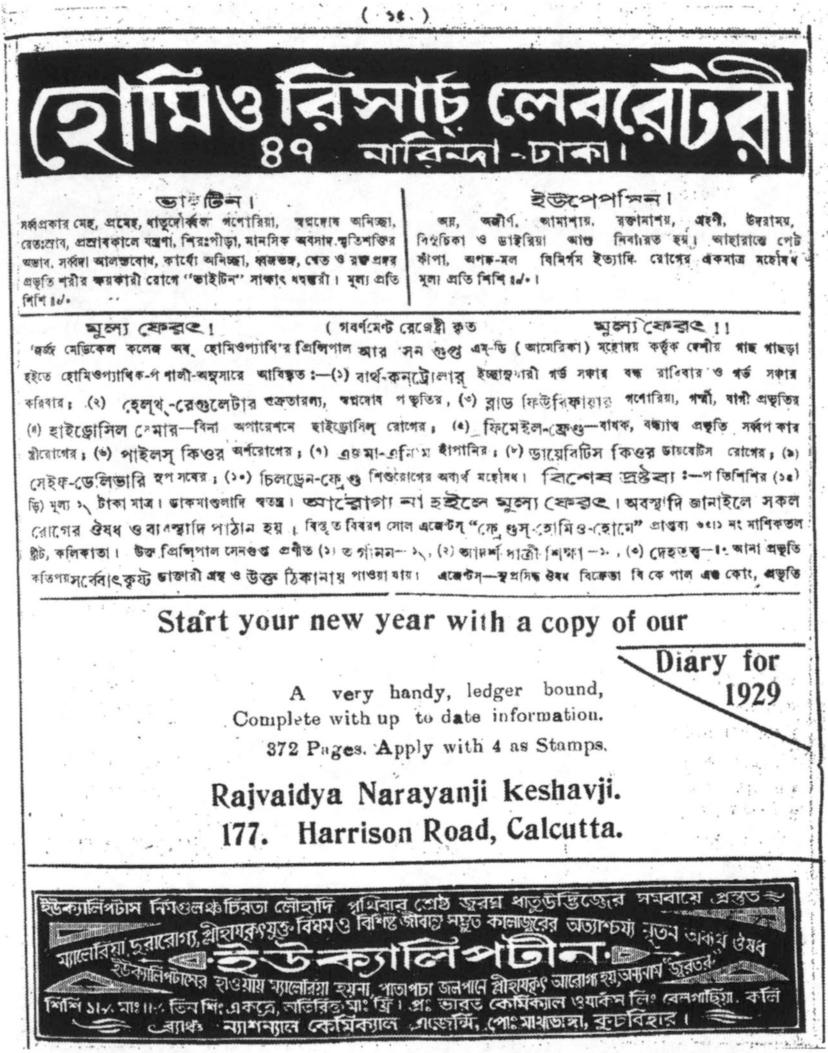

Fig. 3.3 Advertisement for the patent medicine Vytin, and Eupepsin from Homoeo Research Laboratory, Narinda, Dacca district in the Bengali journal *Grihasthamangal*, 1, 10 (1928), 399. Reproduced from the collection of the Archives of the Centre for Studies in Social Sciences, Calcutta.

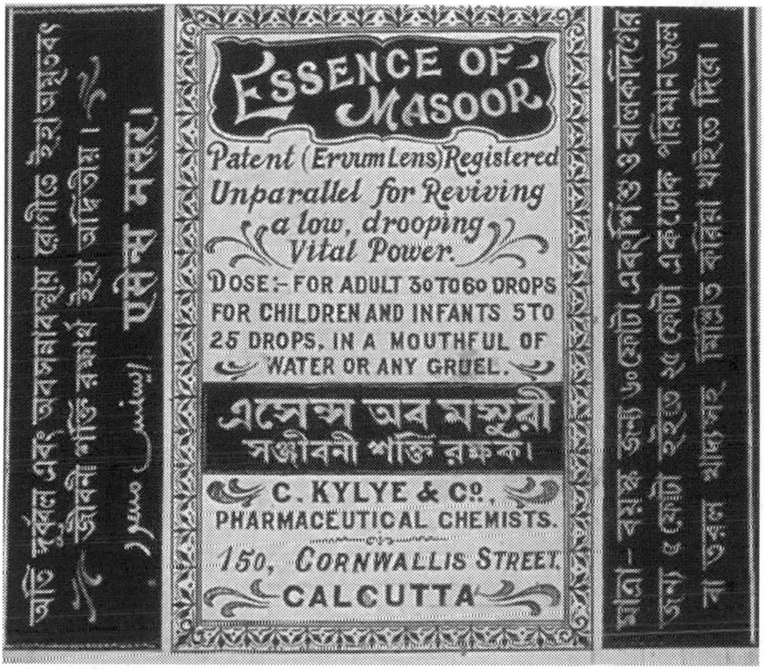

Fig. 3.4 Advertisement for the patent tonic 'Essence of Masoor' by the Calcutta-based homoeopathic firm C. Kylye and Company. Reproduced from the collection of the Archives of the Centre for Studies in Social Sciences, Calcutta.

1940, advertisements for the Hahnemann Publishing Company also promoted patent drugs like 'Jvorona', 'Alfalfa Tonic' and 'Masoori Essence'.[175]

Among other explanations, these advertisements emphasised that the urban firms had changed their opinion of patent drugs since such products suited the tastes and the economic constraints of Bengal's vast rural population. Evidently, the urban authorities on homoeopathy were in dialogue with and drawing upon their counterparts dispersed across the *mofussil*.

Conclusion

The sustained engagement with the theme of 'translation' that is evident in the homoeopathic literature reveals translation as an inventive

[175] 'Advertisement of Jvarona of Hahnemann Publishing Company' in *Hahnemann*, 23, 5 (1940), 8.

process involving interpretation, explanation, appropriation and omission, among other operations. It also indicates the creative tension involved in the negotiation of meaning across languages and locales, which chimes in with the growing corpus of scholarship on colonial science translations. These works illustrate how acts of translation were inevitably mired in 'questions of linguistic tradition, cultural purity, and modernity itself, these debates played out against the background of colonial rule'.[176] Bengali translators with proclaimed aims of vernacularising homoeopathy at once reified western science and English language as global, universal categories, while simultaneously contesting that status by rendering it local and indigenous.

Discussions around 'incommensurability of knowledge' were addressed by homoeopathic authors in ways that caused the 'politics of neologism' to congeal with growing 'anxieties over a denationalised Bengali language'. Tracing the impact of translation in the entwined realms of language and science, I have reflected upon the inroads made into the Bengali vocabulary by a range of English words (often with supposedly German roots) and terminology. Of these, the more recurrent and significant were those including 'homoeopathy', 'Organon', 'vital force', 'Hahnemann', 'drug proving', 'chronic disease' and 'law of similars'. Simultaneously, attempts were also being made to translate and adapt far too many English (foreign) words to Bengali. Efforts at such scientific translations were allegedly generating a prose that was Bengali only in its form, alphabet and verbs. The meaning and interpretation of such words and the context and location of the translators became critical in such circumstances. Thus 'homoeopathy' became '*amiya-patha*', 'potency' was interpreted and translated as '*shakti* ', the Sanskrit verse '*samah samang samayati*' was written to be a close translation of the Latin phrase '*similia similibus curantur*', and Hahnemann was sometimes associated with the healing prowess of the Hindu God Hanumana. The chapter has dwelt on the associated displacements in meanings and their implications in hierarchising languages and cultures.

To be sure, existing literature has suggested how translations of science often acquired displaced, different and even 'enchanted' meaning in colonial India.[177] The homoeopathic discourse on translation, however,

176 Marwa Elshakry, 'Knowledge in Motion: The Cultural Politics of Modern Science Translation in Arabic', p. 702. Also see David Wright, 'Translation of Modern Western Science in Nineteenth Century China, 1840–1895', *Isis*, 89 (1998), 653–73.

177 See Gyan Prakash, 'Translation and Power', *Another Reason: Science and the Imagination of Modern India*, 1999, pp. 49–85; and Prakash, 'Science "Gone Native" in Colonial India', *Representations*, 40, Special Issue: Seeing Science (Autumn 1992), 153–78. Also see Shruti Kapila, 'The Enchantment of Science in India', *Isis*, 101, 1 (2010), 120–32.

illustrates that linguistic hybridity and displacements in meaning and form were not always accidental, but often deliberate and programmatic. To the homoeopathic authors, literal translations of 'science' were often inadequate until they were culturally integrated and transposed within a vernacular context. Accordingly, their translations drew upon religious iconographies to depict Hahnemann, associating him with the healing prowess of Siva or Hanumana; interpreted key homoeopathic tenets such as 'vital force' through religio-cultural references to Indian philosophical understandings on spirituality; and self-consciously invoked a range of familiar and popular tropes. In turn, homoeopathic translations reinforced stereotypes concerning a nationalism-inspired Bengali public culture, which was increasingly Hindu in orientation.

In the production of a vernacularised homoeopathy, the process of translation further posited a western-educated elite as authorities on science. Operating at the interstices of cultures, this western-educated, urban elite often used 'translation' as a means for establishing political and cultural hegemony. However, they also policed the acceptable limit of such localisation and vernacularisation, which exposed inherent class aspirations.[178] Their discussions negotiated between the compulsion to translate and the limits to such translations. Indeed, a collusion between class, language politics and the guardianship of scientific knowledge is made clear from the ways in which the processes of 'translation' excluded various groups, particularly the suburban *mofussil* physicians, unrelated to the big Calcutta families, as improper or illegitimate practitioners of science. 'Authentic homoeopathy' was defined against the insensitive, often inadequate translation of the allopaths/orthodoxy on the one hand and the mindless and 'unscientific' innovations in the *mofussil* on the other.

The discourses around translation posit the 'vernacular' as a relational category. Discussions involving translation hardly remained confined to the Bengali language alone. I have showed that a single act of translation could encompass and implicate a range of languages including German, English, Bengali, Sanskrit and Marathi. The 'vernacular' in this context emerged as a shifting label that could be ascribed to various languages at different points. Thus, English could often be the carrier of vernacular homoeopathy

[178] I have preferred the term 'vernacularisation' rather than 'indigenisation' since the latter is often considered more restrictive, implying efforts to establish homoeopathy as directly part of the Indian tradition, such as the ayurvedic corpus. Chapter 4 engages with the issue more directly.

as much as Bengali or Marathi. In so doing, the chapter is in conversation with recent theorisations that consider the vernacular to be 'a flexible concept – more dependent on the sensibilities it imparts rather than the language'.[179]

Finally, in pursuing recent literature, I raise the possibility of going beyond a twofold model of science translation. Each act of translation, in reality, often remained a moment in a chain of interpretation, involving many languages. Translations operated beyond the paradigm of 'original and translated', which were continuously reworked in processes of translation.[180] Drawing upon the insights of Paul de Man, who sees translation as a process that 'shows in the original a mobility, an instability, which at first one did not notice', current researchers are pushing towards establishing translation as essentially multiple in nature.[181] Careful study of homoeopathic translations in Bengal reveals most acts of translation as a point in a continuous chain of interpretation, often involving many languages across a global network of science popularisers. Digging through metatextual layers, one often finds major journals and texts like them being used in turn as sources of ideas in yet further texts and interpretations. Viewed from this perspective, Hahnemann and his texts emerge not as an unchanging standard, but rather as 'part of an extended system of meanings, references and significations'.[182] This further complicates the conventional 'displacement' model of perceiving the reception of western science in the colonies that often assumes a given, preformed 'science'. Not recognised as 'scientific medicine' by mainstream European medical authorities, nor endorsed by the colonial state at least until the early twentieth century, homoeopathy, in fact, garnered much of its scientific status in the realm of popular print, through processes of multiple translations.

[179] For a development of this concept, see Raziuddin Aquil and Partha Chatterjee (eds.), *History in the Vernacular* (New Delhi: Permanent Black, 2008), pp. 1–19.

[180] Interesting new work is being done on how translations destabilise the original, the supposedly classical and the vernacular, and how they influence one another. Ronit Ricci's work on translations of Islam in South and Southeast Asia explicates the ways in which Arabic was vernacularised, while the local Southeast Asian languages were often Arabicised. See Ronit Ricci, *Islam Translated: Literature, Conversion and the Arabic Cosmopolis of South and South East Asia* (Chicago: University of Chicago Press, 2011), p. 17.

[181] Drawing upon Paul de Man's essay 'Conclusions: Walter Benjamin's 'The Task of the Translator', Marwa Elshakry builds up this point in her book on Arabic translations of Darwin. See Marwa Elshakry, *Reading Darwin in Arabic*, pp. 5–6.

[182] Ibid.

4 Healing the Home
Indigeneity, Self-Help and the Hindu Joint Family

> 'Homoeopathy is our own Vedic property which has recently come back to us dressed in western attire. If we make it our own, with time it will be most efficient in maintaining the power, health and resources of independent "swaraj" India.'[1]

> ' . . . if the householders had to visit a doctor or a kaviraj on every domestic complaint, it would be extremely taxing on the familial budget.'[2]

> 'It is more than probable that the Indian flora contains specimens which would best be adapted to cure diseases peculiar to this country. Will there not be found, in that very same country, specimens of men, ready to subject themselves to proving of the drugs of their own soil?'[3]

In the tenth volume of the journal *Hahnemann* published by the Hahnemann Publishing Company, 'amateur' physician Kunjalal Sen, a retired clerk by profession, contributed an autobiographical account of his personal journey of learning homoeopathy. The article, titled 'Abishvashir Homoeo Mantre Deekha' or 'The Conversion of an Unbeliever to Homoeopathy', narrated how Sen introduced homoeopathic drugs within his domesticity. As the self-proclaimed 'head' of an extended Hindu joint family, he was impressed by the inexpensive and 'magical' cure of his youngest son from what was suspected as a severe case of typhoid.[4] The physician who cured his son advised Kunjalal to read the Homoeopathic *Organon* on his own. Intrigued, Sen eventually ended up reading the *Organon*, the *Materia Medica* and other fundamental texts under the physician's guidance. The result, in his own words, was the following:

[1] Kalikumar Bhattacharya, 'Ashar Alok' ('Light of Hope'), Hahnemann, 7, 2 (1924), 80.
[2] Anonymous, 'Atma Nirbharata'('Self-Sufficiency'), *Swasthya*, 3, 7 (1899), 204–5.
[3] Ibid.
[4] Kunjalal Sen, 'Abishvashir Homoeo Mantre Deekha' ('Conversion of an Unbeliever to Homoeopathy'), *Hahnemann*, 10, 6 (1927), 295–300.

> Before I took refuge in homoeopathy, within my big joint-family, every year there were a few cases of typhoid, bronchitis or pneumonia. Western allopathic treatment of such diseases drained off huge amount of money . . . once a small child was detected with pneumonia and was treated allopathically . . . what a treatment it was! . . . That case of pneumonia used up all my hard-earned money and left the child weakened for life. Since converting to homoeopathy, I have been able to prescribe gentle, indigenous drugs myself for worse instances of pneumonia and typhoid. They have all recovered without any permanent damage caused to their health. Besides, since I introduced homoeopathy, such frequent illness has almost stopped visiting our household. Before converting to homoeopathy, we followed the allopathic treatment and our monthly familial budget on drugs alone was around Rs. 20. Now, unless it is a case of surgery we do not need doctors at all. Not only that, women can look after themselves and I can look after the health of even my neighbours, friends and distant relatives with the power of the small globules.[5]

Hidden within the personal narrative of Kunjalal Sen are some of the central themes that help decipher homoeopathy's distinctive appeal within colonial households. In many ways, Sen's account is reflective of the multifaceted anxieties plaguing middle-class Bengali domesticity at the turn of the twentieth century. Concern over domestic health was intricately tied to questions of familial resource and economic management within the extended Hindu household. Equally, the article suggests a tension among ordinary householders who had to choose between expensive western modes of medico-rational practice, and the available 'indigenous' knowledge, to ensure healthy living. Mastering homoeopathy at home, through extensive reading of key texts such as *Organon*, provided Kunjalal with a means to confront these challenges head-on. One can hardly miss the triumphant note in Sen's account as he narrates how he came to grips with issues of domestic health, women's health, strain on the familial economy and unwarranted wasteful westernisation all at once.

Pervasive as the abovementioned accounts were, unpacking some of the anxieties helps us situate homoeopathy's unique position within colonial domesticity. Looking into homoeopathy's domestication, I explore specifically the rich gamut of domestic health manuals published mostly by the leading homoeopathic firms. Along with these manuals, widely circulating homoeopathic journals, too, included steady streams of articles on themes of domesticity, targeting women or specifically the '*grihastha*' (i.e. householder). The term '*bhadralok*' has been the most commonly used category in South Asian historiography with relation to the English-educated, modernising – though not necessarily affluent –

[5] Ibid., pp. 299–300.

middling to upper stratum of society. The homoeopathic manuals stand out for their focus on the figure of the '*grihastha*', or the middle-class male in strictly his familial context (i.e. as the householder).

I have shown in Chapter 3 that through efforts to 'translate' homoeopathy, the vernacular print market reiterated homoeopathy's status as a German science with western scientific credentials compatible with ancient Indian philosophy. Here I explore the simultaneous strands of vernacular discussion specifically pertaining to domestic health, which argued for homoeopathy's ancient Indian origin. Even when they acknowledged the European roots of homoeopathy, authors of domestic health manuals often championed it as the most effective indigenous remedy for Indians over the archaic and increasingly outdated ayurveda. The vigorous championing of homoeopathy's indigeneity needs to be studied against the backdrop of growing concern over westernisation of Indian families as well as a snowballing mobilisation by ayurveda and unani advocates, particularly in north India, since the early years of the twentieth century. Existing literature delineates the efforts by vaidic and unani practitioners to garner state support for 'indigenous' medicine that culminated in the formation of the All India Vaidic and Unani Tibbi Conference by 1910.[6]

Along with concerns over indigeneity, I explore more generally the homoeopathic intervention in the pervasive discourse on quotidian domestic health. As is known, the institution of family was the central focus of a larger nationalist concern with the preservation of Indian identity in the face of westernisation of values and lifestyle – family was repeatedly highlighted as the blueprint, the foundational unit and spiritual core of the emergent nation.[7] Central to this literature was a concern for the declining health of the Indian people. Works on sexuality and gender have looked at the ways in which medicine and scientific reform mediated issues of ideal domesticity, conjugality and health practices including reproductive

[6] See Kavita Sivaramakrishnan, *Old Potions, New Bottles: Recasting Indigenous Medicine in Colonial Punjab, 1850–1945* (Hyderabad: Orient Longman, 2006), pp. 113–21; Rachel Berger, *Ayurveda Made Modern: Political Histories of Indigenous Medicine in North India, 1900–1955* (Basingstoke: Palgrave Macmillan, 2013), pp. 106–27; and Neshat Quaiser, 'Science, Institution and Colonialism: Tibbiya College of Delhi – 1889–1947' in Uma Das Gupta (ed.) *Science and Modern India: An Institutional History, c. 1784–1947* (Delhi: Pearson Longman, 2010).

[7] For a comprehensive discussion of the link between debates on Bengali domesticity, and the civil-political society of the emerging nation, see Dipesh Chakrabarty, 'The Difference: Deferral of (A) Colonial Modernity: Public Debates on Domesticity in Colonial Bengal', *History Workshop*, 36 (1993), 1–36; and Partha Chatterjee, *The Nation and Its Fragments: Colonial and Postcolonial Histories* (Princeton, NJ: Princeton University Press, 1993), pp. 116–34.

health.[8] These interesting works have opened up discussions on the myriad facets of the nationalist discourse on the intersections of health, body and national sovereignty.

Simultaneously, the nationalist popular print culture of the time exhibited a growing concern over the structure and vitality of the traditional Indian family, characterised as the 'joint family' or the '*ekannoborti poribaar*'.[9] Authors raised an alarm about the impending disintegration of the traditional Hindu joint family in the face of colonial rule. Colonialism, English education and the westernisation of social values were identified as critical factors engendering a crisis in what was highlighted as the 'eastern Hindu' life traditionally lived within the joint family. Such texts agonised over an excessive westernisation resulting in an extravagant, indulgent lifestyle that weakened the foundation of traditional family structure. They prescribed efficient management of economy by shunning foreign goods and ideas – an idea that especially gained currency after the years of *swadeshi* nationalism. Since R. C. Dutta formulated the thesis of 'economic drain'[10] through colonialism, this notion had been repeated endlessly in the nationalist literature and had became a common trope in the vernacular press by the 1870s.[11] Unsurprisingly, the 'economic drain' thesis transposed itself powerfully onto the anxious discourses on the future of joint families.

I contend that authors advocating homoeopathy strategically intervened in these apparently disparate discourses, and wove them together, in order to uphold the practice of homoeopathy as an ideal 'indigenous' remedy for nationalist apprehensions pertaining to the decline of health and disintegration of joint families. Homoeopathy was written about as the most cost-effective, competent and 'indigenous' solution to domestic health problems. It rendered lay householders, including women, self-reliant in terms of health and promised to empower the reformist Bengali household with a uniquely western doctrine with distinct indigenous roots. Homoeopathy's greatest strength lay in ensuring in the perpetuation of a joint familial situation by rationing wasteful expenditure. Bengali

[8] Charu Gupta, *Sexuality, Obscenity, Community: Women, Muslims and the Hindu Public in Colonial India* (Ranikhet: Permanent Black, 2005). Also see Maneesha Lal, 'Purdah as Pathology: Gender and the Circulation of Medical Knowledge in Late Colonial India', in Sarah Hodges (ed.), *Reproductive Health in India: History, Politics, Controversies* (New Delhi: Orient Longman, 2006), pp. 85–114; and Joseph Alter, 'Celibacy, Sexuality and the Transformation of Gender into Nationalism in North India', *The Journal of Asian Studies*, 54, 1 (1994), 45–66.

[9] See for instance Anonymous, 'Bange Ekannabarti Paribar' ('Joint Family in Bengal'), *Grihasthali*, 1, 4 (1884), 94–6.

[10] R. C. Dutta, *The Economic History of British India* (London: Kegan Paul, 1902).

[11] Manu Goswami, *Producing India: From Colonial Economy to National Space* (Chicago: University of Chicago Press, 2004), p. 227.

domesticity, moreover, was projected not only as the site for the consumption of indigenous drugs but also for its production.

As distinct from self-centred, Europe-induced, individualised consumption, use of homoeopathy signified an acceptable, indigenous form of consumption compatible with the commitment towards a moral economy of family. Beyond the mere materiality of drugs, consumption and even production of homoeopathy within the household was perceived as an embodied way of living – an efficient disciplining mechanism to reform colonial domesticities through biomoral regulations. In explicating this proposition, the chapter also contends that the homoeopathic discussions on domesticity idealised and reified the Hindu joint family as traditional and timeless. The disjunction between the romantic celebration of the joint family and its actualisation becomes apparent if one remembers that the homoeopathic entrepreneur families vigorously championed the cause of the nucleated family while discussing issues of personal inheritance (as shown in Chapter 1), while their publications on domestic health, discussed here, chimed in with the wider nationalist anxiety around preserving the timeless joint family.

Innovating the Indigenous

By the early years of the twentieth century, the concept of 'indigeneity' was a politically loaded, emotive issue in India. The years of *swadeshi* nationalism had set up a backdrop whereby idioms of *swadeshi* (literally meaning home-grown/indigenous) were linked to ideas of *swaraj* (i.e. political sovereignty). Existing works show that a welding of *swadeshi* and *swaraj* was the ideological core of late nineteenth-century economic nationalism.[12] There was an increased effort to delineate and authenticate indigeneity also in the sphere of medico-scientific knowledge and culture. A recent spate of research on ayurveda and unani has examined their respective late nineteenth-century claims to the status of India's authentic indigenous medical tradition vis-à-vis modern medicine.[13] Rachel Berger and Kavita Sivaramakrishnan demonstrate how claims of indigeneity were constituted by urban ayurvedic publicists in colonial north India around issues of language and temporality.[14] The print

[12] Manu Goswami, *Producing India*, pp. 242–76.

[13] Kavita Sivaramakrishnan, *Old Potions, New Bottles*, pp. 114–25; and Guy Attewell, *Refiguring Unani Tibb: Plural Healing in Late Colonial India* (New Delhi: Orient Longman, 2007).

[14] Rachel Berger, *Ayurveda Made Modern*, pp. 75–9; and Kavita Sivaramakrishnan, 'The Languages of Science, the Vocabulary of Politics: Challenges to Medical Revival in Punjab', *Journal for Social History of Medicine*, 21, 3 (2008), 521–39.

market, including medical advertisements, has been pointed out as a crucial site where ayurvedic notions of indigeneity were fundamentally negotiated and publicised for the wider public.[15]

In Chapter 3 I noted how epistemological equivalence was being claimed between homoeopathic doctrine and ancient Indian philosophy, centred around the power of the invisible, minute spirit. Practitioners and authors in vernacular print contended that such equivalence rendered German homoeopathy culturally translatable to Indian languages and ethos. Here I discuss parallel strands of contested genealogies and origin myths, all of which trace out antique Indian origins of homoeopathy. These assertions included engagements with simultaneous publications that claimed ayurveda as part of an authentic Indian classical past. My discussion is informed by the literature that has studied the historical construction of labels like 'indigenous' and 'classical' through myriad registers such as language, music and gender identity.[16] The existing historiography, which simply notes the indigenisation of western sciences in India, merits the addition of nuance. Surinder M. Bharadwaj, for instance, had argued that the terms of homoeopathy's indigenisation in India derived from its remarkable affinity with the therapeutic principles of ayurveda.[17] I refrain from taking such 'affinities', 'overlaps' or 'equivalence' between two medical traditions for granted. Such assertions of homoeopathy being 'indigenous' and 'natural' to the Indian context were consciously and recurrently propounded in the vernacular print by practitioner-turned-authors making careers out of writing on homoeopathy. The negotiations in print helped homoeopathy delineate a unique identity for itself, of being simultaneously modern and traditional, of being western, yet with entrenched Indian roots.

In the manuals advocating homoeopathy, ayurveda was often recognised as the authentic, traditional medical knowledge of India. Yet, even as they acknowledged ayurveda's rich heritage, the homoeopaths invariably drew attention to the pathetic condition of ayurvedic knowledge in British India. The article 'Bharatbarshe Homoeopathy' or 'Homoeopathy in India' in the journal *Hahnemann*, for instance, began by describing the

[15] For a historiographical discussion, see Projit Bihari Mukharji, 'Symptoms of Dis-Ease: New Trends in the Histories of Indigenous South Asian Medicine', *History Compass*, 9 (December 2011), 893–4.

[16] See Eric Hobsbawm and Terence Ranger (eds.), *The Invention of Tradition* (Cambridge: Cambridge University Press, 1992); and Lata Mani, *Contentious Traditions: The Debate on Sati in Colonial India* (Berkeley: University of California Press, 1998).

[17] Surinder Bharadwaj, 'Homeopathy in India' in Giri Raj Gupta (ed.), *The Social and Cultural Context of Medicine in India* (Delhi: Vikas, 1981), pp. 31–54. Also see Donald Warren, 'The Bengali Context', *Bulletin of the Indian Institute of the History of Medicine*, 21 (1991), 17–51.

lost glory of an ancient Indian civilisation in which ayurveda had flourished.[18] Such texts lamented the fading importance of ayurveda under the impact of mindless imitation of the West under the influence of colonialism. It was argued that although ayurvedic knowledge was particularly suitable for Indians, there was an increasing dearth of experienced and reliable physicians. The article 'Rog o Paschatya Sabhyata' or 'Disease and Western Civilisation' pointed out that 'presently, ayurveda is in such a state that no one can be sure if there will be any existence of it another century from now as there has been a drastic decrease in the number of physicians. Among those who still practice, there are hardly any outstanding physicians left'.[19]

Ayurveda was declared particularly out of step with the modern world and its diseases. In a series of articles in the journal *Chikitsha Sammilani*, the homoeopaths elaborated on the inadequacies of ayurveda in contemporary society.[20] In his article on the homoeopathic treatment of fever, physician Haranath Ray argued that 'under foreign domination there has been tremendous change in our social context and with the advent of several new diseases there is dire need of modern medical knowledge. We cannot take it for granted that the way the Susrut, Charak, Bhagbat and Dhanwantary devised ayurveda, will be as effective in all times and in all social contexts'.[21]

Under these circumstances, the homoeopaths emphasised that the failing reputation of ayurveda necessitated the intervention of western medicine. However, they cautioned against the apparent benefits of modern western civilisation, saying their gifts were almost always underpinned with debilitating disadvantages. As an author satirically remarked, 'just as western rule has enabled us to cover long distances very fast, so also it has made sure that we are covering our life span in a shorter time period and retiring from this world very fast'.[22] Unsurprisingly, the homoeopaths condemned the consumption of western drugs advocated by western allopathic treatment. The strong drugs used in the colder climate of the west were considered unsuitable in the hot climate of India.[23] It was

18 G. Dirghangi, 'Bharatbarshe Homeopathy' ('Homoeopathy in India'), *Hahnemann*, 3, 11 (1920), 401.

19 M. Chakrabarti, 'Rog o Pashchatya Sabhyata' ('Disease and Western Civilisation'), *Hahnemann*, 3, 6 (1920), 217.

20 See, for instance, Shashibhushan Mukhopadhyay, 'Baidya Chikitshak er Ashumparnata' ('Inadequacies of the Kavirajes'), *Chikitsha Sammilani*, 8 (1891), 269–72.

21 Haranath Ray, 'Homoeopathy Mowt e Jvar Chikitsha' ('Homoeopathic Treatment of Fever'), *Chikitsha Sammilani*, 3 (1886), 222.

22 M. Chakrabarti, 'Rog o Pashchatya Sabhyata' ('Disease and Western Civilisation'), p. 215.

23 Ibid., pp. 215–17.

pointed out that allopathic treatment often involved the use of alcohol and was therefore incompatible with Indian constitutions. Thus, the author of the text *Rog o Arogyo (Disease and Cure)* argued that 'the strong allopathic drugs are causing havoc to our people. The alcohol mixed strong drugs that are suitable for the daily-meat-eating powerful people of the west are too much for the vegetarian and amicable people of the east'.[24]

Homoeopathy, in this context, was upheld as the most obvious choice for Indians. Highlighting its modern, western roots, the homoeopaths elaborated on the reasons why homoeopathy still had legitimate claims to indigeneity. At one level, as I have shown with the works of translation in Chapter 3, an underlying equivalence was claimed between the inherent homoeopathic principles and Hindu philosophy. Given the proximity of his ideas to the Hindu tradition of thought, it was considered a pity that Hahnemann was not in reality born in India. It was said time and again that since 'Indians believe in the power of infinite, imperceptible and imponderable spirit or "paramatma"', therefore 'India is the real land of homoeopathy'.[25]

But beyond the issue of equivalence, other authors directly contended that homoeopathy had a claim to ancient Indian heritage comparable to that of ayurveda. These writers asserted that 'the main principle of homoeopathy was actually inherent within the large ayurvedic corpus'.[26] Ironically, in their effort to highlight ayurveda's relevance, the vaidic authors too frequently identified the remote Indian past as the 'authentic' origin of homoeopathy. In a representative long article written in 1885 in the journal *Chikitsha Sammilani*, Kaviraj Madhusudan Roy explicitly asserted, 'the law which has made Hahnemann world famous had originally been invented by the now-fallen Aryans'.[27] Vaidya Raj Surajit Dasgupta Bhishak Shastri made identical assertions in his text *Rog o Arogyo (Disease and Cure)*, which was originally a lecture delivered at the twelfth session of the Mymensingh Ayurved Sabha. Mentioning the divine origin of ayurveda and discussing its greatness, Shastri stated that the principle of 'similars' on which homoeopathy was based, was included in ayurveda as a viable curing principle. He argued that the Sanskrit verse '*somoh somong samayati*' or '*sadrisa sadrisen shamyoti*' in ayurveda denoted

[24] Surajit Dasgupta, *Rog o Arogyo* (*Disease and Cure*) (Mymensingh: Surajit Dasgupta, 1925), pp. 19–32.

[25] G. Dirghangi, 'Bharatbarshe Homeopathy' ('Homoeopathy in India'), p. 406.

[26] Ibid., p. 407.

[27] Madhusudan Roy, 'Abadhoutik ba Sadrisa Chikitsha' ('Abadhoutik or Homoeopathic Treatment'), *Chikitsha Sammilani*, 2 (1885), 146–61.

the exact same meaning as the Latin phrase '*similia similibus curanter*' later made famous by Hahnemann.

Such ayurvedic claims were hardly contested by writers propagating homoeopathy. In a range of texts dealing with homoeopathy's past and its claims of belonging to India, they referred to these assertions by ayurvedic practitioners and expressed solidarity with such a position. Through complicated historical narratives, several early twentieth-century homoeopathic texts argued that the fundamental tenet of homoeopathy was indeed inherent in ayurveda. A typical text like *Susrut o Hahnemann* published in 1906, for instance, developed a detailed account of the historical origin and trajectory of ayurveda and homoeopathy.[28] Referring to Indian civilisation and ayurveda as the oldest body of medicine, the author described how such doctrines travelled west primarily with the spread of Buddhism. On reaching Greece, some of the ayurvedic tenets were translated to Latin by the Romans that influenced Hippocrates. It was argued that these 'historical truths' explain why homoeopathy truly has deep roots in India. The author of *Susrut o Hahnemann* asserted that although the possibility of cure by similars was included in ayurveda, it was not elaborated in a 'systematic and disciplined manner' before Hahnemann.[29] These homoeopaths in colonial Bengal acknowledged that the greatness of Hahnemann lay in developing the fundamental principle already given in ayurveda into a coherent body of knowledge. Through their participation in discussions on contentious historical pasts, the perpetrators of homoeopathy claimed to irrefutably establish homoeopathy's *indigenous* roots. In his 1924 article 'Light of Hope', author Kalikumar Bhattacharya conclusively wrote, 'homoeopathy is our own Vedic property which has recently come back to us dressed in western attire. If we make it our own, with time it will be most efficient in maintaining the power, health and resources of independent "swaraj" India'.[30]

To substantiate these claims, the homoeopathic practitioners made sincere, consistent efforts to demonstrate the proximity and compatibility between homoeopathy and ayurveda. In a remarkable display of medical pluralism, these authors made repeated attempts to synthesise the fundamental features of the two doctrines. In a manual titled *Sadrisa Byabastha Jvar Chikithsa* (*Homoeopathic Treatment of Fever*), published in 1871, for example, the author highlighted the importance of consulting ayurvedic texts for the most relevant classification of Indian fevers, which is

[28] Surendra Mohan Ghosh, *Susrut o Hyaniman* (Calcutta: Bengal Medical Library, 1906), pp. 2, 6–11.

[29] Ibid., pp. 6–11. [30] Kalikumar Bhattacharya, 'Ashar Alok' ('Ray of Hope'), p. 80.

unavailable in European texts.[31] He stated that his manual has been prepared by synthesising the knowledge of such classification from the ayurvedic texts of Susrut and Madhab, with the treatments suggested in the texts of European homoeopathic giants like Tsar, Gaurency and Kent, to prescribe the most effective remedy.[32]

Attempts at synthesis had myriad manifestations. Appropriate and disciplined diet was considered a critical aspect of homoeopathic cure. Accordingly, a number of manuals carefully discussed the food that was to be consumed in various stages of treatment. The manual *Pathya – Nirbachan (Selection of Diet)* stated explicitly that, 'since homoeopathic drugs are very subtle and gentle, they cannot function half as efficiently with adverse substances. Therefore, it is crucially important in homoeopathy, much more than in all other forms of healing, to be vigilant of the food habit and lifestyle of the patient'.[33] Such regulations were often imbued with distinctly nationalist resonances. It was pointed out that the homoeopathic drugs worked best with indigenous food. Emphasising the importance of the freshness and quality of '*deshiya khadya*' or indigenous food over western imported food and milk, the author of *Homoeopathy Mowt e Saral Griha Chikitsha (Simple Domestic Treatment According to Homoeopathy)* stated, 'for these reasons western diet is incompatible with homoeopathic healing'.[34] In the third chapter of his manual *Pathya Nirbachan (Selection of Diet)* written in 1925, homoeopath H. N. Mukhati discussed the ayurvedic notion of '*tridosha*' or the three bodily humours '*bayu*', '*pitta*' and '*kaph*'.[35] He argued that 'it is advisable to adopt the ayurvedic idea of diet along with homoeopathic drugs as the former is ideally suited for our country'.[36] It is important to note that such trends of assimilation and proclaimed 'harmonisation' of the principles of both doctrines continued on the part of the homoeopaths. A culmination of this trend may be seen in the book *The Science of Tridosha*, written by homoeopath Benoytosh Bhattacharya in the 1950s. Here, Bhattacharya held that 'in order that this dynamic system may be made full use of, it is absolutely necessary that the Tridosha methods should be applied to homoeopathy for the benefit of mankind'.[37]

[31] Harikrishna Mallik, Preface, Sadrisa Byabastha Jvar Chikitsha (Homoeopathic Treatment of Fever), Berigny and Company's Bengali Homoeopathic Series Number II (Calcutta: J. G. Chatterjee and Co's Press, 1871), page number not cited.
[32] Ibid. [33] H. N. Mukhati, *Pothyo Nirbachan* (*Selection of Diet*) (Dacca, 1925), p. 7.
[34] Anonymous, *Homoeopathic Mowt e Saral Griha Chikitsha* (*Simple Domestic Treatment according to Homoeopathy)*, 7th edition (Calcutta: Batakrishna Pal and Company, 1926), pp. 1–2.
[35] H. N. Mukhati, *Pothyo Nirbachan* (*Selection of Diet*), 1925, p. 17. [36] Ibid.
[37] Benoytosh Bhattacharya, 'Preface' in *Science of Tridosha* (Calcutta: Firma K. L. Mukhopadhyay, [1951]1975), page number not cited.

Frail Families, 'Endangered Grihasthas'

Based on their claims of indigeneity, homoeopaths participated in ongoing nationalist discussions on the crisis of the institution of family. By the turn of the twentieth century, various Bengali sociomedical journals and contemporary social anthologies were raising the alarm about the crisis of domesticity and disintegration of Indian familial structure. These included journals dealing with issues relating to everyday domesticity and the home (for example, *Grihastha, Grihasthamangal*); those broadly dealing with health and medicine (for example, *Svasthya, Bhishak Darpan, Chikitsha Sammilani*) or journals dedicated exclusively to themes of women and household (for example, *Mahila, Antahpur, Bangamahila*). The themes and explanations of impending domestic crisis elaborated in this literature were the very ones picked up by the homoeopaths in their own manuals and journals dedicated exclusively to homoeopathy. Citing homoeopathy's indigenous roots, unique features and compatibility to Indian situations, these texts highlighted it as the ideal remedy over ayurveda to tide over any crisis.

The nationalist literature on families celebrated the traditional Hindu joint family while lamenting its potential disintegration in the face of an imposed modernity initiated by British rule. A wide range of writings compared and differentiated between familial experiences in the East and the West. A representative article in the journal *Grihastha,* characterised the Hindu Bengali social existence as a 'collective' as opposed to the 'individualistic' western families.[38] It contended that it was difficult to perceive a Hindu to be completely dissociated from his extended kinship network.[39] Given such an idea, several authors, like the author of an article titled 'Bange Ekannabarti Paribar' or the 'The Joint-Family in Bengal' in the journal *Grihasthali,* argued that the joint family was the natural familial set up in Bengal.[40] Long unbroken historical trajectories were claimed for the joint family from the time of the Hindu epics, the *Ramayana* and the *Mahabharata.*[41] It was held that as opposed to the individualised life in the west, the collective social existence of the Hindus often transcended the immediate family to include even other social commitments, like those towards fellow caste members.[42] Indeed, in highlighting the collective nature of Hindu family life, the texts identified

[38] Radhakamal Mukhopadhyay, 'Madhyabitta Srenir Durobostha' ('Wretched Condition of the Middle Class'), *Grihastha* [Ben: Ashadh], 1913, p. 573.
[39] Ibid.
[40] Anonymous, 'Bange Ekannabarti Paribar' ('Joint Family in Bengal'), pp. 94–6.
[41] Ibid.
[42] Radhakamal Mukhopadhyay, 'Madhyabitta Srenir Durobostha' ('Wretched Condition of the Middle Class'), p. 573.

a unique tie of affection and love that characterised eastern families. They held that the concept of family in the east was inspired by a positively higher ideal of living involving qualities of 'sharing, compassion, respect and love' as well as 'obedience, sacrifice, selflessness'.[43] Such an ideal entailed sacrificing even one's own life for the happiness of others in the family.[44]

These anxious reflections on the 'family ideal' inevitably invoked issues of familial economy. Most authors agreed that the 'eastern' notion of happiness was not necessarily contingent on family fortunes. The article 'Sukhi Paribar' or 'Happy Family' in the journal *Mahila* thus asserted, 'our ideal of happy family is different ... family to us is a divine institution ... hence real happiness is not contingent on wealth'.[45] On the contrary, eminent social commentators like Bhudeb Mukhopadhyay in his authoritative anthology *Paribarik Prabandha* (*Essays on Family*) elaborated on the economic advantages of the joint familial set up.[46] Mukhopadhyay argued that in the absence of the European Poor Law or the life insurance system in India, the eastern joint familial arrangement provided immunity against financial problems.[47] It was further argued that poverty and pecuniary constraint was one of the major factors that had prompted the emergence of the joint family.

These texts were unanimous in their explanation of and concern about the dangers threatening the institution of joint family in India. The corrupting influence of an essentially western modernity was identified as the root cause disturbing the Indian familial fabric, as well as producing diseased Indian bodies. Western ideas were understood to be causing dislocation in the fundamentals of everyday life including child rearing, food habits, medication and education, which in turn brought about widespread ill health. A representative article titled 'Baje Kharach' or 'Unjustified Expenditure' in the journal *Grihasthamangal* lamented,

> the Indians seemed to have made up their mind regarding the fact that everything western – the ways, customs, social norms, systems are all good, while everything indigenous is bad. All things they [the westerners] do are scientific while everything Indians ever did is superstitious ... by denying indigenous weather, food,

[43] Anonymous, 'Bange Ekannabarti Paribar' ('Joint Family in Bengal'), p. 95; and Bhudeb Mukhopadhyay, *Paribarik Prabandha* (*Essays on Family*), 3rd edition (Hooghly: Budhoday Jantra), 1889, p. 183.

[44] Nirupama Devi, 'Ekannabhukta Paribar er Ashanti Nibaran er Upay Ki'? ('What are the Ways to Pacify the Problems in a Joint Family?'), *Antahpur*, 6, 9 (January 1904), 197.

[45] Anonymous, 'Sukhi Paribar' ('Happy Family'), *Mahila*, 9, 8 (March 1907), 207.

[46] Bhudeb Mukhopadhyay, *Paribarik Prabandha* (*Essays on Family*), 1889, pp. 182–3.

[47] Ibid., p. 183.

clothes, recreation, music etc and trying to emulate the English in all these spheres, we are being weak, coward, unhealthy and poor by the day.[48]

An alarming increase in human need, coupled with intense consumption and extravagance, was characterised as an obvious fallout of this gratuitous westernisation. The contemporary age was suggested to be in the '*bhog marg*' (i.e. in a stage that could be defined solely in terms of consumption).[49] '*Bilash*' or luxury and '*bhog*' or consumption were identified as the two most potent evils of the western, modern lifestyle. Preserving the indigenous national identity, and judicious management of familial wealth and economy, therefore emerged as crucial themes in most texts. It was contended that the fundamental threat faced by the Indian joint families was economic in nature. Many texts dealt with the theme of major familial tension caused by brothers earning different levels of income. Indeed, Bengali literature of the time is replete with instances of authors elaborating on such themes of disintegration.[50] The authors, in this context, emphasised the importance of thoughtful expenditure and saving. Bhudeb Mukhopadhyay's authoritative tract on the institution of family in late nineteenth-century Bengal, for example, had an entire chapter devoted to 'Artha Sanchay' or 'Codes of Saving'.[51]

Given these ongoing discussions on family, economy and health in the Bengali print culture, the homoeopaths directly addressed the discourse on familial degeneration in Bengal. Consuming homoeopathy, it was argued, took care of the domestic ill health of the people through an efficacious indigenous remedy. Simultaneously, in being extremely affordable, it also remedied the deep-seated economic malaise plaguing Indian families. Directed specifically to the '*grihasthas*' or householders, the homoeopathic texts recurrently emphasised a series of advantages that made homoeopathy indispensable within every household, and preferable to any other form of healing. The consumption of homoeopathic drugs was characterised as 'safe and painless with literally none or very mild side effects'.[52] These drugs were considered so harmless that they 'could be

48 Basanta Kumar Choudhury, 'Baje Kharach' ('Bad Expenditure'), *Grihasthamangal*, 5, 2–3 (1931), 35.

49 Amaresh Kanjilal, *Byaktigato Arthaneeti* (*Personal Economics*) (Calcutta: Samyo Press, 1921), pp. 1–21.

50 Troubles in the joint family were at the heart of a range of novels and stories written by the eminent Bengali author Sarat Chandra Chattopadhyay (1876–1938). Set in colonial Bengal, his texts *Nishkriti* (1917), *Bindur Chhele* (1913), *Ram er Sumati* (1914), *Mejdidi* and so on, centrally engage joint family crises based in financial management.

51 Bhudeb Mukhopadhyay, *Paribarik Prabandha* (*Essays on Family*), 1889, pp. 186–91.

52 Satyacharan Laha, 'Advertisement' in *Homeopathic Griha Chikitsha* (*Homoeopathic Domestic Treatment*) (Calcutta: Akhil Chandra Shil, 1914), page number not cited.

safely consumed by all – from newborn babies to old people'.[53] Their mild, gentle nature made them suitable for consumption by women too. It was argued that in 'diseases related to pregnancy as well as for infants, even physicians professing other medical systems often prescribed homoeopathic drugs'.[54] In addition, some of the texts highlighted that 'since the Bengalis are becoming debilitated by the day, they can hardly stand the stronger remedies of other heroic therapies. Therefore, the tasty, minute, useful homoeopathic medicines are the most suitable for them'.[55]

Apart from labelling homoeopathic medicine safe, tasty, painless and gentle, the texts eulogised homoeopathy's added advantage of being economical. Not only were the drugs cheaply priced, they were also advertised as long lasting, to the extent that it was believed that 'if kept with care, fresh homoeopathic drugs last for years'.[56] Besides, a very small amount of the drug needed to be consumed at a time.[57] Thus it was pointed out that 'whereas a simple allopathic fever mixture for a week prescribed by other physicians costs a patient around Rs. 4–5, a homoeopathic drug worth Re. 1 can easily cure 5–6 such patients'.[58]

Moreover, the texts argued that the greatest advantage associated with the practice of homoeopathy was the virtue of being self-reliant in terms of one's health. A range of homoeopathic domestic manuals pledged to make amateur physicians out of all ordinary householders so that they would be sufficiently competent to take care of their own selves and their families. Homoeopathic manuals promised to invest the *grihasthas* with enough curative power to make the figure of the expensive allopathic physician redundant in everyday life. Written for the 'endangered *grihasthas* and the literate women', these texts promised to be 'easy guides to various diseases, their special symptoms and the relevant drugs'.[59] Texts like *Garhasthya Svasthya o Homoeopathy Chikitsha Bigyan* or *Domestic*

[53] Anonymous, 'Advertisement of Improved Homeopathic Griha Chikitsha' *in* Benimadhab Dey and Company Almanac (Calcutta: Benimadhab Dey and Company, 1896–97), page number not cited.

[54] Anonymous, 'Preface' *in* Homeopathy Mowt e Adorsho Griha Chikitsha (*Ideal Domestic Treatment according to the Homoeopathic Method*) (Calcutta: The Standard Homeopathic Pharmacy, 1914), page number not cited.

[55] Raimohan Bandopadhyay, *Homeopathic Griha Chikitshak* (*Homoeopathic Family Physician*) (Calcutta: Gurudas Chattopadhyay and Sons, 1926), Dedication page.

[56] Anonymous, *Homeopathic Mowt e Saral Griha Chikitsha* (*Simple Domestic Treatment According to Homoeopathy*), 1926, pp. 13–14.

[57] Anonymous, 'Advertisement of Improved Homeopathic Griha Chikitsha' in *Benimadhab Dey and Company Almanac*, 1896–97, page number not cited.

[58] Anonymous, 'Letter to the Editor', *Svasthya*, 4, 8 (1900), 238.

[59] Jagachandra Raya, 'Preface', *Garhasthya Svasthya ebong Homeopathic Chikitsha Bigyan* (*Domestic Health and Homoeopathic Medical Science*) (Calcutta: Harendranath Roy, 1917), page number not cited.

Health and Homoeopathic Medicine mentioned that these texts were specifically written for lay householders by purposely excluding 'complicated scientific explanations'.[60] The homoeopathic domestic chest or box was highlighted as the most prominent, visible symbol of the self-sufficiency associated with the consumption of homoeopathy, as Fig. 4.1 suggests. Most texts advertised a range of boxes of various shapes and contents, which, along with the domestic medicine manuals, were considered essential in enabling the householders to treat themselves. Sarat Chandra Dutta's *Primary Guide to Homoeopathy* promised that, 'with the said medical chest and a prescriptive manual, those who know absolutely nothing about medicine can also treat general cases'.[61] Most of the domestic manuals, like *Homoeopathic Griha Chikitsha* written by Satyacharan Laha in 1914, guaranteed that their readers would become practising physicians of homoeopathy through meticulous reading.[62]

Together these texts demonstrated a fracturing of homoeopathy's professional identity and domain of expertise. Homoeopathy was written about as a science that could be mastered at home. In a deeply pedagogic tone, the manuals promised to make an amateur physician out of every lay householder.[63] The manuals included careful details of how to diagnose and detect symptoms of various diseases, furnished minute instructions on how and in what frequency one needed to change drugs and also acted as guides on how to adjust the doses.[64] Most of the texts were careful about their design. The preface to *Shishu Rog Samhita (Compendium of Children's Disease)* by Narayan Chandra Basu, for instance, justified the author's placing disease histories first, saying that this organisation would be most useful for the readers while treating their children.[65] Some of the domestic manuals, like

60 Ibid.

61 'Advertisement of Indian Homeopathic Hall', in Sarat Chandra Dutta, *Primary Guide to Homeopathy or the Companion to the Family Medical Chest* (Calcutta: Homeopathic Medical Hall, 1899).

62 Satyacharan Laha, 'Advertisement' in *Homeopathic Griha Chikitsha* (*Homoeopathic Domestic Medicine*) (Calcutta: Akhil Chandra Shil, 1914), page number not cited.

63 'Advertisement of Indian Homoeopathic Hall' in Sarat Chandra Dutta, *Primary Guide to Homoeopathy or Companion to the Family Medical Chest*, 1899.

64 For instance, see Mahendranath Ghosh, *Soudaminir Dhatri Shikkha ebong Garbhini o Prashuti Chikitsha* (*Guidelines on Midwifery, Pregnancy and Reproductive Health Enunciated by Soudamini*) (Calcutta: Bharat Mihir Jontro, 1909).

65 Narayan Chandra Basu, 'Preface' in Shishu, *Rog Samhita* (*Compendium of Children's Disease*) (Calcutta: Sadhana Library, 1922), page number not cited.

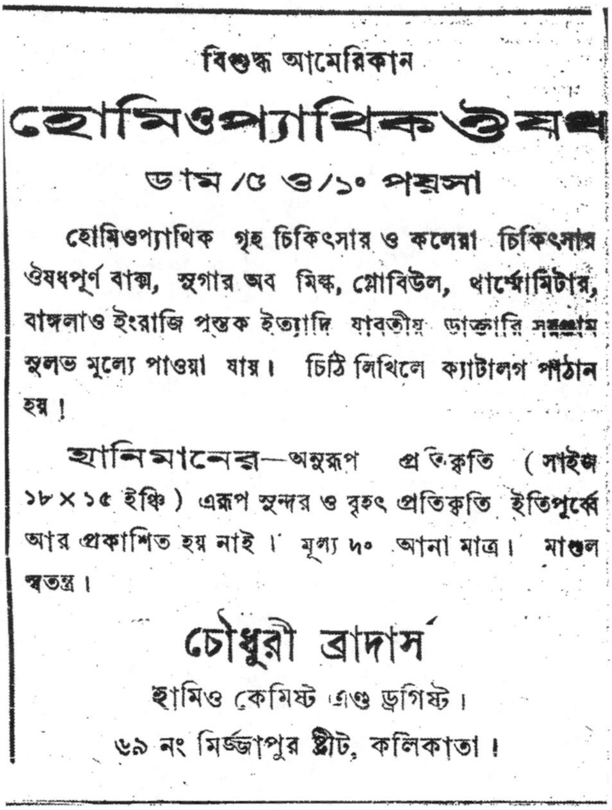
বিশুদ্ধ আমেরিকান
হোমিওপ্যাথিক ঔষধ
ডাম /৫ ও /১০ পয়সা
হোমিওপ্যাথিক গৃহ চিকিৎসার ও কলেরা চিকিৎসার ঔষধপূর্ণ বাক্স, সুগার অব মিল্ক, গ্লোবিউল, থার্ম্মোমিটার, বাঙ্গলা ও ইংরাজি পুস্তক ইত্যাদি যাবতীয় ডাক্তারি
সুলভ মূল্যে পাওয়া যায়। চিঠি লিখিলে ক্যাটালগ পাঠান হয়!
হ্যানিমানের—অনুরূপ প্রতিকৃতি (সাইজ ১৮ × ১৫ ইঞ্চি) এরূপ সুন্দর ও বৃহৎ প্রতিকৃতি ইতিপূর্ব্বে আর প্রকাশিত হয় নাই। মূল্য ৵০ আনা মাত্র। মাশুল স্বতন্ত্র।
চৌধুরী ব্রাদার্স
হোমিও কেমিষ্ট এণ্ড ড্রগিষ্ট।
৬৯ নং মির্জ্জাপুর ষ্ট্রীট, কলিকাতা।

Fig. 4.1 Representative advertisement for homoeopathic boxes and accompanying manuals for domestic consumption by the firm Chowdhury Brothers, *Grihasthamangal*, 2, 11 (1928), 5. Reproduced from the collection of the Archives of the Centre for Studies in Social Sciences, Calcutta.

Homoeopathic Griha Chikitsha written by Satyacharan Laha, even guaranteed that their readers would become practising physicians of homoeopathy through meticulous reading.[66] These assurances of empowerment by homoeopathy, however, were often criticised by others. For instance, an article titled 'Chikitshay Her Pher' or 'Variations in Treatment' in the allopathically inclined journal *Bhishak*

[66] Satyacharan Laha, 'Bigyapon or Advertisement' in *Homoeopathic Griha Chikitsha* (*Homoeopathic Domestic Treatment*), 1914, page number not cited.

Darpan, powerfully argued for the relevance of specialisation in medicine.[67] Homoeopathy's role in diffusing the notion of professionalisation was particularly condemned. It was noted, with irony, that homoeopathy was so much in conversation with the ideas of independence, *swaraj* and boycott that 'the *grihastha* has stopped consulting the physicians regarding matters medical, they are guided by the advice from their wife, or may be even servants, conversant in homoeopathy!'[68]

The texts, thus, evidence a deep traffic and overlap between the nationalist anxieties around domesticity and the homoeopathic promises of relief. The virtues of '*shwabolombita*' (i.e. self-reliance) and '*mitabyayita*' (i.e. sense of judicious spending), were shown to be intricately related.[69] Hence, overtly nationalist texts like *Byaktigato Arthaneeti (Personal Economics)* argued that the economic problems of the nation had to be essentially negotiated in the '*nityo jibon*' or everyday life of its people within their domestic spaces.[70] Such texts often recommended homoeopathic knowledge as ideal for taking care of the health of the family without the intervention of physicians.[71] 'Atma Nirbharata' or 'Self-Sufficiency' – an article published in the journal *Svasthya* in 1901, pointed out that if the householders had to visit a doctor or a *kaviraj* for every domestic complaint, it would be extremely taxing on the family budget.[72] Familial economy and notions of self-help in this sense were considered integrally related.

Given the advantages claimed for homoeopathy, the homoeopathic authors further asserted that it was only natural that the homoeopathic family medical guides were extremely popular in Bengali families plagued with economic crisis induced by colonial rule. As the introduction to the seventh edition of the manual *Homoeopathic Mowt e Saral Griha Chikitsha* or *Simple Home Treatment according to Homoeopathy* noted, 'that we are compelled to publish repeated editions of this book so often, clearly indicates that it is widely accepted by all'.[73] Similarly, writing in 1926, the author of the manual *Homoeopathic Family Physician* confidently hoped that the 'book will circulate just like an almanac, among poor Indians as well as among the rich residing in palaces'.[74] Indeed, the

[67] Ramesh Chandra Ghosh, 'Chiktshay Her Pher' ('Variations in Treatment'), *Bhishak Darpan* (September 1911), pp. 340–7.
[68] Ibid., p. 341.
[69] Amaresh Kanjilal, *Byaktigato Arthoneeti* (*Personal Economics*) (Calcutta: Samyo Press, 1921), pp. 1–21.
[70] Ibid. [71] Ibid. [72] Anonymous, 'Atma Nirbharata'('Self-Sufficiency'), pp. 204–5.
[73] Anonymous, 'Introduction', *Homeopathic Mowt e Saral Griha Chikitsha* (*Simple Domestic Treatment According to Homoeopathy*), 1926, page number not cited.
[74] Raimohan Bandopadhyay, *Homeopathic Griha Chikitshak* (*Homoeopathic Family Physician*), 1926, Dedication page.

texts unanimously argued that the greatest advantage associated with the practice of homoeopathy was the virtue of being self-sufficient in terms of one's health. It was framed as the most appropriate response to the nationalist anxiety related to loss of self-respect and an attitude of dependency that allegedly characterised the Indians.

It is hardly surprising that in the tirade against wasteful westernisation, homoeopathy upheld itself as the indigenous solution against western allopathy, especially with regards to maintaining familial economy. The homoeopathic texts unequivocally condemned the Bengali fascination with expensive allopathic drugs, arguing that consumption of allopathy signified the larger trend of extravagance set in motion by western modernity.[75] These texts lamented that the Bengali *grihasthas* were easily carried away by the allopathic drugs imported from Britain and that allopathic treatment made them indulge in injections on the slightest pretext and conduct unnecessary tests for simple diseases like fever. The cheap price of homoeopathic drugs in comparison to both allopathy and *kaviraji* was emphasised. By virtue of its indigeneity and the sense of economy that it promoted, this literature often upheld homoeopathy as 'natural' – almost as cheap and essential as the elements of nature. In view of its cost, it was compared with wind, water, food and other elements essential for living that had been provided free of cost by nature. As an article entitled 'Homoeopathy Aushadh er Mulya' or 'Price of Homoeopathic Drugs' in the journal *Hahnemann* stated, 'although it costs a little to collect the plants and to prepare the drugs, yet so minute are the doses, each patient may be cured with as little as one paisa'.[76] Homoeopathy was perceived as the only form of treatment that could erase the existing social distinctions between the rich and the poor.[77]

It was further pointed out that not only the drugs, but homoeopathic publications too were extremely cheap and denoted value for money. Thus, a typical advertisement for the homoeopathic manual *Chikitsha Darpan* stated, 'the book is all of 1250 pages, divided into seventeen chapters. Not bearing profit in mind its price has been fixed at a level which is accessible by everyone'.[78] Consumption of homoeopathy was regarded as economical not only for every family but for the nation as

[75] Nilmani Ghatak, 'Allopathy r Moho' ('The Allure of Allopathy'), *Homoeopathy Paricharak*, 2, 5 (August 1928), 165–8.
[76] M. Chakrabarty, 'Homoeopahy Oushadh er Mulyo' ('Price of Homoeopathic Drugs'), *Hahnemann*, 5, 8 (1923), 419.
[77] Ibid., p. 419.
[78] 'Advertisement of Chikitsha Darpan' in Anonymous, *Homoeopathic Mowt e Saral Griha Chikitsha* (*Simple Domestic Treatment According to Homoeopathy*), 1926.

a whole. Thus, the article 'Homoeopathy Sombondhe Du Ekti Kotha' or 'One or Two Words about Homoeopathy' in the journal *Hahnemann* noted,

> Allopathic drugs have been introduced by the English rulers and they earn millions of rupees by selling those drugs in India. Homoeopathy has been introduced much later and independently of the English. The drugs are primarily imported from America and Germany. Besides, initiatives are being taken to produce them indigenously with Indian flora and fauna.[79]

Necessary Tool for 'the Ideal Hindu Wife'

Any nationalist discussion on domestic reform and the future of families within the nation could hardly leave aside the 'women's question'. As has been established by a range of scholars, despite the goals of reform and the promise of emancipation, the patriarchal, nationalist discourse on women demarcated the home as their ideal space. Embodied as the true essence of the nation's culture and spirituality, the role of women was predominantly seen as that of a '*grihalakshmi*' or the goddess of home.[80] Operating within this larger schema, the homoeopathic literature proposed homoeopathy as a 'necessary tool' for women to assert their position within the familial confines. Consumption of homoeopathy promised to ensure female autonomy and authority in important ways. More significantly, women's voices and their own agency in debates on reform have emerged as crucial questions. In the late 1990s Lata Mani's important scholarship exposed the patriarchal nature of the Sati debate surrounding questions of tradition and modernity. Since then, others like Mrinalini Sinha have been exploring whether and to what extent the organised voice and actions of women themselves were instrumental in shaping the colonial domestic ideal.[81] The homoeopathic discourse relating to gender adds to the investigation of these important questions.

In the interwoven discourses of health, economy and the future of the joint family, women equipped with homoeopathy were framed as the most trusted custodians of the Bengali extended household. As such,

[79] N. C. Ghosh, 'Homoeopathy Sombondhe Du ekti Kotha' ('Few Words on Homoeopathy'), *Hahnemann*, 21, 7 (1938), 508.

[80] See Partha Chatterjee, 'Nationalist Resolution of Women's Question' in Kumkum Sangari and Sudesh Vaid (eds.) *Recasting Women: Essays in Indian Colonial History* (Brunswick: Rutgers University Press 1990), pp. 233–53. Also see Dipesh Chakrabarty, 'The Difference: Deferral of (A) Colonial Modernity: Public Debates on Domesticity in Colonial Bengal', pp. 1–36.

[81] Mrinalini Sinha, 'Lineage of the Indian Modern: Rhetoric, Agency and the Sarda Act in Late Colonial India' in Antoinette Burton (ed.), *Gender, Sexuality and Colonial Modernities* (London and New York: Routledge, 1999), pp. 207–19.

many manuals gave instructions on how homoeopathy could serve as an efficient tool for Hindu women in judicious management of the family's health and its resources. Homoeopathy was advocated as the ideal means for a woman to serve her husband and his family. A typical example is *Grihinir Hitopodesh (Advice for the Wife),* written by Hemangini Ghosh Dastidar in 1917.[82] Composed in the form of a prolonged conversation between a newlywed wife and her mother-in-law, the manual offered detailed instructions on becoming 'an ideal Hindu wife'. It resonated with the ideal of self-less service – an essential part of holding a large family together. Keeping one's husband and his family happy was presented as the greatest virtue of female life. Indeed, such manuals emphasised that, 'a woman's greatest duty lay in keeping her husband and God satisfied'.[83] The second part of the book was wholly dedicated to teaching homoeopathy to the new wife, since 'it is essential for every woman to possess some medical knowledge to run the family. Respectable women should know homoeopathy. It is most effective in diseases related to women and children and enables wives to take care of their families most efficiently'.[84] The text engaged extensively with various homoeopathic drugs and their usage. It even recommended using homoeopathy interchangeably with other indigenous folk healing practice or '*totka*', which were transmitted between female members of families across generations.[85] Such texts thus promised to empower women to take complete charge of the familial health in absence of the *grihastha*.[86]

Besides taking care of the other members of the family, women were also encouraged to be cautious in looking after themselves. It was argued that women's ill health disrupted the smooth functioning of families, not least because women's health was directly associated with that of the children they bore.[87] Concern over excessive westernisation and strain on family resources intersected with notions of the ideal woman's role in the family. It was lamented that women refrained from engaging in any domestic duties, as erstwhile they did, and indulged instead in luxury. The article 'Common Ailments of the Women in Bengal and their Causes' in the journal *Indian Homoeopathic Review* stated,

[82] Hemangini Ray Dastidar, *Grihinir Hitopodesh* (*Advice for the Wife*) (Srihatta: Karimganj Press, 1917), pp. 5–17.

[83] Ibid., p. 23. [84] Ibid., p. 23. [85] Ibid., p. 33.

[86] Khetranath Chattopadhyay, 'Advertisement' in *Homoeopathic Griha Chikitsha (Homoeopathic Domestic Treatment)*, 1st edition (Calcutta: People's Press, 1887). Also see Anonymous, *Homoeopathic Mowt e Saral Griha Chikitsha (Simple Domestic Treatment according to Homoeopathy)*, 1926, pp. 26–7.

[87] Anonymous, 'Bharat Mahilar Svasthya' ('Health of Women in India'), *Antahpur*, 4, 7 (1901), 149–51.

we are gradually doing away with the little opportunities that our ladies used to have of breathing fresh air or getting the rays of the sun on them in the shape of fetching water or bathing in the river, and though the poorer inhabitants of country-places may still retain these customs in a small scale, the comparatively richer ones consider it simply derogatory to indulge in any of these vulgar practices. Their only recreation consists of – a midday nap, or rather to be more accurate . . . nap, novel and gossip.[88]

This discourse on women's health, luxury and indulgence was evidently linked with the broader anxiety concerning the draining of family expenses and on the celebrated virtues of self-sufficiency. An article in the journal *Antahpur*, for instance, candidly stated, 'if the women of our generation get rid of their laziness and get involved with household duties, then the family can be run with much less expenditure and their health remains intact. The household would also be bestowed with divine blessings'.[89]

The issue of reproductive health was fundamental to nationalist reform. Sarah Hodges points out that angst about national degeneration and women's health was quintessentially an eugenic project, which equated a healthy mother with a healthy future nation.[90] The homoeopathic literature highlighted how marriage and procreation were related to the advancement of the father's lineage or '*bangsha*'.[91] Indeed, a popular manual on women's health like *Soudamini r Dhatri Shikkha ebong Garbhini o Prashuti Chikitsha (Guidelines on Midwifery, Pregnancy and Reproductive Health Enunciated by Soudamini)* urged its readers to look at every individual pregnancy as a potential contribution to the cause of the nation. It asserted that,

Women who bear child are immensely fortunate. Who can predict that their pregnancies would not bear great men like Maharshi Debendranath Tagore, Dharmabeer Keshab Chandra Sen, Samajbeer Ramgopal Ghosh, Jnanbeer Iswarchandra Vidyasagar, Daanbeer Kalikrishna Thakur . . . Natyabeer Girishchandra Ghosh and Ranabeer Rana Pratap Singha? Who can say they will not give birth to religious minded women like Ahalya, Rani Bhabani or Rani Swarnamoyee?[92]

[88] S. Goswami, 'Common Ailments of Women in Bengal and Their Causes', *Indian Homoeopathic Review*, 20, 1 (January 1911), 12.
[89] Anonymous Hindu Female, 'Mahilar Svasthya' ('Health of Women'), *Antahpur*, 6, 3 (1903), 57–61.
[90] Sarah Hodges, 'Indian Eugenics in an Age of Reform' in Sarah Hodges (ed.), *Reproductive Health in Colonial India: History, Politics, Controversies* (Hyderabad: Orient Longman, 2006), pp. 115–38.
[91] Hemangini Ray Dastidar, *Grihinir Hitopodesh* (*Advice for the Wife*), 1917, p. 18.
[92] Mahendranath Ghosh, *Soudaminir Dhatri Shikkha ebong Garbhini o Prashuti Chikitsha* (*Guidelines on Midwifery, Pregnancy and Reproductive Health Enunciated by Soudamini*), 1909, pp. 25–6.

By invoking figures associated with the so-called 'Bengal Renaissance' and adding the epithet of *beer* or courageous/warrior with each name, these manuals showed signs of being implicated in the muscular and chivalrous forms of the larger Hindu nationalist project.

Given the fundamental significance of reproductive health, the westernisation of the process of childbirth was another site of nationalist debate. Contemporary concern over the age-old, traditional childbirth process can be delineated into several categories, including insanitary conditions, illiterate midwives and high rates of mortality.[93] And it is also important to remember the raging colonial discussions on the system of '*purdah*' and the British equation between *purdah*, pollution and defilement.[94] On the other hand, however, western medicine's diktat of hospitalisation for childbirth faced stark cultural resistance from Indians. Indians, male and female alike, presented strong cultural resistance to exposing their bodies to the male English gaze.[95]

In this cultural turf war between modernity and tradition governing norms of reproduction, homoeopathy intervened with its culturally ambiguous identity. Homoeopathic authors reiterated notions of Indian modesty and the 'natural shyness' of respectable Hindu women, even arguing that Indian women were so coy that they 'preferred dying than exposing their body parts to unknown male doctors'.[96] By the decade of 1870–80, teaching medicine professionally to women in Medical Colleges was a topic of controversy, and homoeopaths were vocal in their objections against exposing women to professional medical education.[97] The article 'Stree Chikitshak' or 'Female Doctors', published in the journal *Hahnemann*, raised issues of ethics and morality in connection with the idea of women conducting dissection of nude human bodies.[98] It accused the government of not providing adequate infrastructure to ensure separate lectures for female students, since it was ethically incorrect for women to attend the lectures with men. Reading and

[93] Supriya Guha, 'The Best Swadeshi: Reproductive Health in Bengal' in Sarah Hodges (ed.), *Reproductive Health in Colonial India*, pp. 139–63.

[94] Maneesha Lal, 'Purdah as Pathology: Gender and the Circulation of Medical Knowledge in Late Colonial India, in Sarah Hodges (ed.), *Reproductive Health in India: History*, Politics, *Controversies*, 2006, pp. 85–114. Also see Maneesha Lal, 'The Politics of Gender and Medicine in Colonial India: The Countess of Dufferin's Fund, 1885–1888 ', *Bulletin of the History of Medicine*, 68, 1 (1994), 29–66.

[95] David Arnold, 'Touching the Body: Perspectives on the Indian Plague, 1896–1900', Ranait Guha (ed.) *Subaltern Studies V* (Delhi: Oxford University Press, 1987), pp. 55–90.

[96] Anonymous, 'Deshiya Dhatri' ('Indigenous Midwife'), *Hahnemann*, 2, 9 (1884), 161–3.

[97] Geraldine Forbes, *Women in Colonial India: Politics, Medicine and Historiography* (Delhi: Chronicle Books, 2005), p. 113. The book singles out Jamini Sen as the only woman who could continue her professional career

[98] Anonymous, 'Stree Chikitshak' ('Women Physician'), *Hahnemann*, 1, 4 (1883), 49–52.

learning homoeopathy at home, through the self-help homoeopathic manuals was promoted instead as the ideal solution, especially with relation to childbirth. Indeed, asserting homoeopathy's indigenous roots, such texts discussed how homoeopathic drugs assured painless, natural deliveries commensurate with the comfort ensured by modern medicine. It was argued that the application of suitable homoeopathic drugs 'works like a charm and spares women from difficult operations'.[99] Texts like *Thakurma (Grandmother)* – written as advice given by a grandmother to her granddaughter on the essentials of being an 'ideal woman' – stated that even in cases of complicated pregnancies, if doctors were not available, 'one should simply add a drop of homoeopathic Pulsatilla 30 in water and give that to the pregnant woman at regular intervals. It will inevitably lead to easy delivery'.[100] Manuals on reproductive health gave graphic details of the various phases of delivery and gave assurances against the need for any trained physician. It was held that physicians were necessary only in those exceptional cases where a defective child was born.[101]

These discussions inevitably extended to the issue of rearing healthy children. Conceived as the future citizens of the emerging nation, children remained the focus of a range of nationalist texts like *Grihadharma (Codes of the Household)*, which dealt with notions of appropriate upbringing of children for the good of the nation. Commenting on the fallen status of Indians at the hands of the British, this book urged every mother to bring up her child in a way that they could look after their 'relatives, society and the nation' and 'make contributions towards his race'.[102] The third section of the book, titled 'Lalon Palon' or 'Rearing of Children', included the opinions of famous contemporary homoeopaths including Pratap Chandra Majumdar, Chandrashekhar Kali, Jagadish Lahiri and others on child health.[103] The discourses on women's health, childcare and reproductive health remained deeply entangled with one another in the homoeopathic literature. It was held that the care of the child in reality 'begins, not at the time of birth but *in utero*. It is essential to guard the health, mental and physical, of the mother during pregnancy, if the best possible child is to be

99 M. M. Khatun, 'Homoeopathy r Abyartho Sandhan' ('The Guaranteed Cure of Homoeopathy'), *Hahnemann*, 20, 3 (1937), 158–60.

100 Manmathanath Chakrabarti, *Thakurma* (*Grandmother*) (Calcutta: Indian Art School, 1912), pp. 23–5.

101 Mahendranath Ghosh, *Soudaminir Dhatri Shikkha ebong Garbhini o Prashuti Chikitsha* (*Guidelines on Midwifery, Pregnancy and Reproductive Health Enunciated by Soudamini*), 1909, p. 298.

102 Bidyabati Saraswati Abiar (ed.), *Griha Dharma* (*Religion of Domesticity)*, 2nd edition (Calcutta: Hitabadi Press, 1910), pp. 2–3

103 Ibid., Preface to the 2nd edition, pp. 6–7.

born'.[104] Hence, discussions on child health frequently elaborated on various homoeopathic drugs effective in various stages and symptoms of pregnancy.[105] They also pledged to provide the most efficient treatment and handling in postnatal care of children beginning with the washing of the child.[106] The texts provided for the appropriate drugs for an extensive range of possible postdelivery disorders.

In identifying mindless modernisation as a fundamental reason behind increasing child mortality, the homoeopaths reiterated their diatribe against crass westernisation. In his book *Infantile Liver*, homoeopathic physician L. M. Pal lamented that, 'probably no other civilised nation witnesses so many untimely deaths in children'.[107] Pal identified the liver as the most vulnerable organ lying at the root of most suffering of children.[108] He was convinced that out of the false vanity of exhibiting their westernised lifestyle and affluence, middle-class Bengali women often continued the liquid milk diet for their children until they were two to three years of age. He argued that with age the liver began secreting liquid suitable for digesting solid food. At such a stage, if the child was still fed with liquid alone, the liver function was significantly hampered. He emphasised, 'when there was no advent of this crass civilisation in our country, this disease was nowhere to be found. It is seen recently in the last fifty years when we have learnt to emulate the English civilisation'.[109] The author prescribed independent indigenous solutions to such problems. He was a strong critic of the idea of depending on westerners for the solution of all the problems of Indians, including bodily unease.

Heralding it as the ideal 'indigenous' remedy, the texts elaborated on the possible use of homoeopathy as a substitute for certain forms of indigenous, folk knowledge or *totka*, transmitted within families across generations. A text on the traditional role of women in familial health explicitly stated, 'the earlier generation of women were specialists in child health. This is because prior to the advent of homoeopathy no one ever consulted a physician for treating children'.[110] Several commentators on women's health, homoeopaths and others, concurred that homoeopathy

[104] Douglas M. Borland, 'Homoeopathy and the Infant', *The Hahnemannian Gleanings*, 5 (1934), 80–1.

[105] Ibid., pp. 81–3.

[106] See Mahendranath Ghosh, *Soudaminir Dhatri Shikkha ebong Garbhini o Prashuti Chikitsha* (*Guidelines on Midwifery, Pregnancy and Reproductive Health Enunciated by Soudamini*), 1909.

[107] L. M. Pal, *Infantile Liver*, Calcutta: Hahnemann Publishing Company, 1935, pp. 1–3. Also see Anonymous, 'Jvar Tattva O Shishur Akal Mrittyu' ('Theories of Fever and Untimely Deaths of Children'), *Hahnemann*, 4, 5 (1921), 161–70.

[108] L. M. Pal, *Infantile Liver*, 1935.

[109] Ibid., pp. 18–26.

[110] Lalmohan Chakrabarty, 'Preface' in *Paribarik Chikitshay Grihini* (*Role of the Wife in Domestic Treatment*) (India: Dhaka Shakti Press, 1925), page number not cited.

was the most suitable form of medical treatment in the domestic arena, especially for women – it could be aligned with the modes of womanly caring that existed prior to the depredations of 'western living' and the harsh treatments associated with allopathy.

Nevertheless, the issue of women's agency remained a tricky one. In extending Lata Mani's contention about the patriarchal nature of debates around reform and the 'women's question', Mrinalini Sinha has identified the passing of the Sarda Act or the Child Marriage Restraint Act in 1929 as a crucial moment reflecting the organised women's voice in late colonial India.[111] She, and others including Sarah Hodges, have highlighted the significance of the women's groups and their journals like *Stri Dharma* in the passing of the Act, and other associated developments that invented new subject positions for women in consolidating 'a new nationalist modernity'. Targeting exclusively women readers, at one level, the homoeopathic discussions on women's health claimed to create a robust public platform for voicing women's issues. Such a platform promised to provide the most uninhibited responses to all queries that women might possibly have regarding their body and its functions. While discussing menstruation, for instance, homoeopathic manuals included, in minutest detail and with pictures, anatomical description of internal organs during menstruation.[112] They discussed the various possible menstrual dysfunctions and derangements at length. These discussions included descriptions of private, intimate details like the various forms of menstrual blood including their colour and smell, or the different kinds of unease related to breasts, their sizes and shapes.[113] Through such discussions homoeopathy asserted its claim in the most intimate world of femininity. In their attempt to reach out to women, the homoeopaths often devised certain novel strategies. Often the *materia medica*, with the names of various drugs and their symptoms, as seen in Fig. 4.2, was written in the form of a poem.[114] Women were advised to remember these verses by heart, and to use them from memory when required.[115]

[111] Mrinalini Sinha, 'Lineage of the Indian Modern: Rhetoric, Agency and the Sarda Act in Late Colonial India' in Antoinette Burton (ed.), *Gender, Sexuality and Colonial Modernities*, 1999, pp. 207–19.

[112] Krishnahari Bhattacharya, *Homoeopaty Mowt e Stree Rog Chikithsa* (*Homoeopathic Treatment of Female Diseases*) (Calcutta: Medical Library, 1886), p. 4–7.

[113] For instance, see Mahendranath Ghosh, *Soudaminir Dhatri Shikkha ebong Garbhini o Prashuti Chikitsha* (*Guidelines on Midwifery, Pregnancy and Reproductive Health Enunciated by Soudamini*), 1909.

[114] See, Ambikacharan Rakshita, *Homoeopathic Oushadh Shorashak* (*Sixteen Rules for Homoeopathic Drugs*) (Calcutta, 1909). See also Rajanikanta Majumdar, 'Bheshaja Shatak' ('Compendium of Hundred Drugs'), *Grihasthamangal*, 1, [Ben: Baisakh-Chaitra] (1927), p. 17.

[115] Ibid., Majumdar, p. 17.

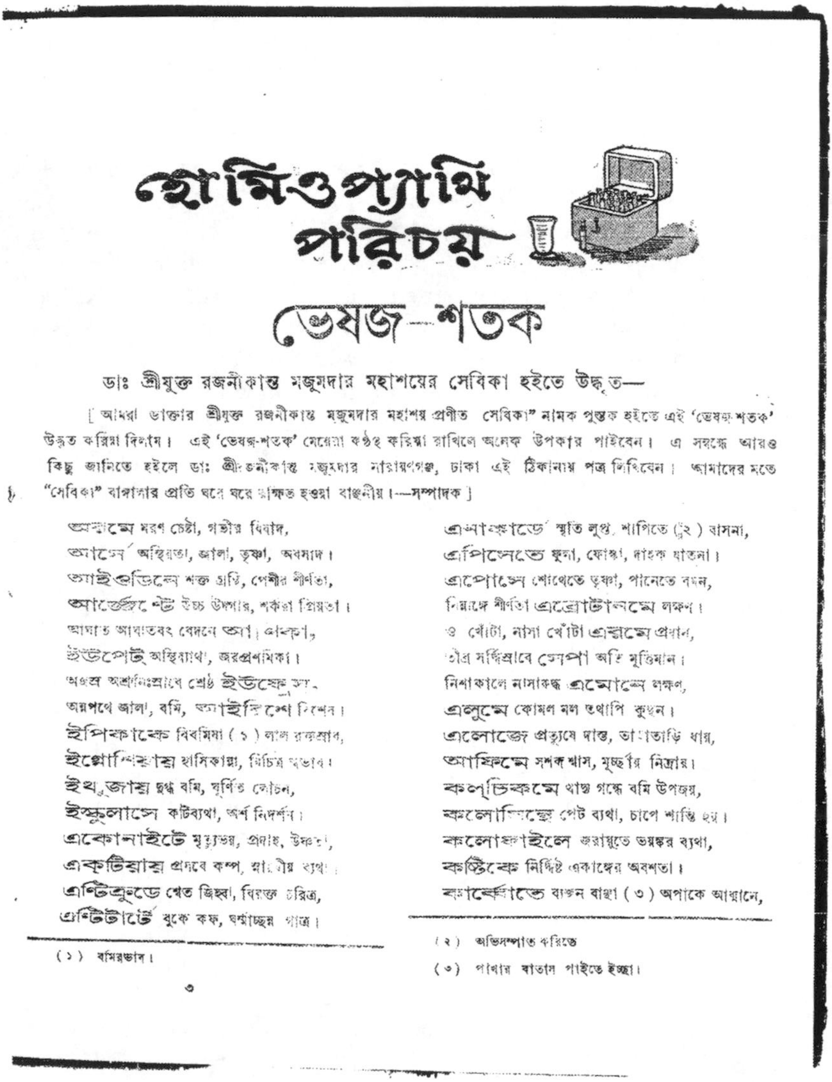

হোমিওপ্যাথি পরিচয়

ভেষজ-শতক

ডাঃ শ্রীযুক্ত রজনীকান্ত মজুমদার মহাশয়ের সেবিকা হইতে উদ্ধৃত—

[আমরা ডাক্তার শ্রীযুক্ত রজনীকান্ত মজুমদার মহাশয় প্রণীত "সেবিকা" নামক পুস্তক হইতে এই 'ভেষজ-শতক' উদ্ধৃত করিয়া দিলাম। এই 'ভেষজ-শতক' মেয়েরা কণ্ঠস্থ করিয়া রাখিলে অনেক উপকার পাইবেন। এ সম্বন্ধে আরও কিছু জানিতে হইলে ডাঃ শ্রীরজনীকান্ত মজুমদার নারায়ণগঞ্জ, ঢাকা এই ঠিকানায় পত্র লিখিবেন। আমাদের মতে "সেবিকা" বাঙ্গালার প্রতি ঘরে ঘরে রক্ষিত হওয়া বাঞ্ছনীয়।—সম্পাদক]

অরামে মরণ চেষ্টা, গভীর বিষাদ,
আর্সেনে অস্থিরতা, জ্বালা, তৃষ্ণা, অবসাদ।
আইওডিনে শক্ত গ্রন্থি, পেশীর শীর্ণতা,
আর্জেন্টে নাইট্রে উচ্চ উদ্গার, শর্করা প্রিয়তা।
আঘাত আঘাতবৎ বেদনে আর্ণিকা,
ইউপেটে অস্থিব্যথা, জ্বরপ্রশমিকা।
অজস্র অশ্রুনিঃস্রাবে শ্রেষ্ঠ ইউফ্রেসিয়া,
অন্নপথে জ্বালা, বমি, আইরিসে [illegible]।
ইপিকাকে বিবমিষা (১) লাল রক্তস্রাব,
ইগ্নেশিয়ায় হাসিকান্না, বিচিত্র স্বভাব।
ইথুজায় দুগ্ধ বমি, ঘূর্ণিত লোচন,
ইস্কুলাসে কটিব্যথা, অর্শ নিদর্শন।
একোনাইটে মৃত্যুভয়, প্রদাহ, উৎকণ্ঠা,
এক্টিয়ায় প্রসবে কম্প, স্নায়বীয় ব্যথা।
এণ্টিক্রুডে শ্বেত জিহ্বা, বিরক্ত চরিত্র,
এণ্টিটার্টে বুকে কফ, ঘর্মাচ্ছন্ন গাত্র।

(১) বমিরভাব।

এনাকার্ডে স্মৃতি লুপ্ত, শাপিতে (২) বাসনা,
এপিসেতে ফুলা, ফোস্কা, দাহক যাতনা।
এপোসে শোথেতে তৃষ্ণা, পানেতে বমন,
নিম্নাঙ্গে শীর্ণতা এব্রোটানমে লক্ষণ।
[illegible] খোঁটা, নাসা খোঁটা এরামে প্রধান,
তীব্র সর্দিস্রাবে সেপা অতি মূর্তিমান।
নিশাকালে নাসাবদ্ধ এমোনে লক্ষণ,
এলুমে কোমল মল তথাপি কুন্থন।
এলোজে প্রত্যুষে দাস্ত, তাড়াতাড়ি ধায়,
আফিমে সশব্দ শ্বাস, মূর্চ্ছার নিদ্রায়।
কল্চিকমে খাদ্য গন্ধে বমি উপজয়,
কলোসিন্থে পেট ব্যথা, চাপে শান্তি হয়।
কলোফাইলে জরায়ুতে ভয়ঙ্কর ব্যথা,
কষ্টিকে নির্দ্দিষ্ট একাঙ্গের অবশতা।
কার্ব্বোভেজে ব্যঞ্জন বাঞ্ছা (৩) অপাকে আধ্মানে,

(২) অভিসম্পাত করিতে
(৩) পাখার বাতাস পাইতে ইচ্ছা।

৩

Fig. 4.2 Excerpt from the text *Beshaja Shataka*, a compendium of a hundred drugs written in poem form for women published in the Bengali journal *Grihasthamangal*, 2, 1 (1928), 6. Reproduced from the collection of the Archives of the Centre for Studies in Social Sciences, Calcutta.

Often books were published as conversations between various female members of the household, most notably between the different wives and the mother-in-law. These texts cumulatively ended up projecting the figure of an idealised woman, who diligently practised homoeopathy in the home and who could serve as a role model for other Bengali middle-class women. These ideal types were sometimes the wives of the very same eminent homoeopaths whose model virtues were celebrated in obituaries published in homoeopathic journals. As was shown in the obituary article 'Homoeopathy Sebika r Parolokgamon' or 'Death of a Maid in Service of Homoeopathy', printed in the journal *Homoeopathy Paricharak*, the sphere of practice of Kiran Shashi Devi – wife to homoeopath Kalikumar Bhattacharya – was not always delimited by her own domesticity. Following their illustrious husbands, these women also dedicated their lives to the 'service of homoeopathy'.

Yet, this overwhelming engagement with women's issues should not blind us from recognising the almost wholesale absence of women's own voices from the homoeopathic archive. *Grihinir Hitopodesh (Advice for the Wife)*, written by Hemangini Ghosh Dastidar in 1917, features among the few glaring exceptions. A representative example of this absence of woman's own voice in the archive is the series of manuals framed around the fictitious character 'Soudamini', the supposed wife of a famous city-based homoeopath. In being self-sufficient, confident, literate and committed to social good, the character of Soudamini resonated with the woman *vaid* Yashoda Devi of northern India who has attracted scholarly attention, except that Soudamini was a fictitious character.[116] The Soudamini series of manuals elaborated the exploits of Soudamini as she visited her native village. Written as conversations between Soudamini and various village women, these manuals depict the free services that she offered to the female members of the village across hierarchies of caste and class. A hugely popular manual which went through three rapid editions, the story of Soudamini was also written in a distinctly pedagogic mode. It highlighted how an exclusive community of women was built around the personality of Soudamini as she disseminated free and effective medical knowledge among women beyond her immediate family. And although they illustrated the promise of a woman-centric network of homoeopathic transmission across Bengal, this series of manuals was authored by Calcutta-based male physician Mahendranath Ghosh.

[116] See Charu Gupta, 'Procreation and Pleasure: Writings of a Woman Ayurvedic Practitioner in Colonial North India', *Studies in History*, 21, 1 (2005), 17–44.

Ideal Domesticity and Its Threat: Prostitutes and Venereal Disease

Just as certain type of women were upheld as role models, however, others were designated as outright threats to both domesticity and health. Indeed, the new reformed woman of late colonial India was defined against an array of 'others', judged according to the categories of race, religion and class.[117] While the middle-class, Hindu undertone of the homoeopathic discourse is evident, it is the moral othering of the lowly women outside the marital framework that becomes most obvious in the discussions on health, gender and domesticity. A common trope in the late nineteenth-century social commentary alerted the readers to the immorality and sexual promiscuity that was pervasive among Bengali males, and which risked the peaceful sanctity of the familial space.

As the preface to the fourth manual of *Berigny and Company's Bengali Homoeopathic Series* suggested, 'the men in our country, either due to bad company in youth or as result of contagion or due to various other temptations ... suffer from venereal diseases'.[118] While complimenting the ideal-women encountered in the foregoing section, these texts demarcated a sphere of the 'bad women', marginal to the domestic space (i.e. the prostitutes or the 'dangerous outcastes' who nonetheless had the power to contaminate it).[119] Indeed, the eugenic core of the nationalist project was deeply committed to the control and proper channelling of sexuality within society.[120] Scholarship has only recently begun reflecting on the myriad vernacular discourses on eugenics, and are mostly focused on exploring the Hindi public sphere of North India.[121] Apart from the reproductive health manuals discussed in the previous section, there were specifically sexological advice manuals from homoeopathic authors who were convinced of the significance of eugenics, especially

[117] See Mary Hancock, 'Gendering the Modern: Woman and Home Science in British India' in Antoinette Burton (ed.), *Gender, Sexuality and Colonial Modernities*, 1999, pp. 149–62; and Charu Gupta, *Sexuality, Obscenity, and Community: Women, Muslims and the Hindu Public in Colonial India* (Delhi: Permanent Black, 2001), pp. 222–306.

[118] Harikrishna Mallik, 'Introduction', Sadrisa Byabostha Chikitsha Dipika *(*Glossary for Treatment According to the System of Similars), Berigny and Company's Bengali Homoeopathic Series Number III (Calcutta: Berigny and Company, 1870), page number not cited.

[119] The term has been borrowed from the exhaustive work on Bengali prostitutes by Sumanta Banerjee, *Dangerous Outcaste: Prostitutes in Nineteenth Century Bengal* (Calcutta: Seagull, 1998).

[120] Sanjam Ahluwalia, *Reproductive Restraints: Birth Control in India, 1877–1947* (New Delhi: Permanent Black, 2008), p. 305.

[121] Luzia Savary, 'Vernacular Eugenics? Santati-Sastra in Popular Hindi Advisory Literature (1900–1940)', *South Asia: Journal of South Asian Studies*, 37, 3 (2014), 381–97.

within the home. Discussions on sexology, venereal disease, reproduction and healthy self-reliant domesticity were inevitably interrelated. With its special promise with regard to moral disciplining, homoeopathy was considered indispensable not only to holding the moral fabric of the family together, but also to bolstering ideal conjugality and ensuring healthy progeny.

Immorality and promiscuity were seen as a regular, quotidian crisis. The article 'Jouna Samasya Samadhan er Ingit' or 'Hints towards Solving Sexual Problems' in the journal *Hahnemann* noted: 'Presently, the problem of sexuality is as widespread as that of shortage of food and poverty. It is difficult to discern which is a greater menace to familial peace and the health of different members. These problems are very closely related if one looks at them from the perspective of the norms of ideal domesticity.'[122] These homoeopathic texts drew the attention of their readers to an ever-growing demand for remedies for various sexual and venereal disorders among the Bengali male population. The article 'Homoeopathy Mowt e Jouna Byadhi Chikitshar Ingit' or 'Hints to Curing Sexual Ills with Homoeopathy' in the journal *Hahnemann*, regretted that the author was receiving too many letters from patients with sexual disorders to have the time to respond to them individually.[123] He was therefore forced to write an article in *Hahnemann* to reach out to many patients at once. He further noted that the cases were so diverse in their nature, orientation and symptoms, that they defied the standard prescriptions stated in the authoritative books on sexuality.[124]

The homoeopaths argued that it was impossible for social reformers to prevent people from engaging in sexual excess simply by lecturing and advising against it.[125] To them, sexual instinct was a natural, biological and even necessary human instinct. The manuals dealing with the cure of venereal diseases, therefore, contained wide-ranging discussions on the notions of sexuality, deviance, morality and their relationship with the changing institution of family. The two-volume manual *Sachitra Rati Jantraidir Peera: Sexual and Venereal Ills and Evils* is a representative text. It delineated in detail several familial structures that came into practice over time.[126] The author listed different familial formations like

[122] Bijoya Kumar Basu, 'Jouna Samasya Samadhan er Ingit' ('Hint towards Solving Sexual Problems'), *Hahnemann*, 22, 1 (1939), 26.

[123] R. Biswas, 'Homoeopathy Mowt e Jounabyadhi Chikitshar Ingit' ('Hints towards Curing Sexual Ills with Homoeopathy'), *Hahnemann*, 21, 10 (1938), 613.

[124] Ibid.

[125] Jnanendra Kumar Maitra, *Sachitra Rati Jantradi r Peera: Sexual and Venereal Ills and Evils*, Vol I (Calcutta: Maitra and Sons, 1923).

[126] Jnanendra Kumar Maitra, *Sachitra Rati Jantradi r Peera: Sexual and Venereal Ills and Evils*, Vol II, 1923, pp. 61–5.

the 'consanguine family', where men and women from the same lineage engaged in sexual acts. This was followed by the '*punaluan*' structure, after which the 'pairing' system came into vogue. By discussing the evolution of the notion of sexuality and corresponding ideas about 'family', the author arrived at his principal thesis. He argued that the modern notion of conjugality among monogamous couples was a very recent phenomenon. Since men were more numerous, he held, this particular idea of family centred around the father's lineage was devised keeping in mind the most effective distribution of paternal property.[127] The homoeopathic authors recognised the importance of families with monogamous couples. However, they were also acutely aware of the fact that men have had a longer history of engaging in sexual acts beyond marriage and procreation.[128] They rationalised that vestiges of such instincts persist, and prostitution as an industry thrives. Despite such rationalisation, however, they identified such trends as deeply troubling for 'modern' families. Syphilis and gonorrhoea, in this context, were identified as the two most threatening diseases. The readers were repeatedly reminded of the fact that 'gonorrhoea and syphilis – both are deeply entrenched in Bengali society, cohabiting with prostitutes is the main cause of both the diseases and such prostitutes are sources of much instability for the familial bonds'.[129]

The manuals condemned the inclination of Bengali *grihasthas* to conceal venereal diseases arguing that such a tendency towards 'concealing external manifestations' inevitably resulted in an aggravation of the disease, which often led to 'eternal suffering'.[130] The *grihasthas* were warned against the grave ramifications of this for their 'wife and future children who are forced to suffer'.[131] Furthermore, the silence and moral taboo around these diseases were identified as the biggest social obstruction to curing them. The author of *Sexual and Venereal Ills and Evils*, pointed out how the moral and social taboos associated with such ills forced sufferers to be secretive of their unease, and to rely upon 'advertisements of patent drugs promising miraculous cure of hidden diseases'.[132] These advertisements in almanacs, newspapers and other forums were decried as frauds that were essentially 'a means for filthy profit-making by abusing the physical

[127] Ibid., p. 63. [128] Ibid., pp. 64–5. [129] Ibid., p. 66.

[130] Jnanendra Kumar Maitra, *Sachitra Rati Jantradi r Peera: Sexual and Venereal Ills and Evils*, Vol I, 1923, Dedication page.

[131] Harikrishna Mallik, 'Introduction', *Sadrisa Byabostha Chikitsha Dipika* (*Glossary for Treatment According to the System of Similars*), *Berigny and Company's Bengali Homoeopathic Series Number III*, 1870, page number not cited.

[132] Jnanendra Kumar Maitra, 'Preface', *Sachitra Rati Jantradi r Peera: Sexual and Venereal Ills and Evils*, Vol I, 1923, page number not cited.

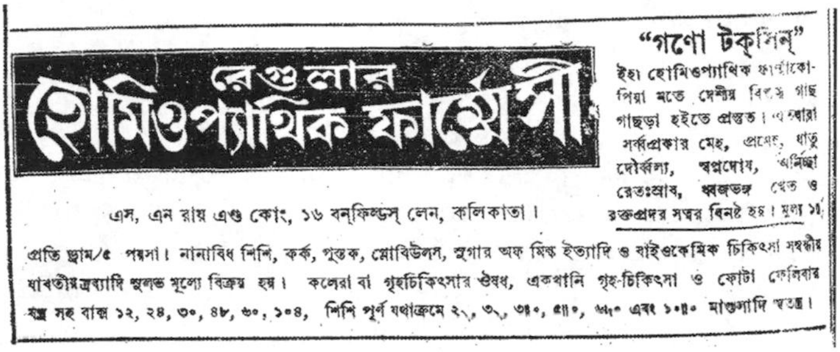

Fig. 4.3 Advertisement for the drug Gono-toxin by the Regular Homeopathic Pharmacy for home-based treatment of venereal disease, published in the Bengali journal *Grihasthamangal*, 2, 11 (1928), 2. Reproduced from the collection of the Archives of the Centre for Studies in Social Sciences, Calcutta.

weaknesses of people'.[133] Issues of morality, taboo and propriety also prevented these diseases and their remedies from being discussed even in medical schools and colleges, with the result that doctors did not seem to possess the expertise necessary to deal with these cases.[134] The homoeopathic manuals and journals, in this context, promised to fulfil the social duty of providing the most up-to-date scientific cure of such diseases (see Fig. 4.3).

Homoeopathic manuals argued that all other forms of treatment were ineffective against these maladies. Allopathy, according to them, could only provide for general sedatives and tonics: 'sedatives helped controlling the sexual impulses while tonics contributed to the overall health of the patient'.[135] Homoeopathy, in contrast, had an extensive list of drugs and cures specific to various symptoms. It was argued that unlike other systems, homoeopathy never recommended quick-fix cures with the use of injections. As was discussed in Chapter 3, homoeopathy in its diagnosis relied almost solely on the symptoms of the individual patient, and this was highlighted as its greatest advantage. Thus, the author of *Sexual and Venereal Ills and Evils* stated, 'the present symptoms and the past history of an individual is the guide in selecting homoeopathic drugs. It is never the case that two people suffering from the same disease have identical symptoms. Therefore, unlike any other form of treatment,

[133] Bijoy Kumar Basu, 'Jouna Samasya Samadhan er Ingit' ('Hint towards Solving Sexual Problems'), p. 26.
[134] Jnanendra Kumar Maitra, 'Preface', *Sachitra Rati Jantradi r Peera: Sexual and Venereal Ills and Evils*, Vol I, 1923.
[135] Ibid., p. 14.

a homoeopath will never be able to prescribe the same drugs for two similar cases'.[136]

It was further noted that mental symptoms occupied a central role in the homoeopathic treatment of sexual problems. The author of the article 'Homoeopathy Mowt e Jounabyadhi Chikitshar Ingit' or 'Hints towards Curing Sexual Ills with Homoeopathy' affirmed, 'Sexual problems are often manifestations of mental problems'.[137] Citing several case studies, the author stated that the names of a disorder like spermatorrhoea or impotency meant nothing for homoeopaths, since for them the key to the remedy lay in discovering the exclusive, specific symptoms.[138]

Apart from symptoms, the homoeopaths also put serious emphasis on dosage. In discussing the relative advantages of homoeopathy, it was argued that in case of certain diseases like syphilis, the chief curative substance (i.e. mercury) remained the same in all forms of treatment including allopathy, *kaviraji* and homoeopathy.[139] However, the extra-large doses prescribed by allopaths and others frequently resulted in further suffering for the patient. The mild, minute doses of homoeopathy in contrast ensured, 'that the patient's body was exempted from paying a painful penalty for taking drugs'.[140] The biggest 'benefit' and 'advantage' of homoeopathy in these diseases remained the painless nature of recovery that it ensured. Besides, the homoeopathic repertoire was far more extensive and included drugs 'whose use is never seen in allopathy, and in all likelihood, they have not heard of them'.[141] The manuals included elaborate *materia medica* exclusively for venereal diseases.[142]

Discussions in these manuals about the homoeopathic cure for venereal diseases incorporated commentaries on sexuality and deviance in contemporary society. While they acknowledged prostitution as one of the biggest menace to Indian domesticities, they argued against the forceful control of prostitution by the state. On this issue, they cited the example of the German state which attempted in vain to ban prostitution by police force.[143] The materiality of the homoeopathic drug itself was also considered insufficient in dealing with the widespread problem of immorality and the resultant venereal diseases. As such, the texts unequivocally

[136] Ibid., p. 126.
[137] R. Biswas, 'Homoeopathy Mowt e Jounabyadhi Chikitshar Ingit' ('Hints towards Curing Sexual Ills with Homoeopathy'), p. 614.
[138] Ibid., p. 618.
[139] Jnanendra Kumar Maitra, *Sachitra Rati Jantradi r Peera: Sexual and Venereal Ills and Evils*, Vol I, 1923, p. 157.
[140] Ibid., p. 69. [141] Ibid., p. 69.
[142] Jnanendra Kumar Maitra, *Sachitra Rati Jantradi r Peera: Sexual and Venereal Ills and Evils*, Vol II, 1923, pp. 1–47.
[143] Ibid., pp. 74–6.

prescribed a moral regimen and discipline, requiring them as complements to the drugs. They formulated a moral universe for their readers. Consumption of drugs was presented as only one part of the disciplining guided by moral proscriptions. An advertisement in the second edition of Hahnemann Publishing Company's *Dhatu Daurbalya* or *Seminal Weakness* stated that the book was a perfect balance of discussions on ethical advice and homoeopathic drugs for sexual diseases.[144]

Predictably, the institution of marriage was regarded in high esteem in these literatures. Families structured around monogamous married couples were praised as having the most desirable form. The homoeopaths regarded marriage as the most 'civilised and effective' way to retain 'true health and spirit'.[145] It was noted earlier that marriage and the proliferation of familial lineage were considered integrally related. Accordingly, and referring to the threats faced by the family institution from venereal diseases, the texts highlighted the potential dangers to monogamous marriage from venereal diseases. It was argued that these conditions had the potential to tarnish 'not only the reputation of the lineage but also the conjugal happiness of couples'.[146] The women within the families, who could be contaminated by their husbands, were shown to be particularly vulnerable to these diseases. In an engaging article titled 'Syphilis and Its Relations to Marriage' the author stated that usually 'she [the wife] is liable to very dangerous late lesions, and her power of transmitting the poison is much greater and more long lasting than that of the male'.[147] The homoeopathic literature affirmed these diseases as capable of infecting the child and threatening 'the disappearance of that particular lineage and race'.[148]

The prescribed regimen within the texts, therefore, included instructions for living in an ethically sound conjugality. Every couple had to be aware of the essentials of eugenics, and Bengali girls and boys should also be made aware of them 'at home and in schools and colleges'.[149] The texts disciplined their readers not only about the frequency with which one could practice cohabitation for a healthy family life, but also

144 'Advertisement of Dhatu Daurbalya' in *Hahnemann*, 22, 1 (1939), 11.

145 Jnanendra Kumar Maitra, *Sachitra Rati Jantradi r Peera: Sexual and Venereal Ills and Evils*, Vol II, 1923, pp. 76–7.

146 Jnanendra Kumar Maitra, *Sachitra Rati Jantradi r Peera: Sexual and Venereal Ills and Evils*, Vol I, 1923, p. 61.

147 Anonymous, 'Upodangsho o Bibaho' (Syphilis and Marriage'), *Hahnemann*, 3, 1 (1885), 26.

148 Anonymous, 'Jvar Tattva O Shishur Akal Mrittyu' ('Theories of Fever and Untimely Deaths of Children'), p. 214.

149 Jnanendra Kumar Maitra, *Sachitra Rati Jantradi r Peera: Sexual and Venereal Ills and Evils*, Vol II, 1923, pp. 72–3.

about the prescribed number of times that couples of various age groups should practice intercourse. They further detailed the most suitable time of the day for such sexual acts.[150] They even included a *materia medica* exclusively for physical unease resulting from cohabitation.[151] Readers were warned against frequent cohabitation as it could result in loss of strength in men, even leading to impotency.[152]

Contemporary Bengali medical print is ridden with anxiety over the potential depletion of seminal fluids.[153] Existing scholarship has dealt with regulations and norms of sexuality set by the nationalist patriarchy in constituting the ideal Hindu wife.[154] The homoeopathic texts shared such concerns, while also connecting the eugenic anxiety with the concerns over familial economy and budget. This is evident from homoeopathic texts that discouraged frequent cohabitation since it increased the possibility of frequent impregnation of the wife. These texts cautioned the *grihasthas* that too many children often meant paying less attention to them individually, while also implying a strain on the familial budget. It was argued that, 'it is important to comfortably bring up the child who is forced to arrive as a result of the parents seeking pleasure'.[155]

Cohabitation without pregnancy was acceptable. The book *Sexual and Venereal Ills and Evils* extensively discussed all prevalent forms of contraception from rubber sheaths to patent medicine or quinine solutions.[156] However, the author expressed his reliance on *sangyam* or 'self-control' and 'will power' as the most effective measure. Reminding the householders of the necessity of cultivating an ethical way of life, he advised the husbands to 'concentrate all the force of their mind upon the more peaceful, devotional, sacrificial aspect of their love, rather than upon its more passionate and physical side'.[157] Certain homoeopaths even pointed out the importance of addressing the increasing lack of religiosity among the Hindus as compared to Christians and Muslims.[158] Cultivation of

[150] Ibid., pp. 82–4.
[151] R. Biswas, 'Homoeopathy Mowt e Jounabyadhi Chikitshar Ingit', pp. 618–19.
[152] Jnanendra Kumar Maitra, *Sachitra Rati Jantradi r Peera: Sexual and Venereal Ills and Evils*, Vol I, 1923, p. 24.
[153] Projit Bihari Mukharji, *Nationalizing the Body: The Medical Market, Print and Daktari Medicine* (London and New York: Anthem Press, 2011), pp. 213–50.
[154] See Tanika Sarkar, *Hindu Wife, Hindu Nation: Community, Religion and Cultural Nationalism* (Delhi: Permanent Black, 2001). Also, see Charu Gupta, Sexuality, Obscenity, and Community, 2001, pp. 123–96.
[155] Jnanendra Kumar Maitra, *Sachitra Rati Jantradi r Peera: Sexual and Venereal Ills and Evils*, Vol II, 1923, p. 86.
[156] Ibid., p. 101–11. [157] Ibid., p. 116–17.
[158] Anonymous, 'Jvar Tattva O Shishur Akal Mrittyu' ('Theories of Fever and Untimely Death of Children'), pp. 211–13.

religiosity was considered relevant to stimulating a morally sensitive way of being.

Apart from advising a monogamous, controlled and morally upright conjugal life, the homoeopathic manuals also advocated a disciplined and regulated way of living. They strongly advised against alcohol and every other form of intoxication and suggested a simple diet. It was argued that strong food or drink clashed with the mild doses of homoeopathic drugs and was an impediment to their smooth functioning.[159] It was asserted that the homoeopathic drugs worked best when one led a composed, balanced and disciplined life.[160] Consumption of alcohol was especially discouraged in a range of articles, which enumerated the evils of alcohol in the body and its harmful interactions with homoeopathic drugs.[161] Those who found it difficult to get rid of their habit were advised to have a small quantity of indigenous liquor, as it was relatively less harmful.[162] To some authors, 'vegetarianism and practice of celibacy are often more effective than any drug in curing venereal disease'.[163] It was argued that '*jibon jatrar pronali*' or the conduct of everyday life held the key to an ideal domesticity.[164]

So much importance was attached to the conduct of everyday life that the manuals even insisted on the need of such discipline on the part of the physicians themselves.[165] In an interesting article titled 'How I Attained My Long Life' published in the journal *Hahnemann*, the author Piyari Mohan Mukhopadhyay identified his own disciplined lifestyle, along with consumption of homoeopathy, as the secret to his long life of ninety-plus years.[166] An obituary article in the same journal highlighted that Piyari Mohan, a close friend of both Rajendralal Datta and Mahendralal Sircar, had conducted an extremely disciplined lifestyle.[167] The article emphasised that he never consumed any other

159 Jagachandra Raya, *Garhasthya Svastha ebong Homoeopathic Chikitsha Bigyan* (*Domestic Heath and Homoeopathic Medical Science*) (Calcutta: Harendranath Roy, 1917), p. 176.

160 Anonymous, *Homoeopathic Mowt e Saral Griha Chikitsha* (*Simple Home Treatment According to Homoeopathy*), 1926, pp. 14–16.

161 For instance, see Anonymous, 'Surapaan' ('Drinking Alcohol'), *Hahnemann*, 1, 12 (1883), 177–81. Also see Haranath Ray, 'Madyapan Jonito Rog' ('Diseases Relating to Drinking Alcohol'), *Chikitsha Sammilani*, 4 (1887), 26–8.

162 Jagachandra Raya, *Garhasthya Svastha ebong Homoeopathic Chikitsha Bigyan* (*Domestic Heath and Homoeopathic Medical Science*), 1917, p. 176.

163 R. Biswas, 'Homoeopathy Mowt e Jounabyadhi Chikitshar Ingit' ('Hints for Treating Venereal Disease According to Homoeopathy'), p. 614.

164 Ibid., p. 614.

165 Akhil Chandra Ray, 'Jouna Samasya Samadhan Sambandhe Du Ekti Kotha' ('One or Two Words on the Treatment of Venereal Diseases'), *Hahnemann*, 23, 7 (1940), 29, 32.

166 Piyari Mohan Mukhopadhyay, 'Amar Deeghayu Labh er Karon' ('How I Attained My Long Life'), *Hahnemann*, 21, 7 (1938), 411–13.

167 'Editorial', *Hahnemann*, 21, 7 (1938), 422–3.

drug other than homoeopathy in his lifetime and enjoyed a remarkably long and healthy life.[168]

Swadeshi Homoeopathy: Domesticity as the Site for Production

Quotidian practice of homoeopathy was thus seen as the proposed indigenous remedy for the crisis-ridden, ailing domesticity in Bengal. Regular consumption of homoeopathy was held to be commensurate with the values and ethics representing the emergent nation. It was widely noted that both nationalism and homoeopathy shared the specific virtues of self-sufficiency: self-rule or '*swaraj*', and self-reliant economy or '*swadeshi.*'[169] Since the early twentieth century, homoeopaths intermittently pointed out that despite its emphasis on self-reliance, India was largely dependent on the supply of homoeopathic drugs from abroad. Hence homoeopathic literature on domestic health increasingly encouraged its consumers to be attentive to the processes of production. This appeal was directed primarily to the same householders or the Bengali *grihasthas* who had been encouraged to consume homoeopathy since the mid-nineteenth century. The texts emphasised the crucial role that every household could potentially play in the experiments related with the preparation of drugs. One finds an unmistakable resonance with the Gandhian ideology of production and consumption around '*khadi*', except that it was now adopted even in the production of scienticised commodities.[170]

Through their publications, the homoeopaths elaborated on the incentives to experiment with indigenous or local plants of India. The process of discovering new drugs or 'proving' was considered a critical aspect of homoeopathic knowledge. As the author of the tract *Bharat Bhaishajya Tattwa: Materia Medica of Indian Drugs* pointed out, apart from the homoeopathic law, the other crucial contribution of Hahnemann was the methodology of testing drugs on the healthy

[168] Ibid., pp. 422–3.

[169] '*Swadeshi*', literally meaning 'indigenous', was a specific strand of nationalist ideology that emphasised confronting the colonial rule through the development of Indian economy. *Swadeshi* was committed to the ideology of self-sufficiency, primarily in the economic realm. Strategies of the *swadeshi* movement involved boycotting British products and the revival of domestic products and production processes. For a comprehensive history of *swadeshi*, see Sumit Sarkar, *Swadeshi Movement in Bengal, 1903–08* (Delhi: People's Publishing House, 1973).

[170] For a discussion on the relation between Gandhian ideology of spinning Khadi and nationalism see Susan S. Bean, 'Gandhi and Khadi: The Fabric of Indian Nationalism' in Annette B. Weiner and Jane Schneider (eds.), *Cloth and Human Experience* (Washington: Smithsonian Institution Press, 1989), pp. 355–76.

human body.[171] Indeed, it was argued that testing and proving drugs on healthy individuals as opposed to 'clinical verification' was a distinct feature that set homoeopathy apart from other medical systems, notably allopathy.[172] Drug proving essentially involved ingestion of different forms of vegetation in a specified manner, by healthy individuals. The 'provers' had to maintain a record of all the minute reactions that were generated in their body following such ingestion. The knowledge of their reactions to various quantities of consumed vegetation was considered critical to preparing homoeopathic drugs from the plants. The authors regretted the fact that while many Bengali householder-physicians adopted the homoeopathic law in their practice, they remained deficient in their efforts towards the other important aspect of homoeopathy (i.e. proving), especially of Indian plants.

There is a body of scholarship on the sustained imperial interests in indigenous botanical resources as part of 'knowing' and ruling India.[173] However, more recent scholarship, such as Projit Bihari Mukharji's work, has opened up the study of the transition from the initial imperialist-orientalist engagements with Indian botanical knowledge, to the rising nationalist interest in Indian plants.[174] Although more interested in exploring the contested identity of plants as well as the 'politics of retro-botanising', Projit's work, nonetheless, hints at the ways in which the emotive logic of economic nationalism manifested itself in a heightened sense of nationalism around the production of 'indigenous drugs'.[175] With the rapid Indianisation of the scientific establishment in post-First World War India, the decade of the 1920s saw an unprecedented spike in the number of scientists in Indian laboratories who were working with indigenous plants. Not all of these were medicinal plants. Many were the potential source of dyestuff, but many others were investigated for their

[171] Pramada Prasanna Biswas, 'Note to Indian Physicians', Bharat *Bhaishajya Tattwa: Materia Medica of Indian Drugs* (Pabna: Hahnemann Medical Mission, 1924), page number not cited.

[172] See Pramada Prasanna Biswas, 'Letter to the Editor', *Hahnemann*, 7, 7 (1924), 332. See also by the same author, *Bharat Bhaishajya Tattwa: Materia Medica of Indian Drugs*, 1924, pp. 466–7.

[173] For a comprehensive study, see Kavita Philip, *Civilising Natures: Race, Resources and Modernity in Colonial South India* (Hyderabad: Orient Longman, 2003). Also see David Arnold, *Tropics and the Travelling Gaze: India, Landscape and Science, 1800–1856* (Seattle: Washington University Press, 2006).

[174] Projit Bihari Mukharji, 'Pharmacoloy, Indigenous Knowledge and Nationalism, Few Words from the Epitaph of Subaltern Science' in Mark Harrison and Biwamoy Pati (eds.), *The Social History of Health and Medicine in Colonial India* (London: Routledge, 2008), pp. 195–212.

[175] Projit Bihari Mukharji, 'Vishalyakarani as E. Ayapana: Retro-Botanizing, Embedded Traditions and Multiple Histories of Plants in Colonial Bengal, 1890–1940', *Journal of Asian Studies*, 73, 1 (2014), 65–87.

potential medicinal uses. Likewise, Guy Attewell's work illustrates that the issue of plant heritage was an integral part of the Islamic revivalist agenda around unani medicine explicated most prominently in the All India *vaid* and unani conferences of the 1910s and 1920s.[176] In conversation with these ongoing developments in high nationalism and among distinguished medico-scientific professionals, the Bengali homoeopaths then extended the discussion on indigenous plants within the bounds of everyday domesticity. Their texts envisioned each household and its backyard as a potential laboratory of homoeopathic drugs. Ordinary householders or the *grihasthas*, with no professional training, were argued to be capable of producing and positively contributing to the repertoire of homoeopathic knowledge and pharmacopoeia. In so doing, these texts diffused the professional/amateur divide yet again, also in the realm of drug production.

The authors issued a clarion call for their fellow homoeopaths and readers to address the problem of foreign dependence by engaging in extensive experimentation and 'proving' with Indian vegetation. A letter to the editor of the journal *Hahnemann* in 1925 stated this urgency, by saying that proper proving of indigenous plants would be beneficial not only for Indians but for the entire world.[177] Directly referring to the growing nationalist ideology of '*swadeshi*' and self-reliance, the authors held that the production of indigenous drugs should be the logical culmination of the cult of swadeshi nationalism.[178] The authors reminded their readers of the difficulty faced in procuring homoeopathic drugs during the First World War. Published in 1924, the *Materia Medica of Indian Drugs* stated that 'it was impossible to get drugs from Germany during the war. Simple drugs like Aconite, Bryonia and Belladonna that are prepared from German plants were difficult to procure. The American dealers supplied those drugs at their will at the end of the war'.[179] Early twentieth-century homoeopaths further argued that the imported drugs fell short of curing peculiarly Indian diseases. They emphasised, as Fig. 4.4 suggests, the manifold usefulness of drugs made of indigenous vegetation over the imported ones. Sarat Chandra Ghose, a biographer of Mahendralal Sircar, for instance, noted in his work, 'it is daily marked by us that the plants growing in a particular locality bear a remarkable affinity to the temperament and constitution of the individuals inhabiting

[176] Guy Attewell, *Refiguring Unani Tibb*, 2007, pp. 171–91.
[177] Anonymous, 'Letter to the Editor: Alochona'('Discussion'), *Hahnemann*, 8, 5 (1925), 234.
[178] Anonymous, 'Atma Nirbharata' ('Self-Sufficiency'), *Svasthya*, 3, 7 (1899), 35–7.
[179] Pramada Prasanna Biswas, 'Note to Indian Physicians', *Bharat Bhaishajya Tattwa: Materia Medica of Indian Drugs*, 1924, page number not cited.

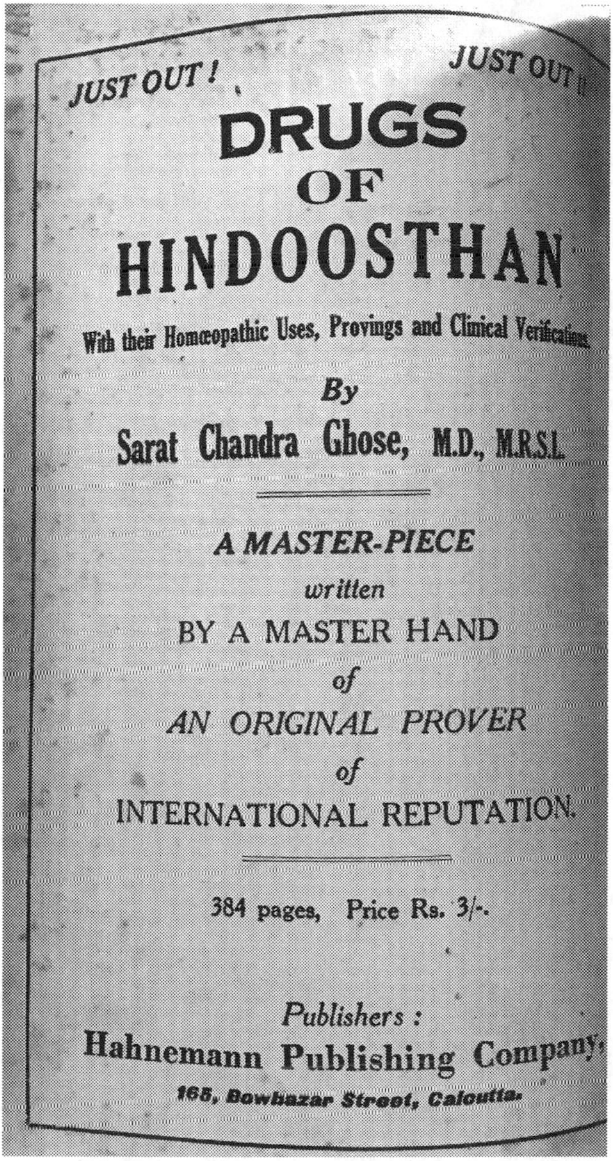

Fig. 4.4 Advertisement for a representative homoeopathic text on the indigenous drugs of India, advocating domestic homoeopathic proving. *Hahnemannian Gleanings*, 9 (May 1938), 13. Credit: Hahnemann Publishing Company Private Limited, Kolkata.

that locality. It is, therefore, apparent that Indian drugs will be found most suitable to our constitution'.[180]

These texts recommended the 'discovery' of newer remedies through experiments with indigenous substances. Celebration of the 'indigenous' or *swadeshi* was indeed a compelling feature in shared discussions on homoeopathy, family and nationalism. The proving of indigenous plants was upheld as an effective way to overcome dependence on the West and to cultivate self-sufficiency for Indians. The December 1928 editorial of the journal *Homoeopathy Pracharak*, for instance, proudly noted that the homoeopathic drugs prepared out of indigenous plants were selected for the exhibition marking the following session of the Indian National Congress, the biggest nationalist party in colonial India.[181]

Lay householders were encouraged actively to participate in experiments directed towards producing newer homoeopathic drugs with 'indigenous' vegetation. They were urged to come forward in an endeavour to complete an Indian *materia medica* of homoeopathic drugs.[182] It was declared that such a 'daunting task' would require the participation of the 'thousands of amateurs, patrons and practitioners of homoeopathy'.[183] As an article in the *Calcutta Journal of Medicine* insisted, '[i]t is more than probable that the Indian flora contains specimens which would best be adapted to cure diseases peculiar to this country. Will there not be found, in that very same country, specimens of men, ready to subject themselves to proving of the drugs of their own soil?'[184] Indeed, every individual, every householder, was encouraged to be an 'active' and 'energetic' volunteer, and to participate in whatever capacity they could.[185] It was pointed out that those who could not be physically involved in the direct proving of drugs in their body could still contribute by consuming the drugs after they were proved.[186] They were encouraged to report their reactions to the various doses of a proven

[180] Sarat Chandra Ghose, *Life of Dr. Mahendralal Sircar*, 2nd edition (Calcutta: Hahnemann Publishing Company, 1935), p. 79.

[181] K. K. Ray, 'Editorial: Prodorshoni te Deshiya Homeo Oushadh'('Indigenous Homoeopathic Drugs at Exhibition') *Homeopathy Pracharak*, 2, 9 (December 1928), 366.

[182] Pramada Prasanna Biswas, 'Deshiya Oushadh Sambondhe Aboshyokiyo Kotoguli Kotha' ('Few Useful Words on the Indigenous Drugs'), *Hahnemann*, 8, 7 (1925), 372.

[183] Leopold Salzer, 'On the Necessity of Drug Proving in India', *Calcutta Journal of Medicine*, 2, 5 and 6 (May–June 1869), 177–8.

[184] Ibid.

[185] H. P. Maity, 'Deshiya Beshaja o Tahar Shakti' ('Indigenous Vegetation and Its Power'), *Hahnemann*, 7, 4 (1924), 174.

[186] Pramada Prasanna Biswas, 'Homeopathic Bhaishajya Tattwer Bishesattva o Sustho Manob Dehe Oushadh er Porikkha' ('Peculiarity of the Homoeopathic Materia Medica and Proving Drugs on Healthy Human Bodies'), *Hahnemann*, 6, 10 (1923), 100.

drug. The participation of women was especially sought. Thus, after proving the plant *Atista Indica* and publishing its result in the journal *Hahnemann*, physician Kalikumar Bhattacharya noted, 'before inserting this as an official remedy we need to get it tested in some other humans. Specially to know how it works in female constitution and affects which organs, we have to inspire some women to take up the task'.[187] Participating as a family was also highly recommended, so that many members of the same household were involved. The author of *Bharat Bhaishajjya Tattwa: Materia Medica of Indian Drugs* narrated how members of his big family, as well as other relatives, joined him in his commitment to the task of proving indigenous drugs for malarial fever.[188] By way of preparing the 'ordinary', 'amateur' householders for such tests, the texts included detailed instructions on reading 'relevant parts of the *Organon*, and indicated certain guidelines for the potential lay 'provers'.[189] These provers needed to follow certain routines and regulations in their quotidian life for the period they were engaged in the testing of indigenous plants. The article 'Ashar Alok' or 'Light of Hope', recorded that the *grihasthas* had to practice vegetarianism and celibacy for at least one month prior to the test.[190] During this period of testing, they were required to have a disciplined routine of bathing, eating and sleeping, and were expected to engage in peaceful, religious discussions.[191]

These egalitarian invitations to 'ordinary', 'amateur' people were sometimes debated within the ranks of the homoeopaths themselves. Some authors were doubtful of the viability of involving of lay householders. To them, it was dangerous for a lay person to test any plant and infer its precise medicinal values. They strongly felt that 'some specific knowledge and awareness was necessary for such mass participation in 'knowledge production'.[192] However, authors like Kalikumar Bhattacharya, contributing to the same journals, contested such a viewpoint. In a letter to the editor of the journal *Hahnemann,* Bhattacharya took a strong position against the advocacy of specialised

[187] Kalikumar Bhattacharya, 'Atista Indica Proving er Itibritta' ('Account of Proving Atista Indica'), *Hahnemann*, 4, 9 (1921), 323.

[188] Pramada Prasanna Biswas, 'Note to Indian Physicians' in *Bharat Bhaishajya Tattva: Materia Medica of Indian Drugs* (Pabna: Hahnemann Medical Mission, 1924), page number not cited.

[189] Pramada Prasanna Biswas, 'Homoeopathic Bhaishajya Tattver Bishesattva o Sustho Manab Dehe Aushadh er Parikkha' ('Peculiarity of the Homoeopathic Materia Medica and Proving Drugs on Healthy Human Bodies'), pp. 463–6.

[190] Kalikumar Bhattacahrya, 'Ashar Alok' ('Light of Hope'), pp. 81–2. [191] Ibid., p. 81.

[192] H. P. Maity, 'Deshiya Beshaja o Tahar Shakti' ('Power of Indigenous Vegetation'), *Hahnemann*, 7, 4(1924), 177.

knowledge.[193] In response to an attack by a younger colleague, he cited instances from his own life where his research into new drugs had been guided by time-tested medicinal knowledge gathered among women, and transmitted across the generations of a household.[194] To Bhattacharya, lay, familial participation was of utmost importance, not only in the dissemination of homoeopathic knowledge, but also in its production.[195] However, the texts also admitted the need for adequate caution in the attempts at proving. A letter written in 1925 to the editors of the journal *Hahnemann* had initiated discussions on the precise methods of homoeopathic proving.[196] The letter's author noted that to eliminate any chances of error, it was always advisable to test each plant on multiple groups of people of different ages and constitutions.[197]

These discussions on indigenous vegetation involved a range of plants that were most easily available and 'often grown in the backyards of one's residence'.[198] Of those most extensively experimented and written about were Ocimum (Tulsi), Kalmegh, Papaya and Neem. The authors encouraged ordinary householders to test these mundane, commonplace species of vegetation which one would encounter on a daily basis. The author of the article 'Talks about Homoeopathy' in the journal *The Hahnemannian Gleanings* invited his readers to test 'Marigold (*Calendula officianialis*), known to you as the Gainder; sometimes you decorate your houses with it and make garlands from it'.[199] Deliberately diluting the possibility of any rigid professional/amateur divide, these texts highlighted each Bengali household and its backyard as a potential laboratory for homoeopathic drugs. There were sporadic impulses towards forming formal institutions, especially in the context of experimenting with new drugs. In his biography of Mahendralal Sircar, the physician Sarat Chandra Ghose proudly announced the foundation of the Hindusthan Institute of Indigenous Drug-Proving, stating 'this sort of a society is the crying need of India'.[200] However, such efforts at establishing societies were few and far between, and many of the twentieth-century initiatives almost always faced a dead-end for reasons that will be taken up in Chapter 5.

[193] Kalikumar Bhattacharya, 'Letter to the Editor: Alochonar Prattyuttor' ('Reply to Discusion'), *Hahnemann*, 8, 5 (1925), 239–48.
[194] Ibid., pp. 240–1. [195] Ibid.
[196] Anonymous, 'Letter to the Editor: Alochona' ('Discussion'), pp. 234–8. [197] Ibid.
[198] Pramada Prasanna Biswas, *Bharat Bhaishajya Tattwa: Materia Medica of Indian Drugs*, 1924, p. 1.
[199] J. H. Freebome, 'Talks About Homoeopathy', *The Hahnemannian Gleanings*, 3 (December 1932), 515.
[200] Sarat Chandra Ghose, *Life of Dr. Mahendralal Sircar*, 1935, p. 79.

The author of the article 'Homoeopathy Mowt e Aushadh Porikkha' or 'Drug Testing According to Homoeopathy' complained that there were frequent resolutions towards forming societies or associations to conduct tests that never materialised.[201]

The homoeopaths, in the context of 'proving' familiar plants and testing new indigenous drugs in the lay, familial home, promoted a distinct kind of institutionalisation around the professional journals. They sought active contributions from ordinary readers relating to their experiments with indigenous plants. The readers were encouraged not only to participate in proving, but also to register their names with an established homoeopathic journal before they began doing so.[202] They were asked to report all the relevant information regarding the date, time, amount consumed and the symptoms in their bodies. The journals reported the eagerness of many readers who wrote to them about participating in experiments. Others were reported as expressing interest in consuming the newly proved drugs in illness. Thus, the author of the article 'Ashar Alok' in the journal *Hahnemann* noted that, 'it is a matter of great hope that many people, often as a couple, have proved certain drugs or have shown interest in tasting proved drugs like my quinia indica'.[203] Many readers responded with their feedback on the tested drugs.[204] The journals therefore emerged as a unique forum where professional physicians, amateur authors, lay householders interested in participating in homoeopathic endeavours, as well as ordinary consumers and readers interacted extensively with one another. The authors earnestly encouraged these various genres of readers to write and discuss various facets of homoeopathy including their own experience of consuming drugs. The journals noted that through such reciprocal exchanges, certain drugs became 'popular articles of everyday use'.[205] Experiments with Indian plants were also a medium of assertion for Indian physicians in the homoeopathic pharmacopoeia which circulated globally. The journals equally provided a space for Bengali physicians to advertise their drugs and to assert their presence on international platforms. The 1934 editorial of the journal *The Hahnemannian Gleanings* related at length that physician Sarat Chandra Ghose had been given honorary membership of

[201] S. C. Dey, 'Homoeopathy Mowt e Oushadh Porikkha' ('Drug Testing According to Homoeopathy'), *Hahnemann*, 21, 5 (1938), 272.

[202] Kalikumar Bhattacahrya, 'Ashar Alok' ('Light of Hope'), p. 82. [203] Ibid., p. 81.

[204] See Pramada Prasanna Biswas, 'Advertisement to the First Edition' in *Bharat Bhaishajya Tattva: Materia Medica of Indian Drugs*, 1924, page number not cited.

[205] S. C. Dey, 'Homoeopathy Mowt e Aushadh Parikkha' ('Drug Testing According to Homoeopathy'), p. 278.

the very prestigious Royal Society of Literature of the United Kingdom in view of his 'systematic and original researches in the domain of indigenous drugs'.[206]

Conclusion

I have been tracing the entanglement of homoeopathic writings from the late nineteenth and early twentieth century with the pervasive nationalist angst about the decline of the Hindu joint family owing to unbridled westernisation. I have illustrated how the literature on homoeopathy intervened in the entwined nationalist anguish, both over the future of Bengali families and the deteriorating quotidian health of Bengalis. Consumption of homoeopathy was written about as the most cost-effective, indigenous remedy to the corruptions colonialism had induced to the pristine ways of Indian life. Overlapping ideas on indigenous production and political sovereignty were the ideological core of late nineteenth-century economic nationalism. Homoeopaths framed this politico-economic discourse exclusively in familial terms. With its emphasis on the production and consumption of things 'indigenous' to the home, homoeopathy was to be the precise answer to the nationalist quest for self-help, '*swadeshi*' and economic sovereignty. The Bengali print market crafted homoeopathy as a pragmatically hybrid science – one that was compatible with indigenous ways, yet also equipped with western scientific credentials. In foregrounding the resonance of '*swadeshi* homoeopathy', this account complicates the existing revivalist narratives by illustrating how a hybrid category like homoeopathy was celebrated as the ideal form of indigeneity in a colonial context.

Homoeopathy put forward a unique egalitarian promise of creating democratic citizen-doctors of the future. As the world of manuals and journals reveals, homoeopathy was a science that could be mastered at home, by all, through the simple act of reading and memorising. The notion of professionalisation as understood in twentieth-century India stood fractured and diluted in this discourse. In almost defying the need to learn homoeopathy through professional institutions, it promoted a different form of institutionalisation. Together with the cult of biography writing and an extensive print production generated primarily by the family firms, as demonstrated in earlier chapters, and alongside the advisory literature discussed here, Bengali homoeopathy thrived within a different paradigm of institutions. An overlapping network of

[206] S. K. Das, 'Editorial Notes and Comments', *The Hahnemannian Gleanings*, 5 (August 1934), 332–3.

physicians, manufacturers, drug sellers, publishers, journal editors and writers organised and sustained homoeopathy around the central dynamic of 'family'. Yet, as the twentieth century rolled on, formal institutionalisation of pedagogy and service was inevitable. Next, I turn to negotiations of the aforesaid familial network with the government in the second quarter of the twentieth century in delineating a space for 'authentic' homoeopathy through state legislation.

5 A Homoeopathic Public: Elections, Public Health and Legislation

> '... homoeopathy needed to win the government by its side, failing which it would fade in comparison with its state-supported allopathic or even ayurvedic counterparts.'[1]

> '... some provision should be made to prevent the practice, now prevalent in Calcutta and the *mofussil*, of homoeopathic practitioners adopting letters which imply the possession of registrable (sic) diploma in western medicine while merely correcting this implication by adding in small type the term 'homoeo' or even the letter 'h', eg. L.M.S homoeo or L.M.S.H.'[2]

> 'Allopathic doctors may not find any merit in that system, but so far as millions of patients in Bengal are concerned, they will, I think, freely recognise its merits in view of the benefits they daily derive.'[3]

In the interwar years between the early 1920s and 1941, homoeopathy came to be implicated in various administrative moves involving a series of legislations in Bengal. In August 1941, the nationalist coalition government provided unprecedented official recognition to homoeopathy by setting up a General Council and State Faculty of Homoeopathic Medicine – the first of its kind in British India. The period witnessed changes not merely in colonial health policies and regional state politics but also in the functioning of the entrepreneurial families, who had sustained their interests and investments in homoeopathic drugs, publications and knowledge. These eventful years in Bengal politics saw the growing electoral strength of the Indian parties and the eventual formation of a nationalist government

[1] S. N. Guha, 'Kaj er Kotha' ('Useful Words'), *Hahnemann*, 6, 10 (1923), 437.

[2] W. H. H. Vincent Secretary to the Government of India, Legislative Department to the Secretary to the Bengal Council and Assistant Secretary to the Government of Bengal, Legislative Department. Financial Department Medical Branch, File 2-D/8, Proceedings 18–33 A, December 1915.

[3] *Bengal Legislative Assembly Proceedings*, Vol L. 1, Number 3 (Alipur: Bengal Government Press, August–September 1937), pp. 806–8 [West Bengal Secretariat Library, hereafter WBSL].

in the province in 1937.[4] The state's attitude towards all 'non-allopathic' practices evolved rapidly during a period of instability and transition towards nationalist governance. Medical legislation introduced by the state appeared to be simultaneously dismissive of and accommodative towards homoeopathy. While being critical of the way homoeopathy was practised, such legislation, nonetheless, acknowledged the restricted outreach of state-sponsored medical relief programmes, especially in rural Bengal. There were official deliberations on the necessities of standardising and promoting 'non-allopathic' medicine, and homoeopathy was increasingly being included as an integral part of such deliberations, especially after 1937.[5] This chapter studies the reconfiguration of leading homoeopathic business families into associations, societies and other pressure groups in the face of these politico-legal changes. It also explores the legislation, negotiations and shifting political alliances that shaped homoeopathy as a state-endorsed, 'acceptable' genre of medicine by the mid-twentieth century.

Existing scholarship notes a shift in the colonial state's Eurocentric policy in medicine from the early years of the twentieth century. It has been observed that the severe strain that the First World War placed on the availability of medical services and supplies made it impossible to continue ignoring existing non-state healthcare options.[6] Some have contended that the failure of the state in controlling major epidemic outbreaks through the late nineteenth century propelled changes in colonial policy.[7] Others have highlighted the changes in the administrative structure following the 1919 Government of India Act that initiated a 'diarchy' in major

[4] For an in-depth study of the political history of the period, see Joya Chatterji, *Bengal Divided: Hindu Communalism and Partition, 1932–1947* (Cambridge: Cambridge University Press, 1994). For a study of the political developments in a slightly earlier period, see Tanika Sarkar, *Bengal 1928–1934: The Politics of Protest* (Delhi: Oxford University Press, 1987).

[5] Indeed, the Homoeopathic Faculty was instituted just after the Ayurvedic Faculty was announced in 1936 but ahead of the formal recognition of any other traditional practices, including unani.

[6] Drawing upon the works of David Arnold and Mark Harrison, Rachel Berger makes this point. See Rachel Berger, 'Ayurveda and the Making of the Urban Middle Class in North India 1900–1945' in Dagmar Wujastyk and Frederick Smith (eds.), *Modern and Global Ayurveda: Pluralism and Paradigms* (Albany: State University of New York Press, 2008), pp. 104–5.

[7] Kavita Sivaramakrishnan, *Old Potions, New Bottles: Recasting Indigenous Medicine in Colonial Punjab (1850–1945)* (Hyderabad: Orient Longman, 2006), pp. 53–70. Kavita holds that the vulnerability and inefficiency of the state in the face of the plague epidemics at the turn of the twentieth century was a trigger for changing health policy.

provinces.[8] The Act initiated a new system of rules wherein administration of 'health' was placed solely under the aegis of the provincial government. The shift in governmental policy simultaneously initiated a drive to standardise and professionalise practices like ayurveda and unani, which were increasingly being labelled, officially, as 'indigenous medicine' in this period. Studies in specific localities including Punjab, United Province and Hyderabad have explored the ways in which ayurvedic and unani advocates were championing the cause of traditional medical knowledge in the face of state regularisation, since the 1910s.[9] These efforts culminated in professionalisation initiatives from within these communities, and also resulted in supraregional conferences and associations, such as the Ayurvedic Mahasammelan and the All India Vaidic and Unani Tibbi Conference, based in Allahabad and Delhi, respectively. Thus, provincial politics and local socioreligious relations were crucial in determining the status of traditional knowledge in the period. However, the notion of 'indigeneity' that emerged from these state-community negotiations often tended to be more capacious and included homoeopathy. Indeed, the story of a western heterodoxy like homoeopathy's formal legalisation within the administrative fabric of the state in this period needs to be plotted within these ongoing broader developments.

Accordingly, here I locate homoeopathy within the currents of provincial politics, the ongoing negotiations between colonial state and traditional medicine in other parts of India, and also the changing relationship of the homoeopathic entrepreneur families with the state. I examine the ways in which these processes produced exclusions and margins. I have previously explored the growing intersections between homoeopathy and a Hindu nationalist ethos. Taking its cue from such overlaps, the chapter studies the processes through which the emergent nationalist state and elite business families negotiated what constituted 'pure', 'acceptable', 'reformed' homoeopathy, compatible with the 'scientific' parameters set by the state. Through such negotiation, homoeopathy was made to fit into the developmentalist, pro-people rhetoric of the government in this period around ideals of economy, indigeneity and mass rural reconstruction. The chapter also follows the unfolding identity politics around

[8] Rachel Berger, 'Ayurveda and the Making of the Urban Middle Class in North India 1900–1945', pp. 104–5.

[9] See, for instance, Kavita Sivaramakrishnan, *Old Potions, New Bottles: Recasting Indigenous Medicine in Colonial Punjab (1850–1945)*, 2006; Rachel Berger, *Ayurveda Made Modern;* and Guy Attewell, *Refiguring Unani Tibb: Plural Healing in Late Colonial India* (Hyderabad: Orient Longman, 2007).

homoeopathy in the interwar period as it was contradictorily framed as both an indigenous 'Hindu science' and a secular scientific practice.

In its formal encounter with state legislation, all 'non-allopathic' medicine was made directly subject to the law and incorporated into the growing bureaucracy as a way to further legislate and secure the health of the population. This ensured, as has been rightly noted, a convergence of the individuated biomoral regimen of the 'indigenous' practices with the biopolitical regimen of the state and its population-level, public health concerns.[10] I extend this argument to closely analyse the various actors and interests involved in enabling this convergence. The changing relationship between the colonial medical administration, the Congress and other regional nationalist parties, the pro-people welfare-oriented electoral mandate, simmering communitarian politics and especially the pharmaceutical interests of the homoeopathic entrepreneurial families, all played a part. This further explicates the flexible, shifting boundaries between of 'science' and non-science as homoeopathy came to be formally legitimised.

Nationalism and a Legislative Framework for 'Non-Allopathic' Medicine

The leading families and their trusted employees reoriented themselves into formal associations and clubs by the 1930s, a process which will be discussed in detail in the chapter. There was a parallel shift in the way in which homoeopathy came to be represented by them in the 1930s – there were pronounced efforts to reach out to the state, to project homoeopathy as an ideal tool for the state's public health apparatus. Along with the changing political landscape, these shifts need to be understood also in the context of a number of twentieth-century pieces of legislation that directly or indirectly implicated homoeopathy.

The period of the 1920s to 1930s was one of significant changes. The nationalist parties, represented most prominently by the Indian National Congress, were in conversation with the colonial state more than ever before. The trend manifested in the 1919 Government of India Act, which allotted certain crucial administrative departments to the provinces, and could be seen to culminate in the 1935 Act that ensured provincial elections. The latter Act opened up the rural electorate in Bengal by reserving an overwhelmingly large number of election seats for the rural constituencies. This Act – coupled with the Great Depression of the 1930s, which markedly affected rural agrarian relations – led to

[10] Rachel Berger, *Ayurveda Made Modern*, pp. 187–9.

what has been poignantly described as the 'emergence of the *mofussil* in Bengal politics'.[11] The countryside, including the huge rural population, came to figure centrally in the nationalist agenda in the 1930s. Meanwhile, the Gandhian programmes around the Civil Disobedience movements in the early 1930s too marked a shift in focus to the rural areas and a departure in Congress organisational activity.[12] However, the limited nature of the Congress' involvement in rural areas in the early 1930s has also been commented upon.[13] Yet, existing histories have emphasised the undeniable centrality of the rural population, especially the lower peasant classes in the electoral agenda of the Congress, which contrasted with its earlier stance of protecting the rights of the landed elites.[14] This was furthered in competition with other regional parties which were gaining rapid prominence, like the Krishak Praja Party (KPP) of Fazlul Haq, whose electoral campaign hinged on an exclusive and emphatic pro-peasant call for radical agrarian reforms with a distinct 'neo-populist rhetoric'.[15] It is indeed revealing that a significant slogan of the KPP campaign in the 1936 Bengal Assembly elections was '*dal-bhat*', or rice and lentils, which was considered 'in Bengal the simplest fare, the basic subsistence requirement of an individual'.[16] The Congress and the KPP were, in fact, in an informal alliance with one another until at least the 1936 elections, which the latter won. The coalition ministry under Fazlul Haq was a combination of parties and groups with divergent ideological orientation and shifting relations with the Congress and the Muslim League. Yet it managed to remain committed to its promise of radical agrarian reforms.

Thus overall, the rhetoric of population, rural construction, mass contact and welfare of the *mofussil* became central themes in mainstream Bengali nationalist formulations of the 1930s. Indeed, 'development' in general had emerged as an essential theme in high nationalist thinking by the decade of the 1930s.[17] As has been pointed out, such nationalist-developmentalist impulses should not be narrowly defined by economic terms, as the ostensibly economic issue of 'development' was linked to wider social and moral questions related to 'progress' and 'welfare'. 'Development' in the 1930s incorporated incongruent and discreet

[11] See Joya Chatterji, *Bengal Divided: Hindu Communalism and Partition, 1932–1947*, 1994, pp. 55–102.
[12] Tanika Sarkar, *Bengal 1928–1934: The Politics of Protest*, 1987, pp. 1–2.
[13] Joya Chatterji, *Bengal Divided*, p. 65. [14] Ibid., pp. 88–96. [15] Ibid., pp. 75–6.
[16] For a discussion of the slogan and its significance in drawing large-scale rural attention, see Paul R. Greenough, *Prosperity and Misery in Modern Bengal: The Famine of 1943–1944* (New York and Oxford: Oxford University Press, 1982), pp. 70–1.
[17] See, for instance, Benjamin Zachariah, *Developing India: An Intellectual and Social History c. 1930–50* (Delhi: Oxford University Press, 2005).

themes of social reform, village uplift, rural reconstruction, constructive work, cooperative farming and credit, self-reliance, improvement and so on.[18]

The growing links between the homoeopathic ethos and nationalist ideologies, particularly *swadeshi*, have been studied already. As the possibility of the establishment of a nationalist government became more apparent in the 1930s, there were tangible changes in the way homoeopathy was interpreted. There was a distinct effort to project it as an ideal tool in governmental administration relating to public health management. While continuing to assert the significance of homoeopathy acting as a catalyst in the regeneration of Indian family, there were simultaneous attempts to move beyond the confines of domesticity. There were conscious efforts to engage with and converse in the language of the emerging nation state, and its concerns around population, rural welfare, public health and development. In the homoeopaths' approach towards reaching out to the masses, one notices an evident overlap with the electoral concerns of the nationalist parties. Such an altered approach needs to be studied in the context of twentieth-century legislation concerning homoeopathy. In addition, one needs to appreciate the historiographic assertion relating to the growing 'economic insignificance of the middleclass Bengalis'.[19] Economic historians have noted the growing competition in the field of private investment and commerce between the European firms and the Marwaris in Calcutta in the interwar period, especially in the 1920s and 1930s.[20] Other than a few exceptions like newspaper companies, the *swadeshi* patriotic firms, quite often run as family enterprises, were suffering from stiff foreign capital competition with multinational companies.[21] The strategic alignment of Bengali homoeopathic enterprise with the vision of the emerging nation state needs to be studied in the light of these broader currents of events over the decade of the 1930s.

Established advocates of homoeopathy had begun appealing to the provincial government to acknowledge homoeopathy as a suitable ally in its growing public health programmes. In their publications, they

[18] Ibid., p. 44. [19] Tanika Sarkar, *Bengal 1928–1934: The Politics of Protest*, 1987, p. 8.
[20] Ibid., pp. 7–8. For detailed discussion on the subject of European competition in private investment, see Amiya Bagchi, *Private Investment in India 1900–1939* (Cambridge: Cambridge University Press, 1972); Rajat K. Ray, *Industrialisation in India: Growth and Conflict in the Private Corporate Sector 1914–47* (Delhi: Oxford University Press, 1979), pp. 5–7; and Amiya Kumar Bagchi, 'European and Indian Entrepreneurship in India, 1900–1930' in Rajat K. Ray (ed.), *Entrepreneurship and Industry in India: 1800–1947* (Delhi: Oxford University Press, 1992), pp. 169–81.
[21] Omkar Goswami, 'Sahibs, Babus and Banias: Changes in Industrial Control in Eastern India', *Journal of Asian Studies*, 48, 2 (1989), 289–309.

referred to the widespread infiltration of the doctrine in Bengali households over the past several decades. The vibrant print culture around homoeopathy was highlighted as the main tool behind the extensive dissemination of homoeopathy across households. In a speech delivered to commemorate Hahnemann's birthday in 1936, which was published in the journal *The Hahnemannian Gleanings* of the Hahnemann Publishing Company, A. N. Mukherjee alluded to the impressive attainments in the field of homoeopathic publications over the years.[22] He pointed out that

> Hundreds of treatises, both in English and in vernaculars, have been published; almost all the classical works from foreign languages have been translated. Side by side there also exist a large number of periodicals, which have proved very helpful in popularising the principles and practice of homoeopathy.[23]

At a national meeting of homoeopaths held in 1938, Jitendranath Majumdar began his presidential speech (published in the same journal) by presenting a collage of various domestic contexts where Bengali householders had 'historically' resorted to homoeopathic drugs.[24] Talking about the remarkable popularity of homoeopathy, these authors boasted that 'nearly fifty percent of the Homoeopathic drugs manufactured by Boericke and Tafel in America are sold in the Indian markets'.[25]

Simultaneously, these authors suggested ways in which homoeopathy could potentially aid the government's extensive public health programmes. The cost-effectiveness of deploying homoeopathy in such governmental endeavours was especially highlighted. For instance, in the article 'Progress of Homoeopathy in India', A. N. Mukherjee asserted, 'the density of the population, the area of square miles and the money spent per capita by the government for medical relief work in India as published in the census report make interesting reading. It clearly shows that the amount spent is very inadequate'.[26] Reminding the readers of homoeopathy's 'special appeal to the people of India who are proverbially poor', Mukherjee argued that 'homoeopathy has made it possible to supplement this (the inadequacy in governmental medical relief) to a great extent and could render further useful services at a nominal cost

[22] A. N. Mukherjee was the principal of Calcutta Homoeopathic College established by Pratap Chandra Majumdar. An associate of the Majumdar family, he emerged as an important voice in the realignment of the entrepreneurial families into associations in this period. Section 3 elaborates on his activities in the period.

[23] A. N. Mukherjee, 'Hahnemann's Birthday Celebration', *The Hahnemannian Gleanings*, 7 (May 1936), 191.

[24] J. N. Majumdar, 'The Sixth All India Homoeopathic Medical Conference', *The Hahnemannian Gleanings*, 9 (February 1938), 49–50.

[25] A. N. Mukherjee, 'Progress of Homoeopathy in India', *The Hahnemannian Gleanings*, 8 (January 1937), 560.

[26] Ibid.

if Government help were forthcoming'.[27] In unprecedented ways, editorials in journals like *The Hahnemannian Gleanings* from the early 1930s began highlighting the potential usefulness of homoeopathy in addressing the government's various public health issues, including combating epidemics.[28] Significantly, these writings tended to demand governmental recognition of homoeopathy as a valid and scientific medical doctrine. Thus, writing in 1936, Jitendranath Majumdar emphasised the importance of securing official validation and formal patronage from the state by aligning with the administrative machinery of the government.[29]

Such homoeopathic optimism was not without basis. From the mid-1930s, there were ongoing discussions at the central legislature regarding homoeopathy's scientific status and potential. In April 1937, a resolution was moved in the Central Legislative Assembly urging the government to recognise the 'introduction of homoeopathic treatment in government hospitals and recognising the homoeopathic colleges in India'.[30] The resolution was passed immediately and was thereafter forwarded to the provinces for their consideration. The leading homoeopathic journals in Calcutta unanimously celebrated the legislative decision as a crucial step towards acknowledging homoeopathy as a necessary resource in governmental health administration.[31] In a jubilant mode, some of them published the whole of the official report detailing this decision of the Government of India.[32] However, doubts persisted about homoeopathy's scientific basis as the central legislature actively debated this issue. Referring to technical details of homoeopathic therapeutics, it was even argued that 'the whole treatment is ultimately reduced to treatment by water . . . '.[33] In the course of the central legislative assembly debates, such issues were addressed and resolved conclusively. In various moments during these debates, homoeopathy's efficacy and economy were predominantly asserted.

[27] Ibid.

[28] For instance, see 'Editorial: New Year's Retrospection and Introspection', *The Hahnemannian Gleanings*, 4, 1 (February 1933), p. 10.

[29] See, for instance, J. N. Majumdar, 'State Recognition of Homoeopathy and Status of Homoeopaths in India', *The Hahnemannian Gleanings*, 7 (May 1936), 178.

[30] *Official Report of the Legislative Assembly Debates of 1937*, Vol 3, Number 10, p. 2935. Republished as 'Resolution Re Introduction of Homoeopathic Treatment in Government Hospitals and Recognition of Homoeopathic Colleges in India', *The Hahnemannian Gleanings*, 8 (August 1937), 301–11.

[31] See, for instance, 'Editorial: Bharat Government Homoeopathic Chikitsha Podhhoti Sombandhe Onumodan' ('Government Acknowledges the Homoeopathic Mode of Treatment'), *Hahnemann*, 20, 1 (1937), 3–4. Also see 'Resolution Re Introduction of Homoeopathic Treatment in Government Hospitals and Recognition of Homoeopathic Colleges in India', pp. 301–11.

[32] Ibid. [33] Ibid., pp. 312–13.

The 1937 central legislation promoting homoeopathy in government hospitals was not completely fortuitous. It had a significant precedent in the 1920 order passed by the governor in Council in Bengal. The Order in Council signed by the secretary to the Government of Bengal specified that 'the dispensary rules should be so altered as to make it possible for district boards to establish, maintain and make grants to dispensaries following systems of medicine other than allopathic'.[34] Existing historiography has noted the growing official tolerance towards the 'indigenous' medicine in this period. As noted in the Introduction to this chapter, historians have analysed this change in the colonial state's stance from various angles, including a focus on the official move towards diarchy in major provinces from 1919 through the Government of India Act. The reforms introduced a new system that brought 'health' (among other departments) fully under the aegis of regional governance. Added to this was the growing mobilisation of ayurvedic and unani proponents for official acceptance since 1910s. Given these distinct factors, provincial administrative policy of these non-state practices became crucial. The reports of the nationalist committees on health policies instituted in the 1940s, like the Bhore Committee Report, also indicate that between 1920 and 1940 the central colonial policies had established a cohesive category in which these non-state, non-allopathic practices could be conceptualised. At the same time, they had also been strictly relegated to the confines of provincial politics and redirected away from the purview of national governance as such.[35]

Thus, following the order passed in 1920, the provincial district boards were encouraged to 'establish, maintain and subsidise non-allopathic dispensaries' and a corresponding set of 'draft rules' for the 'establishment, maintenance and management' of such dispensaries were formulated.[36] In the official discussion regarding the establishment of the 'non-allopathic' dispensaries, private funding was strongly encouraged, apart from the 'grant-in-aid' promised through the district boards. The minister in charge accordingly notified the people of the elaborate

[34] Local Self Government Department Medical Branch Proceedings (Vol July 1921), 'Rules for the Establishment, Maintenance and Management of Dispensaries Following Systems of Medicine Other Than Allopathic', File 2R-1 (1) Proceeding 8 A, March 1920. [WBSA]

[35] Rachel Berger, *Ayurveda Made Modern*, p. 161.

[36] Surgeon General with the Government of India to the Secretary to the Government of Bengal Finance (Medical) Department, Local Self Government Department Medical Branch Proceedings (Vol July 1921), File 2R-1(3) Proceeding 10 A, March 1920p. [WBSA]

rules pertaining to the setting up and management of 'non-allopathic' dispensaries.[37]

This 1920 regulation was followed by the frequent establishment of state-sanctioned homoeopathic dispensaries in the Bengali countryside over the period of the 1920s and early 1930s. The official report for the year 1924 alone recorded the establishment of several homoeopathic dispensaries in the districts of Dacca, Pabna, Burdwan and so on.[38] Indeed, the steady rise in the number of homoeopathic dispensaries was reflected in the annual reports published from 1920. The 'Annual Report on the Hospitals and Dispensaries in Bengal for the Year 1923', for instance, recorded the establishment of twenty-seven homoeopathic dispensaries which treated 46,865 patients, in contrast to thirteen ayurvedic and only two unani dispensaries.[39] In certain cases, the dispensaries declared themselves as resorting to both the ayurvedic and the homoeopathic systems of medicine.[40]

Thus, the provincial government had been accommodative of the so-called 'non-allopathic' therapeutics since the early 1920s. Of such therapeutics, the state was more inclined towards discussing the prospects of ayurveda and homoeopathy, stating them to be more popular than others in Bengal.[41] The optimism of the homoeopathic businesses in the mid-1930s, and their eagerness to align homoeopathy intimately with the state machinery, were premised on this legislation.

Chapters 3 and 4 have dealt with the overlap between the projected homoeopathic ethos and nationalist ideologies in certain distinct registers. They have explored the ways in which homoeopathy's compatibility with an evidently Hindu nationalist sensibility was systematically upheld in the Bengali print market, which maintained an indigenised, traditionalised and largely Hinduised image of homoeopathy. It has also been noted how such publications simultaneously acknowledged the modern,

37 Local Self Government Department Medical Branch, Proceedings (Vol July 1921), File 2-r-1 (13) Proceedings 26 A, Notification No. 1504 Medical, May 1921. [WBSA]

38 Local Self Government Department Medical Branch, Proceedings (Vol 1924), See, for instance, File 1D-70 Proceedings 507–08 B; File 1D-55, Proceeding 229–31 B; File 1D-43 Proceedings 271–73 B.

39 R. Heard Surgeon General, Government of India to the Secretary, Government of Bengal, Local Self Government Department Medical Branch, Proceedings (Vol March 1925), File 1-R-2(II) Number 1–2, 'Annual Report on the Hospitals and Dispensaries in Bengal for the Year 1923', p. 4. [WBSA]

40 Local Self Government Department Medical Branch, Proceedings (Vol 1924), File ID-11 Proceeding 271–78 B. [WBSA]

41 Most official correspondence on the scope of native/indigenous therapeutic practices in Bengal discussed the relative popularity of ayurveda or homoeopathy over unani. See Upendra Nath Brahmachari to the Officiating Secretary to the Government of Bengal Municipal (Medical) Department, Financial Department Medical Branch (July 1913), File 3-M/9 23 Proceeding 33 B. [WBSA]

western, rational face of homoeopathy. Such an indeterminate, liminal, in-between aura around the category 'homoeopathy' was suitably utilised by its chief perpetrators based in north Calcutta. It is important to note that these leading homoeopathic voices over the period of the 1930s selectively drew upon its various attributes to delineate it as a potential public health tool for governance.[42] Particularly in their correspondence with the governmental representatives, as we will see, any association with an explicit religious identity was conveniently underplayed. Instead, they built upon a developmentalist ideal of 'service' and 'relief' in orientating homoeopathy towards an apparently secular nationalist regeneration of the population at large. This was especially true of their interactions with the KPP, which fought and won the Bengal Assembly election on a pro-people mandate, yet, the coalition ministry tended to develop an Islamic overtone at distinct moments through its fluctuating alliance with the Muslim League.[43]

Legislative Regulation, Reform and the Question of Homoeopathic Fraud

The legislative moves to accommodate homoeopathy within the colonial state apparatus were not unconditional. Homoeopathy was hardly ever given a free hand in medical governance. Simultaneously with the inclusive medical acts already discussed, other contemporary pieces of legislation expressed suspicion towards homoeopathic practices. As shown in Chapter 1, through the late nineteenth century the colonial administration remained critical of the 'scandalous' ways in which homoeopathy was allegedly practised. Practice of homoeopathy was considered irregular, unsystematic and incoherent because of a remarkable lack in organisation and formal institutions, especially in relation to pedagogy. Indeed, the state had deep reservations about the ways in which the craft of homoeopathy was acquired and disseminated through print and informal pupillage networks. I have noted already in Chapter 1 the ways in which the alleged homoeopathic irregularities prompted the state to discuss a medical registration act since the 1880s. The state was evidently concerned with the problem of quackery associated with all genres of medicine, and homoeopathy featured centrally in most official correspondence relating to quackery. The criticisms continued and even escalated,

[42] Gary J. Hausman's article on late colonial Tamil Nadu shows the ways in which different groups promoted homoeopathy as part of indigenous and scientific medical traditions. See Gary J. Hausman, 'Making Medicine Indigenous: Homoeopathy in South India', *Social History of Medicine*, 15, 2 (2002), 303–22.

[43] See Joya Chatterji, *Bengal Divided*, pp. 191–219.

culminating in a couple of government legislations being passed in the first quarter of the twentieth century.

The Bengal Medical Bill of 1913 had introduced a medical council and a system of registration whereby only the graduates of government medical institutions, and of institutions recognised by the government, qualified as 'registered practitioners'.[44] The Act thus rendered most of the homoeopathic physicians 'unregistered', since only a handful of them had formal medical training. The unregistered practitioners, homoeopathic or otherwise, were not, however, entirely debarred from practising. Clause 26 of the Act provided a 'penalty upon an unregistered person representing that he is registered'.[45] While the province reeled under the ambiguity relating to the scope of the Act, a second legislation was passed by the Government of India to 'penalise the use of bogus medical degrees'.[46] The Indian Medical (Bogus Degrees) Act, 1915 summarily deemed illegal the grant of degrees by bodies other than institutions which were either established or recognised by the government.[47] The Act, however, related primarily to 'western medical science', which was defined as 'western methods of allopathic medicine, obstetrics and surgery, but do not include the homoeopathic or ayurveda or unani systems of medicine'.[48] As Rachel Berger's and Kavita Sivaramakrishnan's work on the reorganisation of ayurveda in United Provinces (UP) and Punjab demonstrates, the twin issues of 'medical registration' and 'medical certification' stated in the Indian Medical (Bogus Degrees) Act 1915 created considerable confusion, and put limits on the status of *vaids* and *hakims*, whose position came to be determined by complex processes of cultural coding.[49] The provincial medical administration was torn between regulating the number of legitimate *vaids* by making registration valid only for a certain category of practitioners affiliated to the government institutions, while at the same time wanting to increase the number of *vaids* and

[44] J. Donald, Officiating Secretary to the Government of Bengal, Municipal Department to the Secretary to the Government of India, Home Department, Municipal Department Medical Branch February 1913, File 3-M/9 2 Number 47, attached Draft of The Bengal Medical Bill, 1913, p. 15. [WBSA]

[45] Ibid., p. 17.

[46] H. Wheeler, Secretary to the Government of India Home Department to the Secretary to the Government of Bengal Municipal (Medical) Department, Municipal Department Medical Branch May 1913, File 3-M/9 Number 14, Legislation to Penalise the Use of Bogus Medical Degrees, p. 1. [WBSA]

[47] Ibid., p. 2.

[48] W. H. H. Vincent, Secretary to the Government of India, Legislative Department to the Secretary to the Bengal Council and Assistant Secretary to the Government of Bengal, Legislative Department, Financial Department Medical Branch, File 2-D/8, Proceedings 18–33 A, December 1915.

[49] Rachel Berger, *Ayurveda Made Modern*, pp. 118–23; and Kavita Sivaramakrishnan, *Old Potions, New Bottles*, pp. 88–96.

hakims able to produce government certificates that could be accepted when granting leave and wages. Hence, as has been hinted in the existing literature, these regulatory acts, including the Bengal Medical Bill, had simultaneously made it 'pretty evident that while tolerated, the other medical traditions would not be privileged or even considered part of the scientific tradition'.[50]

Indeed, when the Indian Medical (Bogus Degrees) Bill was discussed at the provincial administrative level, the other medical traditions received harshly antagonistic comments from the authorities whose opinions were sought. The majority of such antagonistic remarks in Bengal concerned homoeopathy, which was identified as a particularly significant threat to the practice of 'western medicine'. Prior to the passing of the Act, while the Bill was being discussed, the council of Medical College, for instance, strongly urged that

> Some provision should be made to prevent the practice, now prevalent in Calcutta and the *mofussil*, of homoeopathic practitioners adopting letters which imply the possession of registrable diploma in western medicine while merely correcting this implication by adding in small type the term 'homoeo' or even the letter 'h', eg. L.M.S homoeo or L.M.S.H.[51]

These discussions questioned the standard and credentials of a slowly rising number of homoeopathic institutions which were being set up since the early twentieth century. In his suggestions to the Bill, Rai Kailash Chandra Bose, CIE, LMS, warned the Bengal government about 'several homoeopathic institutions in Calcutta', which

> freely traffic in bogus degrees and diplomas, which strictly speaking are not colourable imitation of the University degrees and as such do not come under the purview of the Criminal Procedure Code, but their moral effect upon the populace is just as bad. They avoid law by the insertion of the letter 'H' before their degrees and diplomas.[52]

Hence, well into the twentieth century, intense administrative doubts prevailed about the ways in which homoeopathy was disseminated. Although the Act did not summarily penalise or debar the ordinary

[50] See, for instance, Rachel Berger, 'Ayurveda and the Making of the Urban Middle Class in North India 1900–1945' in Dagmar Wujastyk and Frederick Smith (eds.), *Modern and Global Ayurveda: Pluralism and Paradigms*, 2008, p. 103.

[51] W. H. H. Vincent, Secretary to the Government of India, Legislative Department to the Secretary to the Bengal Council and Assistant Secretary to the Government of Bengal, Legislative Department, Financial Department Medical Branch, File 2-D/8, Proceedings 18–33 A, December 1915 [WBSA]

[52] Rai Kailas Chandra Bose to The Under Secretary to the Government of Bengal Financial Department, Financial Department Medical Branch, File 2-D/B7 (Number 24, November 1915), p. 12. [WBSA]

homoeopathic practitioner, it identified the vast majority of them as unqualified and unregistered. The government, most importantly, disapproved of the mushrooming of homoeopathic institutions that had begun to grant medical degrees extensively.

However, these bureaucratic discussions simultaneously conceded that 'the present supply of qualified medical practitioners is unable to cope with the need of the country for medical relief'.[53] It was pointed out that 'most of the villages go without any or have to be satisfied with a mere apology of such relief'.[54] In view of this reality, many groups which were consulted in relation to the Bill, like the Indian Association, urged the government to consider 'the question of the protection afforded to qualified men who practice the system of homoeopathy'.[55] It is therefore hardly surprising that within a few years of the passing of the Bogus Degree Act, where the homoeopaths were discussed as a threat to 'western allopathic medicine', the 1920 dispensary regulations welcomed the setting up of homoeopathic dispensaries across the province.

The position of the government in relation to homoeopathy in this period therefore can best be described as ambivalent and hesitant. It was torn between being accommodative and dismissive. While conceding the widespread reach of homoeopathy, it was uncomfortable with the highly informal and 'corrupt' ways in which homoeopathic pedagogy and the emerging institutions functioned. The Calcutta-based entrepreneurial families claiming to represent the legitimate face of homoeopathy internalised the logic of these governmental critiques. In a revealing way, their nationalist portrayal of homoeopathy in this period completely imbibed the reformist, hierarchical bias of the colonial state against the so-called unqualified practitioners. It was precisely against such dispersed and unqualified practitioners of homoeopathy that the leading voices from the entrepreneurial families defined their legitimacy, by invoking a strong rhetoric of 'purification'. The publications of the leading entrepreneurial families in this period engaged consistently with themes of 'reform' and 'purification' to purge the supposedly scandalous and embarrassing miscreants from their trade.

The politics of the families in this period thus exposed an essential tension within their continuing attitudes towards and efforts in promoting homoeopathy. Since the late nineteenth century, they had committed

[53] Pramatha Nath Banerjee, Honorary Assistant Secretary to Indian Association Secretary to the Government of Bengal Municipal (Medical) Department, Financial Department Medical Branch, File 3-M/9 35 (Number 45, September 1913), p. 61. [WBSA]
[54] Ibid.
[55] Financial Department Medical Branch, File 3-M/9 (Nos-14–48 A, November 1913), p. 5. [WBSA]

themselves to a mandate of institutionalising homoeopathy through domestic, familial and affective channels with the aid of the print market. As illustrated in the previous chapters, these leading publishers had encouraged the reading, learning and practice of homoeopathy beyond the bounds of the conventional state-patronised institutions like schools, hospitals and colleges. They had projected an egalitarian vision that invited an equal participation of all future citizens in ensuring the health of the nation through homoeopathic knowledge. Yet, from the 1920s and through the 1930s, the agenda of 'reform' and 'purification' emerged as a central theme in their publications, wherein they took a position against precisely those self-taught, 'amateur', often-suburban and semi-literate practitioners whom the state considered recalcitrant and dangerous. The leading homoeopathic enterprises thus began exhibiting remarkable solidarity with the statist interest in taming such intractable elements, which seemed to have slipped through the disciplining apparatus of the emerging nation state.

The unbridled proliferation of the self-taught, amateur practitioners was, in fact, identified as the most deep-seated problem plaguing homoeopathy in the twentieth century.[56] A range of articles published in the foremost journals including *Hahnemann*, *The Hahnemannian Gleanings*, *Indian Homoeopathic Review*, *Homoeopathy Paricharak*, *Home and Homoeopathy*, as also in other monographs, dealt with this issue as they ridiculed and condemned the trend that allowed men from various eclectic professional backgrounds to acquire an amateurish interest in homoeopathy. The 1923 article 'Kaj er Kotha' or 'Useful Words' published in the journal *Hahnemann*, for instance, sarcastically noted that,

> In our times the lawyers-attorneys, clerks in the courts and offices, the nayeb-gomosthas-amins to the zamindars, clerks in railways and steamers, those dealing with the parcels in these departments, students in various schools and colleges, even the petty shop owners are in effect homoeopathic physicians.[57]

In a similar vein, the article 'Homoeopathic Upadhi Samasya' or 'Problems of Homoeopathic Degrees' noted that, '[n]owadays the station masters become practising homoeopaths while in service. From police

[56] Existing works reflect confusion over the status of the 'lay' and 'self-taught' homoeopaths in other contexts around the same period. See, for instance, Marijke Gijswijt-Hofstra, 'Homeopathy and its Concern for Purity: The Dutch Case in the Early 20th Century' in M. Gijswijt-Hofstra, G. M. Van Heteren and E. M. Tansey (eds.), *Biographies of Remedies: Drugs, Medicines and Contraceptives in Dutch and Anglo-American Healing Cultures* (Amsterdam: Rodopi, 2002), pp. 99–121.

[57] S. N. Guha, 'Kaj er Kotha' ('Useful Words'), p. 434.

officers, *gurus* in *pathsalas* to grocers in local shops all claim equal expertise in homoeopathy'.[58]

As shown in Chapter 3, the *mofussil* was a particular target of the purification zeal that originated in Calcutta. It was argued that the *mofussil* with its large semi-literate population was a fertile ground for nurturing amateur, lay practitioners. The article 'Palligram e Homoeopathy o Tar Durobostha' or 'The Deplorable Condition of Homoeopathy in the Villages' in the journal *Homoeopathy Paricharak*, reflected upon the proliferation of various deadly diseases in the *mofussil*.[59] It wondered whether the overabundance of diseases might have led to the emergence of hundreds of amateur homoeopaths, or the other way round. These authors targeted such practitioners variously as '*bhando*' or 'frauds', 'quacks', '*bhuiphors*' or 'upstarts', 'amateurs' and even 'dacoits'.[60] The deceit involved in projecting oneself as a homoeopathic physician on the strength merely of possessing domestic health manuals and procuring the standard homoeopathic chest was especially criticised.[61] The article 'Gharer Dheki', or 'Internal Problem', specifically castigated the incompetence of the *mofussil* physicians, labelling the bulk of them as 'enemies within'.[62]

The proliferation of amateur practitioners was allegedly associated also with the mushrooming of homoeopathic institutions in the first quarter of the twentieth century. It was held that such institutions were primarily set up by self-taught men of dubious competence. Articles like 'Upadhir Byabsha' or 'Degree Trade', emphatically contended that private homoeopathic schools were being set up with the singular purpose of reaping profit.[63] Commenting on the standard of education in such institutions, the article 'Homoeopathic College' in the journal *Hahnemann* noted with alarm that, 'nowadays it is hardly an exaggeration to suggest that we are beginning to have as many homoeopathic institutions as the number of physicians in the city'.[64] The author held, further, that the relation of 'food and predator' prevailed between the teachers and students in such

[58] K. N. Basu, 'Homoeopathic Upadhi Samasya' ('Problems of Homoeopathic Degree'), *Hahnemann*, 9, 10 (1926), p. 546.

[59] Khagendranath Basu, 'Palligram e Homoeopathy O Tar Durobastha' ('Deplorable Condition of Homoeopathy in the Villages'), *Homoeopathy Paricharak*, 1, 3 (June 1927), 164–6.

[60] Manmatha Nath Gangopadhyay, 'Bisadrisa Chikitshay Sadrisa ba homoeo shabder Obantor proyog' ('Irrelevant Use of the Word Homoeo in Treatment of Dissimilars'), *Homoeopathy Paricharak*, 1, 1 (April 1927), 60–2.

[61] Ibid., pp. 60–2.

[62] Prabal Chandra Chatterjee, 'Gharer Dheki' ('Internal Problems'), *Hahnemann*, 6, 3 (1923), 121.

[63] G. Dirghangi, 'Upadhir Byabsha' ('Degree Trade'), *Hahnemann*, 5, 11 (1922), 553–4.

[64] G. Dirghangi, 'Homoeopathic College', *Hahnemann*, 1, 10 (1918), 308.

schools.[65] The fundamental critique launched against these schools was that in them there remained a complete absence of any standardised, regularised curricula in tune with modern medical knowledge. They were accused of selling degrees in return for an agreed amount of money. Referring to appalling inconsistencies in homoeopathic pedagogy, the journals reported that while some colleges granted degrees at the end of four years, and others at the end of one, yet others simply promised long-distance teaching and examination. A 1923 editorial in *Hahnemann* noted that the newly set up homoeopathic colleges promised degrees within a range varying from two months to two years, and in exchange of money varying from 1 rupee to 100 rupees.[66] Not only degrees, but gold and silver medals too were said to be on offer.[67] This deplorable situation led a number of authors to refer to such institutions as 'degree selling shops'.[68] The distaste of the dominant homoeopathic voices for these small institutions was vented variously, as some of them noted with derision, '[h]opefully in the near future these colleges would sell magic pills for 1 or 2 paise, swallowing which students will get educated in homoeopathy . . . what a fate of a glorious science!'[69]

In a range of articles, these reformist authors blamed the indiscriminate sale of degrees for bringing disrepute to homoeopathy and for promoting quackery.[70] As the article 'Homoeopathic Upadhi Samasya' or 'Problems Relating to Homoeopathic Degrees', contended, such degrees were not respectable simply because there was no way of judging if they were fake or not.[71] The authors lamented that the situation was so grave that it had generated a popular proverb, '*jar nai onno gati, shei pore homoeopathy*', literally meaning 'anyone incapable of attaining a respectable profession could try his hand at homoeopathy'.[72]

Those pushing the agenda of purification simultaneously discussed the importance of negotiating with the government. In view of the legislation passed in the first quarter of the twentieth century, the leading homoeopathic journals regularly published articles that criticised so-called amateur practitioners, while also emphasising the need to secure government support. For instance, the article 'Kaj er Kotha' or 'Useful Words' in *Hahnemann* argued that homoeopathy needed to win the government

65 Ibid., p. 312. 66 'Editorial', *Hahenmann*, 6, 7 (1923), 290.
67 G. Dirghangi, 'Upadhir Byabsha' ('Degree Trade'), p. 554.
68 See 'Editorial', *Hahenmann*, 6, 7 (1923), p. 291. Also see S. N. Guha, 'Kaj er Kotha' ('Useful Words'), p. 437.
69 G. Dirghangi, 'Upadhir Byabsha' ('Degree Trade'), p. 554.
70 G. Dirghangi, 'Homoeopathic College', p. 311.
71 K. N. Basu, 'Homoeopathic Upadhi Samasya' ('Problems of Homoeopathic Degree'), p. 547.
72 S. N. Guha, 'Kaj er Kotha' ('Useful Words'), p. 434.

over to its side, failing which it would fade in comparison to its state-supported allopathic or even ayurvedic counterparts.[73] Indeed, the authors reflected deeply upon the weight of powerful government legislation, even comparing the field of homoeopathic medicine as a veritable 'Kurukshetra',[74] where the government stood for the mighty Kauravas![75] These authors frequently invoked instances where lay homoeopaths fraudulently using false MB (Bachelor of Medicine) degrees were penalised by the government.[76] To the established homoeopathic enterprises, such isolated instances revealed the necessity of appeasing the government rather than antagonising it further.

Several ideas were discussed concerning the agenda of reform. There was serious discussion of the advantages of introducing a centralised board and a premier homoeopathic institution on the model of the Calcutta Medical College.[77] The cry for centralisation was also, evidently, in tune with the government's call for such a move which was slowly being taken up in other provinces. The Board of Indigenous Medicine set up in UP in 1921, and the Delhi Tibbiya College and the Ayurved Vidyapeeth in North India were formed with the aims of centralising and standardising indigenous medical education.[78] Indeed, most recommendations concerned the regularisation of the homoeopathic education through centralised vigilance.[79] The establishment of a centralised examining body was also recommended.[80] It was further pointed out that such a centralised board or organisation could take a leading role in the production of homoeopathic drugs in the country. Referring to the Bengali dependence on the import of crucial drugs from Europe and the United States, these authors argued for this proposed body initiating sustained

[73] Ibid., p. 437.

[74] 'Kurukshetra' is the name of a mythical dynastic battle between the mighty Kauravas and the apparently weaker Pandavas, described in the famous epic *Mahabharata*.

[75] See, for instance, Sashi Bhushan Chattopadhyay, 'Prokrito o Adorsho Homoeopath o Homoeopathy' ('Real and Ideal Homoeopaths and Homoeopathy'), *Homoeopathy Paricharak*, 2, 6 (September 1928), 243–4.

[76] 'Editorial: Homoeopathy Chikitshak er Shasti' ('Punishment of a Homoeopathic Physician'), *Homoeopathy Paricharak*, 2, 5 (August 1928), 185.

[77] See, for instance, K. N. Basu, 'Homoeopathic Upadhi Samasya' ('Problems of Homoeopathic Degree'), p. 549.

[78] See Kavita Sivaramakrishnan, *Old Potions, New Bottles*, pp. 114–23; Rachel Berger, *Making Ayurveda Modern*, pp. 114–25; and Neshat Quaiser, 'Science, Institution, Colonialism: Tibbiya College of Delhi 1889–1947' in Uma Dasgupta (ed.), *Science and Modern India: An Institutional History, 1784–1947* (Delhi: Pearson Longman, 2011), pp. 523–54.

[79] See, for instance, Kalikumar Bhattacharya, 'Samasya o Pratikar' ('Problem and Its Solution'), *Hahnemann*, 7, 1 (1924), 51.

[80] G. Dirghangi, 'Homoeopathic College', p. 314.

investment in research into indigenous plants.[81] In a revealing way the discussions of purification almost inevitably proposed unbridled centralisation of power in the realms of pedagogy and publication, as well as in the production of homoeopathic drugs.

Further, these proposed moves towards cleansing homoeopathy were packaged as essentially nationalist endeavours committed to the welfare of the people. The reforming voices frequently invoked eminent nationalist figures as potential leaders in their endeavour. For instance, the article 'Samasya o Pratikar' or 'Problem and Solution' written in 1924 recommended securing support from widely respected nationalist figures.[82] To the author, Rabindranath Tagore and scientist P. C. Ray were two obvious choices, since both were nationalists of repute who supported homoeopathy. Since Tagore, a 'high class homoeopath' himself, was in China at the time, the author elaborated on the advantages of approaching P. C. Ray. The author expressed himself confident of gaining Ray's support if he could be convinced of the lofty objectives of the reforming agenda, which was for the 'benefit of the nation and the people at large'.[83]

Often enough, these writings in favour of the reform and purification of homoeopathy were also expressions of regional nationalist sentiments. As the article 'Organisation of Homoeopathy and Its Improvement' in the journal *Home and Homoeopathy* argued in 1931, 'Bengal has fallen back considerably from her fraternity in all things pertaining to lead and leadership. Let it once again lead in homoeopathy by being the formulator of a real strong form of action to guide homoeopathic medical education in India'.[84] It was suggested that the homoeopathic fraternity would gain by following keenly the swerves in nationalist politics. Some authors were candid about the potential advantages of aligning overtly with the nationalist parties. The article 'Government o Homoeopathy' written in 1924 thus highlighted the need to pursue the Swarajya Party[85] 'as they are winning in the legislative assembly'.[86] Referring to the fact that their leader Chittaranjan Das was known to personally prefer homoeopathy,

[81] S. N. Guha, 'Kaj er Kotha' ('Useful Words'), pp. 437–8.
[82] Kalikumar Bhattacharya, 'Samasya o Pratikar' ('Problem and Its Solution'), p. 43.
[83] Ibid.
[84] N. M. Choudhury, 'Organisation of Homoeopathy and Its Improvement', *Home and Homoeopathy* (May 1931), 445.
[85] Swarajya Party was a breakaway party formed in 1923 by dissenting Congress men led by C. R. Das. The party worked within the broader ambit of Congress politics for a brief period in the 1920s.
[86] Amulya Kumar Chandra, 'Government O Homoeopathy', *Hahnemann*, 7, 3 (1924), 142.

the author hoped to benefit from the success of the Swarajya Party in the Assembly.[87]

Of Families, Associations and 'Model Institutions'

But who exactly were the leading campaigners for reform? And how were the late nineteenth-century commercial-familial networks reworked in the changing politico-legislative context of the late 1920s and 1930s? Let us take a look at the ways in which the entrepreneurial concerns of family businesses converged with, and were reshaped in response to, the statist agenda of reforming indigenous medicine.[88]

By the early 1930s, of all the entrepreneur families, the Majumdar family and the Bhar family had assumed a central role in reforming homoeopathy. Jitendranath Majumdar, the son of Pratap Chandra Majumdar, and Sarat Chandra Ghosh, the editor of both the journals *Hahnemann* and *The Hahnemannian Gleanings* (published by the Hahnemann Publishing Company owned by Prafulla Chandra Bhar) emerged as the vanguard in restoring homoeopathic purity. Although the other leading entrepreneurial concerns including the M. Bhattacharya and Company, B. K. Pal and Company, and Berigny and Company continued their business primarily around homoeopathic drugs and publications, yet, for a variety of reasons, unlike the Majumdars and the Bhars they failed to retain centre stage in the 1920s and 1930s. Rajendralal Dutta and Mahendralal Sircar, for instance, had died by the early twentieth century. Following the demise of Mahendralal Sircar in 1904, his son Amrita Lal continued to publish the *Calcutta Journal of Medicine* for some years, although he became engrossed in the work of the Indian Association for the Cultivation of Science.[89] However, with the death of Amrita Lal Sircar in 1919, the interest of the Sircar family in homoeopathy slowly petered out. Homoeopathy, as discussed in Chapter 1, comprised a part of the extended entrepreneurial ventures of B. K. Pal and Company. Following Batakrishna Pal's death in the early twentieth century, the company ceased to be a leading voice in the field of homoeopathy, although it did continue its business. Under Batakrishna Pal's son Hari Shankar Paul and others, the company particularly flourished in

[87] Ibid., pp. 142–3. [88] A. N. Mukherjee, 'Progress of Homoeopathy in India', p. 597.

[89] The Indian Association for Cultivation of Science (IACS) was founded in 1876 for the dissemination of scientific education in India. On the involvement of Mahendralal Sircar and son Amritalal Sircar in the IACS, see Arun Kumar Biswas, *Collected Works of Mahendralal Sircar, Eugene Lafont and the Science Movement 1860–1910* (Calcutta: Asiatic Society, 2003).

the manufacturing of other consumer products including soaps, although a comprehensive history of the many commercial ventures of the Paul family, especially in the twentieth century, remains to be written.[90] Meanwhile, the Majumdars and the Bhars endeavoured to reinvent the journals they published as representative voices for the entire homoeopathic community. Sarat Chandra Ghosh, for instance, pledged in a 1933 editorial of *The Hahnemannian Gleanings* to promote unity among the homoeopaths.[91] He was confident that through such acts of organisation and unity the journal would turn into a 'mouthpiece of Bengali Homoeopathy in the era of reform'.[92]

Discussions on the necessity of reform understandably converged with the ways of implementing it. Organising the leadership was considered a part of the purification process. Many of the writings in this period dealt explicitly with efforts to organise the homoeopaths into sharing a common platform. Such efforts in organisation were often juxtaposed with the nationalist reorganisations of the 1930s. For instance, Sarat Chandra Ghosh in his 1935 tome *Life of Dr Mahendralal Sarkar* explicitly noted,

> In the reorganisation of the whole country which is now looming largely before the government and the public, we shall, however, be deprived of our right to occupy our place if we do not, in the first instance organise ourselves into an effective and strong body to do away with all abuses committed by us in the name of homoeopathy.[93]

Since the mid-1920s these writings pointed out the necessity of forming societies and associations in order to organise the homoeopathic fraternity. In an introspective mood, most of these articles expressed the need for a centralised forum with regular meetings, just as the allopaths had.[94] Unlike ayurveda or unani, homoeopathy in India did not have a national front until very late, and was largely dealt with only at the provincial level.

[90] Omkar Goswami, 'Sahibs, Babus and Banias: Changes in Industrial Control in Eastern India', pp. 289–309.

[91] 'Editorial: New Year's Retrospection and Introspection', pp. 10–11; Sarat Chandra Ghosh, as this section will delineate, assumed a central position representing the Hahnemann Publishing Company in this period. He was the author of several biographies published in homoeopathic journals, which Chapter 2 has dealt with. For an overview of his accomplishments in his own words, see Sarat Chandra Ghosh, 'An Open Reply to the Letter Published by One Dr. H. Guha of Dacca on the Homoeopathic Bulletin of July 1932', *The Hahnemannian Gleanings*, 3 (September 1932), 365–77.

[92] 'Editorial: New Year's Retrospection and Introspection', p. 11.

[93] Sarat Chandra Ghosh, *Life of Dr. Mahendralal Sircar*, 2nd edition (Calcutta: Hahnemann Publishing Company, 1935), p. 93.

[94] See, for instance, Anonymous, 'Bhishak Kalima Udghaton' ('Exposing a Fraud Physician'), *Hahnemann*, 8, 7 (1925), 359.

The All India Homoeopathic Medical Association was formed only in 1932.[95] It was formed with the initiative of K. N. Katju and some other practitioners from United Province with support from Jitendranath Majumdar of the Calcutta Majumdar family. W. Younan, a renowned homoeopathic physician of Calcutta, was elected the first president and Jitendranath Majumdar its first general secretary. In the 1930s, the All India Association organised some conferences and lobbied to put pressure on the central legislature for official recognition of homoeopathy as a mode of treatment.

By the early 1930s two other powerful provincial organisations had come into being in Bengal. The first was the South Calcutta Homoeopathic Association, with Sarat Chandra Ghosh (a close associate of the Bhar family) as its president. The other was the Calcutta Homoeopathic Society, which was initially formed by the efforts of Pratap Chandra Majumdar and his son, Jitendranath, in 1909. Chapter 1 has noted that the Calcutta Homoeopathic College was the earliest institution teaching homoeopathy, and was founded by Pratap Chandra Majumdar in early 1880s. It was, in fact, the only attempt at building a formal pedagogic institution by the leading homoeopathic families in the nineteenth century. As reported in the *Indian Homoeopathic Review* edited by the Majumdars, in 1909 'the promoters of the institution (the Majumdar family and a few of their homoeopath associates like D. N. Ray[96]) . . . formed themselves into a committee and registered themselves as the Calcutta Homoeopathic Society'.[97] This Society was rejuvenated in the 1920s as the pursuit of the purification agenda began. The Society held regular meetings to discuss the necessity of reform as well as the utility of having medical clubs and associations. In their regular meetings since the 1920s, both the Calcutta Homoeopathic Association and the Calcutta Homoeopathic Society projected themselves as the sole legitimate voices capable of addressing and resolving the challenges facing homoeopathy.[98]

Figures connected with these associations emerged as the most prominent voices in the period. Apart from Jitendranath Majumdar (who also published as J. N. Majumdar) and Sarat Chandra Ghosh, N. M. Choudhury, the son-in-law of the late Pratap Chandra

[95] Ajoy Kumar Ghosh, 'A Short History of the Development of Homoeopathy in India', *Homeopathy*, 99, 2 (2010), 131–2.

[96] D. N. Ray was a close friend of some of the leading homoeopathic families. Excerpts of his biographies published in the leading journals have been cited in Chapter 2.

[97] 'Editorial: Calcutta Homoeopathic Hospital', *Indian Homoeopathic Review*, 19, 6 (June 1910), 102. Also see 'Editorial: Calcutta Homoeopathic Society', *Indian Homoeopathic Review*, 19, 11 (November 1910), 321–2.

[98] See, for instance, Anonymous, 'Sangbad' ('News'), *Hahnemann*, 10, 1 (1927), 54–6.

Majumdar, was a prominent voice in the meetings. The other important names were those of A. N. Mukherjee and J. N. Ghosh, who followed Jitendranath Majumdar to become presidents of the Calcutta Homoeopathic Society.[99] Both were also influential in running the Calcutta Homoeopathic College. At the same time, the Bengal Homoeopathic Pharmacists Association was formed with J. N. Majumdar as its president.[100] Unlike ayurveda or unani, there has been almost no scholarly work on homoeopathy's history in other provinces and therefore, it is difficult to gauge its mobilisation beyond Bengal. However, it is known that an All India Homoeopathic Medical Association was formed in Calcutta around 1932 with Jitendranath Majumdar as its first general secretary.[101]

Interestingly, the new voices in the 1930s had invariably emerged from the legacies of the older familial networks and establishments. While physician Sarat Chandra Ghosh was patronised by the Bhars of the Hahnemann Publishing Company, he was turned into a spokesperson for the firm in the period. Thus, almost all the meetings convened by Ghosh during this time noted the 'distinguished presence of Prafulla Chandra Bhar, the proprietor of the company and his brother Sudhangshu Mohan Bhar'.[102] However, chiming with the need to regularise education, the leading voices in the period, although invariably patronised by the old familial legacies, had claims not only to formal medical training but also often to foreign degrees. The article 'Dr. A. N. Mukherjee M. D. and Ourselves' in the journal *The Hahnemannian Gleanings*, for instance, detailed the international contacts, degree and laurels earned by A. N. Mukherjee.[103] It also celebrated his service to the journal as a contributing editor and his active role in the Calcutta Homoeopathic Society.

Through regular meetings, conferences and resolutions the two associations indeed posed as the most representative and credible face of homoeopathy, with whom the state could engage. Several conferences in and around Calcutta were organised to discuss the need to unite the community and purify it of the menace of corrupt pedagogical practices.

99 Ibid., pp. 54–6.

100 See 'The Bengal Homoeopathic Pharmacist's Association', *The Hahnemannian Gleanings*, 12 (October 1941), 454.

101 Gary Hausman, 'Making Medicine Indigenous: Homoeopathy in South India', pp. 306–7.

102 See, for instance, 'Editorial: Khulna Jela Homoeopathic Sammelan' ('Homoeopathic Conference at the District of Khulna'), *Hahnemann*, 20, 12 (1937), 661.

103 'Editorial: Dr. A. N. Mukherjee M. D. and Ourselves', *The Hahnemannian Gleanings*, 3 (June 1932), 235. Also see, 'Homoeopathic News: A. N. Mukherjee and Calcutta Homoeopathic Hospital Society', *The Hahnemannian Gleanings*, 8 (February 1937), 49.

Reporting on the first All Bengal and Assam Homoeopathic Conference of May 1931 of which Sarat Chandra Ghosh was the president, Ghosh wrote that the main objective of the conference was to 'bring about unity among the homoeopaths and to elevate the status and position of homoeopathy'.[104] The reform and dissemination of homoeopathy, it was argued, could be enabled by greater association with the official state machinery. Winning governmental support was considered essential not merely for homoeopathy's survival but for its future respectability and authority.

The associations, accordingly, lent their wholehearted support to the Homoeopathic Faculty Bill that was introduced in the Bengal legislative assembly in 1937 by the Congress representative P. Banerji.[105] The Bill sought to establish a centralised provincial faculty to deliberate on matters related to homoeopathy. Since the Congress was the major political party in the province prior to the elections, the leading homoeopathic voices initially attempted to establish direct political alliance with it. The predominantly upper class, Hindu *bhadralok* aesthetics of the Congress party seemed to sit well with the overall politics of the homoeopathic entrepreneur families. Sarat Chandra Ghosh and J. N. Majumdar vigorously supported the Bill in their respective journals. Immediately after the Bill was introduced in the Assembly, Sarat Chandra Ghosh published an article listing the many eminent Bengalis who supported the move.[106] J. N. Majumdar too came in with wholehearted support for the Bill, referring to P. Banerji as 'our member in the Legislative Assembly'.[107] Indeed, the two homoeopathic leaders took every possible step to own P. Banerji as their spokesperson. The January 1938 editorial of *Hahnemann*, for instance, recorded two simultaneous gatherings that took place 'on the same day, at the same time in two buildings virtually across the road', where J. N. Majumdar and Sarat Chandra Ghosh conducted meetings in support of the Bill. In their respective speeches, both the speakers earnestly congratulated the Congress party Assembly member P. Banerji for helping the homoeopathic cause.[108]

The Homoeopathic Faculty Bill, however, suffered an unfortunate fate in the Assembly at the hands of the Krishak Praja Party, which had

[104] Sarat Chandra Ghosh, *Life of Dr. Mahendralal Sircar*, 1935, p. 93.

[105] See 'Editorial: Homoeopathic Faculty Bill, 1937', *Hahnemann*, 20, 4 (1937), 210.

[106] See 'Editorial: Homoeopathic Faculty Bill, 1937', *Hahnemann*, 20, 5 (1937), 269.

[107] J. N. Majumdar, 'The Sixth All India Homoeopathic Medical Conference', p. 51. See 'Editorial: Nikhil Bharat Homoeopathy Sammelan' ('All India Homoeopathic Conference'), *Hahnemann*, 20, 10 (1937), 537.

[108] 'Editorial', *Hahnemann*, 21, 1 (1938), 1–5.

meanwhile assumed power in the province. After a long discussion in the Assembly in 1938, the Bill was finally turned down by H. S. Suhrawardy who was acting briefly as the health minister for the KPP ministry. He acknowledged the Bill as 'an important motion and all are interested in it'. However, hinting at the collaboration between the homoeopathic leaders and the Congress members he stated that 'the honourable mover would be well advised in the interests of the persons, whose cause he is advocating here, to withdraw the bill'.[109] Although conceding the importance and benefits of forming a centralised faculty, Suhrawardy highlighted the problem of widespread 'quackery' associated with homoeopathy as his ground for rejecting the Bill.[110] Rampant irregularities in pedagogy were the main allegation on the basis of which the Bill was ultimately withdrawn from the Assembly. Although the KPP summarily rejected this Bill moved by their major political opponents, the Assembly debates reflected hardly any political animosity. These discussions about the Bill were couched in serious, parliamentary language addressing issues of 'welfare', 'service', 'public health' and the evils of medical malpractice.

In this context, the drive for purification upheld by the Calcutta-based homoeopaths could hardly be considered altruistic. Indeed, along with their call for reform, the leading families, now clustered into associations, exhibited a trend towards diversifying their entrepreneurial zeal to take an interest in the regularisation of homoeopathic pedagogy. While exposing the evils associated with the institutions that were being set up in the early twentieth century, they claimed to establish educational institutions where 'authentic' homoeopathy as expected by the state government would be taught. Writing in 1935, Sarat Chandra Ghosh, for instance, listed the top three credible institutions teaching homoeopathy: the Calcutta Homoeopathic College founded by Pratap Chandra Majumdar; The Bengal Allen Homoeopathic College (whose founder-principal N. M. Choudhury happened to be the son-in-law of Pratap Chandra Majumdar); and the Pratap Chandra Memorial College and Hospital founded by the elder Majumdar's son Jitendranath Majumdar, also known as, J. N. Majumdar.[111]

These institutions were consistently presented as 'model institutions' for disseminating homoeopathy and fighting the 'evils' within the community. Speaking at a meeting of the Calcutta Homoeopathic Society in 1934, president A. N. Mukherjee praised the Calcutta Homoeopathic

[109] *Bengal Legislative Assembly Proceedings*, Vol L. III, Number 4 (Calcutta: Bengal Government Press, September 1938), pp. 65–67. [WBSL]

[110] Ibid., pp. 65–7.

[111] Sarat Chandra Ghosh, *Life of Dr. Mahendralal Sircar*, 1935, pp. 97–8.

College as 'a visible record of this achievement'.[112] It was emphasised that the fundamental difference that remained between the 'model schools' and the others was the formers' engagement, not only in the 'homoeopathic subjects (such as Organon of Medicine, Materia Medica, Philosophy of Chronic Diseases)', but also 'all the auxiliary branches of medicine as Anatomy, Physiology, Pathology, Practice of Medicine, Midwifery, Surgery etc'.[113] Through the meetings organised by the associations, and their publications in the 1930s, the homoeopathic enterprises advertised their schools as the ideal institutions imparting comprehensive medical training to students. Their syllabi were shown to be perfectly in tune with the 'developments in modern medicine including the auxiliary branches of medicine'. As Sarat Chandra Ghosh pointed out in 1935,

> One inevitable disastrous consequence of the homoeopathic schools already opened has been the creation of an impression in the mind of the public that homoeopathy has very little to do with the Science of Medicine and does not require for the understanding of its principles any respectable learning; any knowledge of anatomy or physiology.[114]

It was pointed out that to be considered credible by the government, and to be at par with modern medical developments, the 'model schools' would teach 'all Collateral Sciences in addition to the teaching of Homoeopathic Materia Medica, Philosophy and Therapeutics'.[115] The revised syllabi in such institutions promised to 'take advantage of all modern methods of teaching including the lecture hall, the laboratory, with all obtainable hospital and dispensary facilities and all the laboratory and diagnostic apparatus necessary'.[116]

These 'model institutions' established by the homoeopathic families were considered essential to salvage the situation; to appear 'scientific' and authoritative before the nationalist government. They were upheld also as the 'model' of reform for other institutions already in existence. As N. M. Choudhury, the founder of the Bengal Allen Homoeopathic College pointed out in February 1934, 'in organising homoeopathic education on these lines, it is imperative that some of the well-established institutions should lead the way'.[117] Referring specifically to his own college, he pointed out that it had been 'the product of our

[112] A. N. Mukherjee, 'Hahnemann's Birthday Celebration', p. 193.
[113] N. M. Choudhury, 'Second Andhra Homoeopathic Conference Presidential Address', *The Hahnemannian Gleanings*, 5 (February 1934), 42.
[114] Sarat Chandra Ghosh, *Life of Dr. Mahendralal Sircar*, 1935, p. 89. [115] Ibid., p. 90.
[116] Ibid., p. 91.
[117] N. M. Choudhury, 'Second Andhra Homoeopathic Conference Presidential Address', p. 42.

incessant labour for a decade . . . institutions of this type ought to serve as models for others'.[118]

State Recognition for Indigenous Homoeopathy, 1937–41

The years between 1937 and 1941 proved crucial for the ways in which the homoeopathic associations shifted their alliances between the dominant Congress and the electorally triumphant KPP to secure governmental support. The Homoeopathic Faculty Bill, 1937, as noted in the previous section, was being proposed by the Congress around the time of the first provincial election, which swung in favour of the KPP. Following the rejection of the Bill, the homoeopathic associations were quick to turn from the Congress to establish links with the KPP to secure the position of an acceptable and 'recognised' science for homoeopathy. While the administrative policies of the state had placed homoeopathy in virtually the same status as the traditional medical oeuvre, close negotiations with the government over these few years culminated in its formal recognition as a legitimate practice. The negotiations with the government occurred as much within the legislative assembly as outside it.

The KPP, which had practically come into formal existence on the eve of the elections in 1936, assumed extraordinary prominence in provincial politics between 1937 and 1941 as Fazlul Haq became the first chief minister in 1937 of a KPP-led ministry. Immediately after his assumption of power, the homoeopathic associations veered towards him for patronage and support. Gradually distancing themselves from the Congress leaders, the associations concentrated on establishing contacts with the Haq ministry instead. Later that year, the Calcutta Hospital Society organised a meeting to simultaneously celebrate Hahnemann's birthday and to discuss the 1937 central government legislation that allowed incorporation of homoeopathy in government hospitals.[119] The Society made it a point to invite Fazlul Haq as the Chief Guest who, however, failed to make it to the meeting. The speakers at the meeting discussed the need to build upon the 1937 central government legislation and keenly urged the newly appointed ministry in Bengal to follow the central legislature and take up homoeopathy's cause in the province.

Meanwhile, the Homoeopathic Faculty Bill had been introduced in the Bengal Assembly in September 1937, with the homoeopathic associations collaborating with the Congress party member P. Banerji who introduced the Bill. Since its introduction, the leaders had made conscious efforts in publicising Banerji as working 'at our instance (we

[118] Ibid. [119] Reported in 'Sangbad' ('News'), *Hahnemann*, 20, 1 (1937), 36–7.

purposely use this expression) ... to bring this Bill before the Assembly'.[120] In an editorial in the *Hahnemann*, Sarat Chandra Ghosh gave a detailed account of how he had conceived the Bill with the help of the ex-mayor of Calcutta Santosh Kumar Basu, who convinced P. Banerji of the utility of introducing it.[121] This article amply illustrated that the powerful homoeopathic associations were in fact instrumental in orchestrating the introduction of the Bill in the Assembly, with P. Banerji's assistance.[122] The declared vision of the Bill and the proposed homoeopathic faculty was to 'make homoeopathic education full proof and credible'.[123]

Yet, when the Bill had to be withdrawn on allegations of 'quackery', the homoeopathic associations blamed its failure squarely on P. Banerji. Evidently, they made an immediate and conscious attempt to distance themselves from the Congress party, which had failed to assume power in the province. In an introspective tone, Sarat Chandra Ghosh noted in a 1938 editorial in *The Hahnemannian Gleanings*, '[w]e cannot but find fault with the conduct of Mr. P. Banerjee in this matter. He was the sponsor of the bill ... but unfortunately when the crucial moment arrived and the tie of strength was measured he was found short of our expectations'.[124]

Simultaneously, the associations convened frequent meetings and conferences discussing ways to make homoeopathy credible and useful to the nationalist government. Homoeopathy was projected as the ideal public health tool necessary for a 'neo-populist' KPP government.[125] In their publications between 1937 and 1941 the homoeopathic journals made commitments to serve the government in its programme of eradicating rural ill health. For instance, in a 1939 editorial in *Hahnemann* titled 'Rog, Doridrota o Oshikkhar Birudhhe Bengal Government er Procheshta' or 'The Efforts of Bengal Government in Combating Disease, Poverty and Illiteracy', Sarat Chandra Ghosh reported the launching of a 'National Welfare Unit' by the Bengal government. Describing the lofty ideals of this unit in 'rural reconstruction', the editorial reminded the government that 'the battalion that has gone or the ones that will be sent in

[120] 'Editorial: Fate of the Homoeopathic Faculty Bill', *The Hahnemannian Gleanings*, 9 (October 1938), 502–3.
[121] 'Editorial: Bangiya Byabastha Parishad e Homoeopathy Faculty Bill Prabartan er Sathik Sangbad' ('The Accurate Account of the Introduction of the Homoeopathic Faculty Bill at the Bengal Assembly'), *Hahnemann*, 20, 6 (1937), 320.
[122] Ibid. [123] Ibid., p. 322.
[124] 'Editorial: Fate of the Homoeopathic Faculty Bill', pp. 502–3.
[125] The KPP government has been labelled as such in the historiography. See Joya Chatterji, *Bengal Divided*, p. 78.

future, if they include competent homoeopathic physicians equipped with drugs, can effect large scale good at very low cost'.[126]

Meanwhile, the new nationalist government had begun facing questions within the legislature about their failure to prioritise the 'nation-building departments', like the 'Medical' department. In the budgetary sessions since their assumption of power in 1937, the KPP faced demands that they justify their election to government by ensuring mass rural health. Referring to the bleak rural health situation, various members in the Assembly contended, 'along with the change in government the angle of vision should be changed; otherwise what is the good of ushering a simple change in the form of government, but not in the spirit and sense?'[127] In debates over the medical budgets between 1937 and 1939, the government was reminded of its promised commitment to 'improve and better the poor lot or lessen the sufferings of thousands of villagers who are dying every day without treatment'.[128] Arguing that the 'real nation' lived in villages, the members regularly pleaded for greater allotment of health resources for the villages. It was pointed out that 'the poor cultivators, the growers of raw products, the real producers of wealth are on the verge of ruin due to ill-health and insanitation'.[129]

Against this backdrop, there were mounting pressures within the legislature to formally integrate 'indigenous' practices within the governmental healthcare system. This signified a clear and momentous shift in the government's attitude – the colonial government had refused formal patronage to any form of indigenous medicine ever since the abolition of the short-lived Native Medical Institution in 1835.[130] Yet, some nationalist advocates often ended up echoing the colonial belief in the primacy and unquestioned superiority of western allopathic medicine. Hence, within the Bengal legislature there were recurring suggestions to incorporate 'indigenous' systems as a mere supplement to the western 'scientific' treatment. As Debi Prosad Khaitan argued in the 1937 discussions on the medical budget, 'it is quite true that allopathy has advanced more in science than any other system. But it is equally true

[126] 'Editorial: Rog, Doridrota o Oshikkhar Birudhhe Bengal Government er Procheshta' ('The Efforts of Bengal Government in Combating Disease, Poverty and Illiteracy'), *Hahnemann*, 22, 9 (1939), 563.

[127] *Bengal Legislative Assembly Proceedings*, Vol L. 1, Number 3 (Calcutta: Bengal Government Press, 1937) pp. 802–3. [WBSL]

[128] Ibid., pp. 802–3.

[129] *Bengal Legislative Assembly Proceedings*, Vol L. IV, Number 3 (Calcutta: Bengal Government Press, 1939), pp. 170–1. [WBSL]

[130] Zhaleh Khaleeli, 'Harmony or Hegemony? Rise and Fall of the Native Medical Institution in Calcutta, 1822–1835', *South Asia Research*, 21, 1 (2001), 77–102.

that at least 90% of the people get themselves treated according to the indigenous systems'.[131]

These budgetary discussions dwelt at length on allopathy's many inadequacies to nurse and cure the inhabitants of Bengal's vast countryside. It was repeatedly pointed out that 'in the mufassal the Indian method of ayurvedic treatment may be introduced and homoeopathic dispensaries established, as they are less costly and most useful in rural areas'.[132] In most of these official proposals, homoeopathy featured as part of the discussion on indigenous medicine. In the light of the above considerations, the KPP health minister Tamizuddin Khan too was most supportive of the cause of indigenous medicine. In his 1937 budget speech, he conceded the importance of recognising ayurveda, homoeopathy as well as unani medicine, especially on the grounds of 'people's faith' in them. However, he reminded the audience of the necessity of standardisation before any formal recognition could be granted. Yet, in the same speech the minister gave primacy to registers like 'faith' ahead of considerations of 'science' when a system like homoeopathy was in focus. Of homoeopathy, for instance, he stated in his 1937 speech, 'allopathic doctors may not find any merit in that system, but so far as millions of patients are concerned, they will, I think, freely recognise its merits in view of the benefits they daily derive'.[133] The discussions on the 1939 budget particularly highlighted the importance of indigenous medicine in the context of rural need and allopathic inadequacy. After the speeches made by those urging government patronage of ayurvedic and unani medicine, P. Banerji made a long presentation in favour of homoeopathy. He argued that large-scale investment in allopathic treatment by the government was futile, as it 'does not do good particularly to the constitution of the people of this country'.[134] He also referred to the paltry number of allopathic practitioners in contrast with homoeopathy's rising popularity, especially in the countryside. Finally, he promised that the government could save more 'if the homoeopathic form of treatment is introduced'.[135]

Following the rejection of the 1938 Bill, the spokespersons for homoeopathy focused on negotiating directly with the KPP ministers outside the legislature. The year 1939 saw a string of meetings organised by the associations. A huge gathering, for instance, was organised by the South

[131] *Bengal Legislative Assembly Proceedings*, Vol L. 1, Number 3 (Calcutta: Bengal Government Press, 1937), pp. 804–5. [WBSL]
[132] Ibid., pp. 799–801. [133] Ibid., p. 806–7.
[134] *Bengal Legislative Assembly Proceedings*, Vol L. IV, Number 3 (Calcutta: Bengal Government Press, 1939), pp. 180–1. [WBSL]
[135] Ibid., pp. 180–1.

Calcutta Homoeopathic Association on April 1, 1939 at the residence of its president Sarat Chandra Ghosh, to felicitate the chief minister Fazlul Haq. On behalf of the 'homoeopaths of Bengal', Ghosh presented a deputation to Haq underlining 'the necessity of constituting a Homoeopathic Faculty by the government at an early hour'.[136] The report of this meeting, published in various homoeopathic journals, especially noted the large number of dignitaries from Calcutta including 'eminent allopathic physicians', who attended and expressed their 'solidarity with the motion'.[137] The gathering and the deputation impressed the minister to the extent that in his speech he delegated Sarat Chandra Ghosh the responsibility to 'select members of his association, who would be deputed to confer with him in this matter'.[138]

At the same time, Fazlul Haq had made it clear that he needed to consult his health minister before arriving at any conclusion regarding homoeopathy. The South Calcutta Homoeopathic Association immediately took measures to approach the health minister separately. The association organised another meeting to 'present an address to the Hon'ble Minister of Public Health' Tamizuddin Khan.[139] In his persuasive presentation, Sarat Chandra Ghosh reminded the audience of the 'economy', 'efficacy' and 'popularity' of homoeopathy. Similar justifications, it may be recalled, were put forward in the legislative assembly by P. Banerji to demonstrate homoeopathy's usefulness in public health programmes. Ghosh argued eloquently for the advantages of homoeopathy over both allopathy and ayurveda in terms of economy. He held that the government could save 'at least 70 percent' of their expenditure 'if the patients be treated by homoeopathic medicines'.[140]

In addition to its economic benefits, Ghosh requested Tamizuddin Khan to consider homoeopathy's scientific virtues. He argued that scientific research in modern times by celebrated scientists like Jenner, Pasteur, Lister, Koch and others had ratified the truth of homoeopathy.[141] Ghosh further claimed that 'it is a noteworthy fact that biological works and scientific investigations in various countries

[136] 'Editorial: Reception of the Hon'ble Mr. A. K. Fazlul Huq Chief Minister of Bengal By the Members of the South Calcutta Homoeopathic Association', *The Hahnemannian Gleanings*, 10 (May 1939), 217.

[137] 'Editorial: Manoniyo Pradhan Mantri Fazlul Haq er Sambardhana' ('Felicitation of Fazlul Haq, the Honourable Chief Minister'), *Hahnemann*, 22, 1 (1939), 3–5. Also see 'Editorial: Reception of the Hon'ble Mr. A. K. Fazlul Huq Chief Minister of Bengal By the Members of the South Calcutta Homoeopathic Association', p. 218.

[138] Ibid., p. 218. [139] Ibid.

[140] 'An Address: Presented to Hon'ble Mr. Tamizuddin Khan, Minsiter Public Health, Bengal Government', *The Hahnemannian Gleanings*, 10 (May 1939), 213.

[141] Ibid., p. 211.

from various sources have confirmed the truth formulated by Hahnemann'.[142] The address acknowledged, however, the 'corruption' that had been bred by 'ill-manned and ill-equipped institutions' and their owners by whom 'the noble science of therapeutics is now being prostituted'.[143] A faculty formed by the leading homoeopaths was proposed as the best remedy to salvage homoeopathy from its problems.

Tamizuddin Khan's reply in the meeting was considered a 'landmark' in the career of homoeopathy, since he officially endorsed the formation of a State Homoeopathic Faculty. However, the terms of official governmental patronage carefully elided the question of homoeopathy's scientificity. Instead, it focused on the index of popularity, indigeneity and efficacy in the given situation in India. Khan argued that, '[w]ithout going into comparative merits of the western scientific system of medicine and the indigenous systems, I firmly believe that Homoeopathy is *peculiarly suitable* to Indian conditions and has a bright future in Bengal'.[144] His speech emphasised more the standardised, 'scientific' ways of imparting homoeopathic knowledge. Besides, the logic of indigeneity was especially invoked in the official recognition of homoeopathy. In doing so, and in elaborating on the niche for different forms of medicine, Tamizuddin Khan hinted at the unique secular appeal of homoeopathy, which was apparently unmatched by any other forms of 'indigenous' medicine. He argued that,

> The Tibbi system of therapeutics flourished during the time of Moslem dynasty, Ayurveda reached the climax of position when the Hindu rajas were the sovereigns of the country . . . India is a poor country and as such homoeopathy is the proper system of treatment peculiarly fitted to the existing conditions of India.[145]

Interestingly, the religious allusions associated with homoeopathy were mostly avoided in these private meetings. The KPP government, which had a growing intimacy with the Muslim League, nevertheless maintained a secular rhetoric in their budgetary meetings and Assembly discussions involving the health of the province, as did the Congress. Homoeopathy seemed to fit the Bill for an ideal kind of 'indigenous' therapeutics for all parties. There has been some scholarship on the relation between communal identity politics and medicine, especially around ayurveda and unani. Previous chapters have established how homoeopathy was framed within predominantly Hindu aesthetics and identity over the late

[142] Ibid. [143] Ibid., p. 212.
[144] 'Editorial: Reception of the Hon'ble Mr. A. K. Fazlul Huq Chief Minister of Bengal By the Members of the South Calcutta Homoeopathic Association', p. 220.
[145] Ibid.

nineteenth century. Hence, its formal recognition through a government with close links to the Muslim League is intriguing. However, although communal undertones were evidently attached to ayurveda and unani, especially since the 1920s, Seema Alavi's work on unani shows that not all advocates for traditional medicine were ready to toe that line for publicity.[146] The powerful Azizi family of North India, she demonstrates, were proponents of unani as a 'national medicine', one whose constituency was not narrowly confined to a Muslim *quaum* (community). Besides, the activity of the Congress government in UP, too, demonstrates that even as communalism simmered, particularly in the newly formed institutional spaces for traditional medicine, the actual bills and legislations were devoid of any explicit factionalism. Perhaps, as has been pointed out, the 'gravitas of governance' unmediated by the colonial state was a challenge sombre enough for the provincial governments to quell petty factionalism for the moment.[147] More compellingly, the issue at hand was really the promotion of 'indigenous medicine' to counter the colonial conviction that the power of western biomedicine was the only form of scientific medicine. Besides, especially in the case of homoeopathy, the enduring liminal identity between being at once western and indigenous made it acceptable to the various competing strands of opinion.

Following the announcement of a State Homoeopathic Faculty by Tamizuddin Khan, the homoeopathic journals reported euphoria within the ranks of the associations. Referring to the event as the wonderful achievement of the South Calcutta Homoeopathic Association, *The Hahnemannian Gleanings* pointed out, 'as such this house should be regarded by all homoeopaths as a sacred place – Mandir (i.e. temple) – where they have first heard of the success of the mission'.[148] To expedite the formation of the faculty, Tamizuddin Khan further promised to announce an advisory committee to the government. Predictably, the advisory committee that was announced in the Calcutta Gazette of April 1939 comprised all the individuals who had been vigorously advocating the purification drive induced by the state.[149] Along with Sarat Chandra Ghosh and J. N. Majumdar, it also included A. N. Mukherjee, N. M. Choudhury, J. N. Ghose and

[146] Seema Alavi, *Islam and Healing: Loss and Recovery of Indo-Muslim Medical Tradition* (Basingstoke: Palgrave Macmillan, 2008), pp. 14–16, 242–78.

[147] See, for instance, Rachel Berger, *Ayurveda Made Modern*, pp. 130–8. The point has been made in relation to Congress politics around the status of ayurveda in the United Provinces.

[148] 'Editorial: Reception of the Hon'ble Mr. A. K. Fazlul Huq Chief Minister of Bengal by the Members of the South Calcutta Homoeopathic Association', p. 222.

[149] Ibid.

others.[150] Thus there was a striking overlap between the leading journals, their publishers, the older familial networks of pharmacy owners, leaders of the associations, the government committee and the members of the future faculty. In 1939 and 1940 the leading journals detailed the progress of the committee in drafting the statutes for the state faculty.[151] They regretted the brief interruptions to the cause with the change of ministers when Tamizuddin Khan was succeeded in office by Nawab Habibullah of Dacca.[152] The journals kept urging the committee to work faster on forming the faculty that would 'regulate the standard of instruction in homoeopathic medicine' by holding examinations, granting certificates and maintaining a register of qualified homoeopathic practitioners.[153] The committee further exercised the authority to negotiate and select institutions that would be recognised by the faculty statutes.[154] The July 1940 editorial of *The Hahnemannian Gleanings*, for instance, reported on a scheduled discussion in the committee on making 'the Bengal Allen Homoeopathic College into a public institution prior to its inclusion in the statutes'.[155] The General Council and State Faculty of Homoeopathic Medicine in Bengal were officially founded in August 1941 with the declared mandate of 'stimulating a systematic study of the Homoeopathic system of medicine and of differentiating trained homoeopathic practitioners from the untrained, amateur ones'.[156] The 'statute' outlined the composition of a homoeopathic council where an overwhelming majority of the members were nominated by the 'local government'. The faculty in effect cemented the hold of the closed group of associations on all matters homoeopathic in Bengal, thus turning them into state-endorsed authorities on the subject with full authority to regulate the profession.

[150] Ibid.
[151] See, for instance, 'Editorial: News about the Advisory Committee of the State Homoeopathic Faculty of Bengal', *The Hahnemannian Gleanings*, 11 (July 1940), 334. Also see 'Editorial: Homoeopathic State Faculty Songothon' ('Formation of the Homoeopathic State Faculty'), *Hahnemann*, 23, 9 (1939).
[152] 'Editorial: Bengal Homoeopathic Faculty Sombondhe Sothik Sangbad' ('The Accurate Account of the Introduction of the Homoeopathic Faculty Bill at the Bengal Assembly'), *Hahnemann*, 23, 2 (1939), 113.
[153] 'Editorial: Reception of the Hon'ble Mr. A. K. Fazlul Huq Chief Minister of Bengal By the Members of the South Calcutta Homoeopathic Association', p. 223.
[154] 'Editorial: News about the Advisory Committee of the State Homoeopathic Faculty of Bengal', *The Hahnemannian Gleanings*, 11 (July 1940), 334.
[155] Ibid., p. 334.
[156] 'General Council and State Faculty of Homoeopathic Medicine in Bengal: Government Announcement', *The Hahnemannian Gleanings*, 12, 7 (August 1941), 237.

Resistance and a Homoeopathic Public

The movements for reform within homoeopathy were set not only in relation to colonial medicine and the legislating state, but also multiple strands of opinion within the community. Even during the process of negotiation between the pharmacy-led homoeopathic associations and the government, there were murmurs of dissent about the intrinsic exclusions and alienations of purification. While marking out a privileged domain of mutually acceptable and 'reformed' homoeopathy that qualified for official patronage and recognition, boundaries were redrawn and hierarchies reinforced. Hence, it is especially important to trace homoeopathy's relationship with the public in this period.

Homoeopathic publications since the mid-1920s recorded occasional voices of protest against an alleged alliance between the associations and the state. While accepting the twentieth-century need to be vigilant against the swelling numbers of ill-trained, money-minded lay practitioners, these writings remained critical of the ways in which the problem was sought to be resolved. Mostly written by self-taught homoeopaths, these publications articulated their grievance at being summarily excluded from the newly emerging domain of 'pure' national homoeopathy. The editors of the leading journals, however, registered their differences with such articles that justified 'lay' methods of healing. Almost invariably, the editors put a note before such articles, proclaiming the 'editor and the journal not responsible for the opinion of the author'.[157]

Indeed, a range of writings in the 1920s and 1930s identified the nineteenth-century family-led businesses as the root cause of much of the twentieth-century governmental discomfort with homoeopathy. The article 'Homoeopathy Shebir Asha o Nirasha' or 'The Anxieties of a Servant of Homoeopathy' in the journal *Homoeopathy Pracharak*, for instance, identified 'the greed of business houses' as the fundamental problem plaguing homoeopathy.[158] It pointed out that 'the proprietors of each big homoeopathic pharmacy in Bengal have published a plethora of self-educating health manuals and other such pamphlets'.[159] The author further reminded the readers of the recent investments of

[157] See, for instance, Akhilchandra Roy, 'Homoeopathy'r Mul Tattva Sombondhe Du Ekti Kotha' ('A Few Words on the Fundamental Principle of Homoeopathy'), *Hahnemann*, 22, 11 (1939), 661. Also see Nalininath Majumdar, 'Baro Daktar Rahasya' ('Mystery about Big Doctors'), *Hahnemann*, 8, 8 (1925), 427.

[158] Chintaharan Bandopadhyay, 'Homoeopathy Shebir Asha o Nirasha' ('The Anxieties of a Servant of Homoeopathy'), *Homoeopathy Paricharak*, 2, 8 (November 1928), 296–303.

[159] Ibid.

such businesses in homoeopathic colleges, which were also 'quite profitable'.[160] To him, the indiscriminate sale of homoeopathic boxes and domestic medicine manuals by the big pharmacies signalled the most serious problem. The 1925 article 'Homoeopathy'r Bartaman Abastha', or 'The Present Predicament of Homoeopathy' argued that the extensive sale of such publications engendered an impression that homoeopathy could be mastered and practised by anyone, including 'women and even children'. The author lamented that this attracted many semi-literate, cunning men, on the lookout for easy, amateurish ways of making a living.[161] Such business-induced corruption was projected as the fate of homoeopathy in most countries – a few authors elaborated on similar problems faced by American homoeopathy in the hands of the 'biggest and most trusted American Drug company Boericke and Tafel', which had indulged in the large-scale production of homoeopathic patent drugs.[162]

These dissenting authors were unified in their understanding of homoeopathy as a 'science' that could be mastered at home. However, proper learning of homoeopathy, it was argued, involved meticulous and systematic reading of key texts like *Organon*, and grasping its inherent philosophy.[163] The fatal harm caused by homoeopathic business concerns, it was argued, was the generation of a widespread impression that homoeopathy could be easily accessed through any book and a chest of medicine.[164] It was regretted that 'a therapeutics which is extremely subtle and difficult has been reduced to an easy hobby for one and all'.[165] It was pointed out that the primary duty lay in changing such perceptions in the minds of the educated middle-class Bengalis.[166] It was felt that without a fundamental change of mind-set, no amount of governmental recognition and resolutions could render homoeopathy respectable.[167]

160 Ibid.
161 Nalininath Majumdar, 'Homoeopathy r Bartaman Durabastha' ('The Present Predicament of Homoeopathy'), *Hahnemann*, 8, 12 (1925), 663.
162 Akhilchandra Roy, 'Homoeopathy'r Mul Tattva Sombondhe Du Ekti Kotha' ('A Few Words on the Fundamental Principle of Homoeopathy'), p. 664.
163 Tarak Das Chakrabarty, 'Homoeopathy aj Kon poth e?' ('What is the Future of Homoeopathy'), *Hahnemann*, 23, 11 (1940), 692.
164 Ibid., also see Nilmani Ghatak, 'Lok-Shikkha' ('Lessons for People'), *Hahnemann*, 10, 6 (1927), 285.
165 Anonymous, 'Homoeopathy Chikitshak' ('Homoeopathic Physician'), *Hahnemann*, 9, 6 (1926), 318.
166 Tarak Das Chakrabarty, Homoeopathy aj Kon poth e?' ('What is the Future of Homoeopathy'), p. 693.
167 Ibid., p. 693.

At the same time, such texts, critical about the sudden spurt of professionalisation, spelt out the inevitable inadequacy of institutional pedagogy for a 'science' as homoeopathy. It was pointed out that as 'a symptom-based science', the practice of homoeopathy involved individual reading and consultation of texts 'for life, till one's last days'.[168] Formal institutional settings, in this context, appeared redundant for training as a homoeopath. As the article 'Homoeopathy – Aj Kon Pothe?' or 'What is the Future of Homoeopathy?' elaborated, 'two/three years of education in a college hardly makes one a true homoeopath. Real homoeopathic knowledge is not so easily attainable. It requires lifelong passion for the subject and thorough reading'.[169] Even those associated with the 'mushrooming' homoeopathic colleges frequently shared in this sentiment. A speech delivered at the graduation ceremony of the Hahnemann Memorial College reminded the students of the futility of a formal homoeopathic degree in the practical sphere.[170] Comparing such degrees with 'a useless piece of paper', the speaker urged the audience to remain sincere students of homoeopathy for life.[171] He was confident that only sincere, individualised and informal learning could rescue the lost prestige of homoeopathy, which was often dubbed a 'bogus' or an 'orphan' science.[172] Indeed, a large number of 'self-taught' physicians narrated their experience of successfully treating numerous cases. In a letter to the journal *Hahnemann* in 1940, the author Dharmadas Mandal introduced himself as a 'humble village physician who has neither been to any college nor possesses any degree'.[173] He stated that although a 'sincere follower of homoeopathic texts' and committed to the cause of learning 'pure' homoeopathy, he lacked confidence because of his humble location and funds. Yet, he considered it worthwhile to make the readers aware of the number of cases of mental disease he had been successfully treating in the village Rampur in Burdwan district.[174]

These writings argued in favour of the household-based practice of homoeopathy in contrast to any rigidly regulated formal institutional structure. Such apparently unregulated practice, it was claimed, had

[168] Akhilchandra Roy, 'Homoeopathy'r Mul Tattva Sombondhe Du Ekti Kotha' ('A Few Words on the Fundamental Principle of Homoeopathy'), p. 661.
[169] Tarak Das Chakrabarty, 'Homoeopathy aj Kon poth e?' ('What is the Future of Homoeopathy'), p. 693.
[170] Harendra Nath Mukhopadhyay, 'Homoeopathic Chhatragan er Proti' ('To the Students of Homoeopathy'), *Hahnemann*, 21, 6 (1938), 347.
[171] Ibid., p. 346. [172] Ibid., p. 347.
[173] Dharmadas Mandal, 'Homoeopath er Dak e Saara' ('Response to the Calls of a Homoeopath'), *Hahnemann*, 23, 5 (1940), 289.
[174] Ibid., p. 290.

made homoeopathy what it was – a quotidian household name in Bengal. The article 'School of Medicine in India' published in the journal *The Hahnemannian Gleanings* in 1930 argued, 'homoeopathy is daily gaining ground and that in spite of lacking in state-help ... it may be said that Homoeopathy has already got its entrance into the families of the intelligent and the educated'.[175] These authors alerted the readers to the fact that mere government recognition could hardly ensure or account for the unprecedented dissemination and popularity of homoeopathy within Bengali homes.[176] Authors like R. Biswas writing in *Hahnemann* even as late as 1939 reminded the readers of the immense advantages Bengali families could reap from making men and especially women adept in homoeopathy.[177] For the benefit of families and the larger society he argued: 'I hope that in every village and every household in Bengal the children are inspired to select homoeopathic drugs by reading *Materia Medica* so that they can treat the basic familial ills themselves.'[178] Such proficiency, he insisted, could hardly be acquired through formal training in schools. He contended that the schools could cater to those seeking professional, specialised knowledge by learning details of 'anatomy, physiology and practice of medicine'.[179]

In this context, many of the articles published from the 1920s onwards questioned even the politics of governmental recognition and the associated drive against quackery. The discontent with the move to negotiate with the government was articulated on various counts. For some, resisting the government was a political choice. Authors like Nilmani Ghatak writing in 1922, argued that in an era 'when the Bengalis are so deeply committed to the cause of *swaraj* (self-rule)', it was unacceptable to seek the colonial state's sanction in organising the homoeopathic profession.[180] Others like G. Dirghangi resented the idea of governmental intervention and regulation, arguing that the state would inevitably fail to ensure quality.[181] They argued that the sale or faking of degrees did not endanger homoeopathy exclusively and that such malpractices were inevitable in a free market. Dirghangi reminded the authorities that patients/consumers were the best judges of the quality of products

[175] Nilmani Ghatak, 'School of Medicine in India', *The Hahnemannian Gleanings*, 1, 8 (September 1930), 340.
[176] Tarak Das Chakrabarty, 'Homoeopathy aj Kon poth e?' ('What is the Future of Homoeopathy'), p. 692.
[177] R. Biswas, 'Homoeopathy Balika School' ('Homoeopathic Girls' School'), *Hahnemann*, 22, 7 (1939), 414–15.
[178] Ibid., p. 417. [179] Ibid., p. 417.
[180] Nilmani Ghatak, 'Nijeder Kotha' ('Our Words'), *Hahnemann*, 5, 4 (1922), 184–8.
[181] G. Dirghangi, 'Homoeopathy Parikkha Samiti' ('Homoeopathic Examination Committee'), *Hahnemann*, 4, 12 (1921), 451–9.

associated with homoeopathy.[182] He added, further, that the politics of earning governmental sympathy by cleansing irregularities from the profession was misplaced. He suggested that the 'the cunning business-minded people would get away. If the homoeopathic colleges do not succeed they would publish journals or open up an insurance company or do something else' while the ordinary practitioners would suffer from punitive governmental measures.[183] Finally, some authors drew their readers' attention to the fact that the 'government' was ultimately constituted of people with their own specific agendas and prejudices. Author Nalininath Majumdar argued that even if one believed the good intentions of the government, one needed to appreciate that they are 'lay men in matters related to health', and relied on 'a group of well-paid physicians under whose advice it had to act'.[184] Hence, he urged the readers to be agnostic and not to regard 'governmental recognition' as a sacrosanct end in itself.

These dissenting voices included 'lay' householders inspired by the nationalist vision of self-help, self-taught practitioners committed to the cause of learning and disseminating homoeopathy and often based in the *mofussil*, as well as those urban associates and members of existing homoeopathic colleges, which the proposed faculty sought to categorise as those propagating inappropriate standards of education. By 1940 the advisory committee to the government was busy deciding on the composition and remit of the state faculty. Meanwhile, those excluded from the exclusive state-big business nexus got together to articulate their grievances against the state legislation more vigorously than ever before. Proclaiming themselves 'protestors' against the drive to attract state recognition, they organised protest meetings upholding the cause of the 'self-trained homoeopaths and housewives who had been responsible for propagating homoeopathy so rampantly across Bengal'.[185] Various petitions appeared to convey the voices of the 'general public and the unqualified and semi-qualified homoeopaths in cities and in the *mofussil* '.[186] The presidential address to Howrah Zilla Homoeopathic Sammelan, for instance, elaborated on the reasons to suspect the competence and intentions of the state advisory committee. The speech explicitly stated that 'the selfish, motivated men who have found their way into the

182 Ibid., p. 458. 183 Ibid., p. 459.

184 Nalininath Majumdar, 'Baro Daktar Rahasya' ('Mystery about Big Doctors'), p. 429.

185 N. C. Ghosh, 'Sahar o Mofussil Bashi der Pakkha hoite Homoeopathy o Ashikhita ba Ardha Shikhita Homoeopath Sombondhe Du ekti Kotha' ('From the Inhabitants of Towns and Mofussil a Few Words on the Illiterate or the Semi Literate Homoeopaths'), *Hahnemann*, 21, 2 (1938), 75.

186 Ibid., p. 72.

governmental advisory committees through recommendation and donation can barely cause any improvement to homoeopathy'.[187]

Many excluded and disgruntled voices alleged that the alliance between the associations and the government compromised the original essence of the homoeopathic doctrine. Reformist drives towards regularising and standardising homoeopathic curricula were dismissed as a replication of the allopathic paradigm. The consequent shift in the nature of homoeopathic pedagogy and therapeutics was considered the greatest corruption inflicted upon homoeopathy. The reform agenda of the associations and their 'model institutions', which glorified the relevance of the auxiliary sciences of anatomy, physiology and even bacteriology in teaching homoeopathy, were condemned. Some articles referred to the implicit hierarchies, which were reinforced through the act of governmental recognition. The necessity of homoeopathy, it was lamented, was conceded only in the context of deficient allopathic infrastructure. Otherwise, allopathic superiority was allegedly acknowledged even by those seeking state recognition of homoeopathy.

It was strongly argued that the elaborate efforts towards purging the community of corrupt practitioners ended up diluting the original purity of homoeopathy itself. Some of these authors directly attacked the homoeopathic leaders, such as Jitendranath Majumdar. For instance, the article 'Homoeopathy – Past and Present – in India' expressed regret that experienced physicians 'of name, fame, standing and heritage, not to speak of the exalted position as that of Dr. Majumdar at last favour the idea that "Allopathy is the Science of Medicine"'.[188] Framing the big business-state nexus as a greater evil to the profession than the so-called problem of quackery, these protesting authors pointed out that 'the bogus men do not count much in the field, but the homoeopaths of name and renown do not care to maintain the purity of the pathy'.[189] The self-motivated reform drives of the elite practitioners were considered more injurious to the cause of homoeopathy than the problem of fake degrees and ill-taught practitioners. As author N. Ghatak pointed out, 'it is half-homoeopathy, Allo-Homoeopathy that does the most injury. Those that should uphold and vindicate, do as a matter of fact, lower down and compromise'.[190] Thus, the Calcutta-based elite practitioners and their selfish politics were identified in a range of articles as the principal agents of distorting 'pure' 'Hahnemannian'

[187] J. C. Banerjee, 'Howrah Zilla Homoeopathy Sammelan ('Homoeopathy Conference for the District of Howrah'), *Hahnemann*, 23, 4 (1940), 363.

[188] N. Ghatak, 'Homoeopathy – Past and Present – in India', *The Hahnemannian Gleanings*, 8 (December 1937), 506.

[189] Ibid., p. 506. [190] Ibid., p. 507.

homoeopathy.[191] Author Akhil Chandra Ray seemingly summed up these allegations when he proclaimed, 'the harm that has been caused to homoeopathy by those opposing it completely fades in comparison to the ones induced by its most ardent patrons'.[192]

Conclusion

In the early twentieth century, homoeopathy figured variously in the provincial legislations; as an object of prohibition, policing, disapprobation and appropriation. The gradual entanglement of the family-based business enterprises with the nationalist health agenda for the masses explains homoeopathy's slow incorporation as a governmental public health tool in the late 1920s and 1930s. The formation of the nationalist ministry in the province in early 1937 provided homoeopathy unprecedented visibility in bureaucratic measures, along with ayurveda and unani. Homoeopathy began to be projected as an indispensable tool in the public health agendas of the emergent nation state – a necessary evil that needed to be tolerated and regulated. Though not necessarily lauded as a perfect and 'pure' science, homoeopathy's ubiquitous outreach was widely accepted in government circles. It was shown to represent the radical and novel face of progressive modern science, and often projected as particularly suited to aid the engine of development and reconstruction. Simultaneously, it appeared deeply enshrined within the indigenous traditions of Hindu India. Recent works have hinted at the communal undertones of the apparent secularist values embedded in discourses of indigeneity which were Congress's language of national legitimation.[193] Homoeopathy's Janus-faced identity and cosy intimacies with predominant nationalist-communitarian values, too, are symptomatic of the tensions and contradictions within an emerging 'secular' post-colonial state.

The normative standards of acceptable, necessary and 'recognisable' therapeutics were shaped through a convergence of politico-commercial interventions. Such negotiations took place as much on the floors of the state legislature through official political debates as they did through the medium of private meetings, appeals and deputations. A traffic of interests between state and pharmaceutical business produced the contours

191 See, for instance, Anonymous, 'Amader Atmakahini' ('Our Autobiography'), *Hahnemann*, 9, 7 (1926), 370–6.

192 Akhilchandra Roy, 'Homoeopathy'r Mul Tattva Sombondhe Du Ekti Kotha' ('A Few Words on the Fundamental Principle of Homoeopathy'), p. 665.

193 Rachel Berger makes this point while referring to Benjamin Zachariah's work on nationalism, which contends that indigeneity and secularism were two ideas on which Congress' claims of national legitimacy relied. See Rachel Berger, *Making Ayurveda Modern*, pp. 129–30.

of what constituted 'authentic' homoeopathy, that seemed compatible with the standard scientific parameters of the state. It, as well, constituted state-endorsed official experts or authorities on homoeopathy. Gaining official recognition for homoeopathy depended on the ability of its advocates to successfully negotiate the delicate power balance in provincial politics between the Congress and other regional parties such as the KPP. In studying this process, I also examined the hierarchies which were reinforced, and boundaries that were redrawn, while homoeopathic associations sought 'recognition' from the state. Instead of seeking to judge whether there existed a subaltern realm of homoeopathy, I have remained sensitive to how certain voices within the community were increasingly marginalised and rendered peripheral in the course of the twentieth-century reforms. Homoeopathic pedagogy was considerably restructured, and the vast majority of *mofussil*-based practitioners and self-trained amateurs were rendered illegitimate. Homoeopathic knowledge itself was dramatically redefined through an unprecedented dialogue with the components of allopathic state medicine. Twentieth-century state-acknowledged homoeopathy in Bengal, for example, relied more keenly on bacteriological understandings of the disease than ever before. The curriculum too was more integrated with western auxiliary sciences of anatomy, physiology, pathology and others.

The above trends discussed in the course of this chapter, whereby homoeopathy was identified as a 'necessary evil' which had to be at once castigated, yet tolerated and regulated by the state, are significant. Enunciated between the 1920s and 1941, these tendencies continued into the post-independence period and shaped trajectories of health governance in the nascent Indian nation-state in the decade of 1950s, 60s and after. Indeed, to conclude this penultimate chapter in the book, let me briefly summarise the developments that followed independence until the 1970s, when a Central Council of Homoeopathy was built around the same time as the Central Councils for Ayurveda and Unani were formed.

It is generally agreed that the essential blueprint for national health policy in Independent India was laid down by the Bhore Committee (1946) and the Chopra Committee (1948). Although the latter was far more positive about the role of non-allopathic medicine or 'indigenous medicine' in the Indian healthcare system, recent scholarship contends that the Bhore and Chopra committees' recommendations shared much in common. Both were largely propelled in their decision by what has been variously called a 'biomedical hegemony', 'pharmaceutic episteme' or 'scientific paradigm' that powerfully reinforced a higher scientific status for western state medicine or biomedicine.[194] It has been argued that under a thin veneer of pluralism, complete biomedical hegemony ruled the national policy vision. Elaborating on notions such as 'integration' and 'synthesis', the Chopra Committee's aim was 'for modern medicine to absorb traditional medicine by reinterpreting its principal categories'.[195] In simple terms, indigenous medicine and homoeopathy were recognised as being important for providing healthcare, especially in rural India, but only in a subsidiary capacity to biomedicine. The usefulness of traditional medicine or homoeopathy was acknowledged only as a corollary to recognising biomedicine's limited reach and access. Simultaneously, elaborate plans were drawn up for 'indigenous medicine' to match up to the 'scientific' standards of modern medicine, though processes of scientific standardisation, regularisation and rationalisation of education and research.[196]

To follow up on the Chopra Committee recommendations for standardising non-biomedical practices, the Homoeopathic Enquiry Committee was set up in 1948 by the Government of India. The essential emphasis of the Committee's work was on the scientific standardisation of homoeopathy, especially in relation to pedagogy. Training in western biomedicine was put forward as an essential criterion for homoeopathic specialisation.[197] It was pointed out that the homoeopaths needed to be trained to the same level of medical knowledge as any regular practitioner of medicine, including training in anatomy, physiology and disease-theory. It was held that, along with the shared basic knowledge of anatomy, physiology and the like, all non-biomedical practitioners should then develop a specialisation in their own distinct kind of therapeutics. Thus, the report proclaimed, 'the main difference in the type of training that we have envisaged lies in that the homoeopathic medical student will not learn the therapeutics of the regular system (i.e. biomedicine)'.[198] Besides, the report included a whole set of recommendations on the registration of practitioners and institutes to the provincial State Faculties. There were also discussions

[194] See Madhulika Banerjee, 'Public Policy and Ayurveda: Modernising a Great Tradition', *Economic and Political Weekly*, 37, 12 (2002), 1136; and Dominik Wujastyk, 'The Evolution of Indian Government Policy on Ayurveda in the Twentieth Century' in Dagmar Wujastyck and Frederick Smith (eds.), *Modern and Global Ayurveda: Pluralism and Paradigms*, 2008, pp. 51–60.

[195] Dominik Wujastyk, 'The Evolution of Indian Government Policy on Ayurveda in the Twentieth Century', pp. 65–6.

[196] Madhulika Banerjee, 'Public Policy and Ayurveda: Modernising a Great Tradition', pp. 1136–8.

[197] *Report of the Homoeopathic Enquiry Committee*, Ministry of Health, Government of India (Delhi: Manager of Publications, 1949), pp. 64–73.

[198] Ibid., pp. 23–4.

on setting up, in due course, an exclusively homoeopathic course of study in separate homoeopathic institutes. It was only in the 1970s that this initiative was eventually formalised by the Central Council of Homoeopathy. However, the emphasis on the scientific standardisation of homoeopathy irked a large number of practitioners at the provincial level. Writing on post-colonial homoeopathy in Madras, Gary Hausman quotes a reaction from the Malabar Homoeopathic Association which complained that the 'report smacks at subtle attempts at allopathising the system of homoeopathy.'[199]

The colonial pharmaceutical families did not become entirely irrelevant in the aftermath of independence. Indeed, along with the twin processes of toleration and regularisation, perhaps a third, albeit fading trend of continuity was the role of the colonial pharmaceutical families in the post-colonial history of homoeopathy. Let me recount some instances of the older colonial-era family connections to homoeopathy influencing its post-colonial trajectory. I have already described the processes whereby the representatives of the elite homoeopathic families negotiated their way into Bengal governmental committees and Faculties, to assume positions as provincial official authorities on homoeopathy. As such, their ideas had a bearing on the provincial legislations on homoeopathy between 1937 and 1941. Post-independence, such translation of the familial power into governmental authority could be traced at the national level too. As noted earlier, Jitendranath Majumdar was the secretary to the first All India Homoeopathic Association formed in 1932. Further, he became the secretary of the first All India Homoeopathic Institute formed in Delhi in 1944,[200] and then went on to become a member of the exclusive ten-member strong Homoeopathic Enquiry Committee of 1948.[201] Though the national committee was composed of people from various provinces and professions, it is noteworthy that Dr Majumdar from Bengal and Dr Diwan Jai Chand from Delhi were the only two practising homoeopaths who were members. This committee decided to conduct an extensive survey of the field and visited and spoke to chosen authoritative institutions with proven reputations in homoeopathy. The views of several of the Calcutta-based family firms, including the Hahnemann Publishing Company, M. Bhattacharya and Company, C. Ringer and Company among others were collected, as they were considered 'important pharmacies and publishing houses' even in

199 Gary Hausman, 'Making Medicine Indigenous: Homoeopathy in South India', p. 318.
200 Ajoy Kumar Ghosh, 'A Short History of the Development of Homoeopathy in India', pp. 131–2.
201 Report of the Homoeopathic Enquiry Committee, Ministry of Health, Government of India, 1949, p. 1.

a national context.[202] Their long involvement in homoeopathic pharmaceutical commerce was acknowledged by the committee and their opinion was considered crucial in deciding the future state policy. Such was the reputation of these firms that the 1892 homoeopathic pharmacopoeia published by M. Bhattacharya and Company remained, unofficially, the standard Indian homoeopathic pharmacopoeia right up to the 1970s. It was only in 1971 that the Ministry of Health and Family Welfare began publishing an official multivolume Indian homoeopathic pharmacopoeia.[203]

Finally, the twin processes of toleration and regularisation of non-allopathic medicine, set in motion since the 1920s, are useful for reflecting on the nature of state power in these crucial years of transition from a colonial to a nationalist state. The above discussion showcases an essential continuity between the late colonial state and the new post-colonial nation state in their attitude towards recognising alternative medicine. Just like the colonial state, the independent nation-state, too, upheld the unquestioned supremacy of biomedicine in framing its national policies. Yet, some alternative practices (ayurveda, unani and homoeopathy being the foremost) were tacitly recognised as indispensable for the national health agenda. Even while recognising their importance, the national policy vision marginalised these distinct knowledge epistemologies and disease theories as less-than-science. Besides, in being inclusive and tolerant, the state often left its indelible, powerful imprint on these practices. Through demands of standardisation, formal institutionalisation and purging, these practices were rendered 'acceptable' in the normative standards of the state that often modified their epistemological foundations. As the above account shows, twentieth-century state-acknowledged homoeopathy was more reliant on bacteriological understandings of the disease than ever before. The curriculum in general was more conversant with western auxiliary sciences of anatomy, physiology, pathology and others. Hence, the accommodative stance of the state often ensured discreetly greater degrees of state control and policing. This simultaneous recognition and vilification is resonant with the concept of 'casino capitalism' as deployed by anthropologist Vincanne Adams in her account of the post-colonial history of Tibetan medicine beyond Tibet.[204] Adams shows that the idea of casino capitalism helps explicate

[202] Report of the Homoeopathic Enquiry Committee, Ministry of Health, Government of India, 1949, pp. 34–5.

[203] Stefan Ecks, *Eating Drugs: Psychopharmaceutical Pluralism in India* (New York University Press, 2013), pp. 117–19.

[204] Vincene Adams, 'Randomized Controlled Crime: Postcolonial Sciences in Alternative Medicine Research', *Social Studies of Science*, 32, 5/6, 2002, pp. 659–90.

state action towards alternative medicine that at once criminalises/questions and legalises/recognises such practices. The Indian state, too, at once questioned and legalised homoeopathy, disapproved of its merits, yet standardised it and advocated its proliferation on grounds of contingency, economy and cultural familiarity.

Epilogue: A Familiar Science

What is 'vernacular medicine'? Homoeopathy was translated, domesticated, indigenised and, therefore, vernacularised in Bengal between the 1860s and 1941, when a State Faculty of Homoeopathy was formally established. 'Vernacular medicine' alludes to these multiple processes through which homoeopathy, a heterodox therapeutics with roots in eighteenth-century Germany, was reconfigured in nineteenth- and early twentieth-century Bengal. In the history of homoeopathy in colonial Bengal, the vernacular did not necessarily represent a distinct, preordained sphere. Instead, homoeopathic medicine, to a considerable extent, gave shape to its own vernacular field of operation. The vernacular realm of medicine around homoeopathy consisted of elite medical entrepreneurs, colonial state legislators, provincial politicians debating national health, self-taught physicians and countless domestic, lay practitioners in urban and suburban Bengal. Thus, vernacular homoeopathy was not exclusively a subaltern, nationalist or Bengali-language domain. Rather, as I have shown, it traversed the domains of the western and the indigenous, the elite and the popular, the subaltern and the state. To that extent, the vernacular was more of a product of the colonial encounter rather than an already existing category or domain. This book, therefore, problematises the received notions of the vernacular. While tracking homoeopathy's vernacularisation, it also reminds us of the myriad ways in which the 'vernacular' itself was put together in the colonial period. The interrelated history of the rise of family firms, works of biography, texts in translation, medical manuals and public health debates suggest that homoeopathy and a vernacular domain were co-consolidated.

This epilogue considers whether homoeopathy can be described as a 'familiar science' in colonial Bengal. More generally, it asks whether 'familiar science' could be a useful trope in analysing colonial homoeopathy, and indeed, colonial medicine in other settings. The phrase *familiar science* encapsulates various processes through which diverse medical genres were presented before a colonised audience. The credibility of different medical genres, ranging from biomedicine to ayurveda, was asserted with considerable reliance on the claim that they emanated from abstract scientific principles, and had roots in distant times or places. And yet, significant material and intellectual resources were invested in arguing that these medical genres were also compatible with the immediate experiences, cultural beliefs and economic means of the colonised.

Homoeopathy in colonial Bengal was advertised as part of an established European scientific tradition. David Arnold has drawn attention to homoeopathy's multifarious claims to being the most 'rational' form of medicine in the nineteenth century.[1] It was celebrated by many as rational and scientific since it relied on a universal law (the Law of Similars or 'like cures like'), which was seen as the product of protracted experiments with drugs and people.[2] Its eighteenth-century German roots, which could be traced back to its pioneer Samuel Christian Hahnemann of Saxony and his original text, *The Organon of the Art of Healing*, were repeatedly asserted. Along with Hahnemann, writings by other eminent European and American homoeopaths such as Constantine Hering, James Tyler Kent, Ernest Farrington and Von Bonninghausen were frequently invoked, discussed and translated in the Bengali print market. Further, the Bengali homoeopathic firms projected themselves as being entangled with the west through continuous transactions of drugs, people and pharmaceutical expertise. Contrasting it with western mainstream medicine, homoeopathy was often written about by its advocates in Bengal as a nineteenth-century medical innovation, as a radical, progressive and reformed western science. Yet, it was simultaneously projected as amenable to the everyday life and dominant moral imperatives of the Bengalis. The construction of this supposed familiarity of the Bengalis with homoeopathy acquired different forms.

It was argued that the cheapness and easy accessibility of homoeopathy made it widely popular in Bengal. The colonial health manuals regularly publicised the affordable price and the long-lasting nature of the homoeopathic drugs. It was pointed out that when compared with allopathy, the price of homoeopathic pills appeared to be negligible. A representative article discussing the cheapness of homoeopathy thus

[1] David Arnold and Sumit Sarkar, 'In Search of Rational Remedies: Homoeopathy in Nineteenth Century Bengal' in Waltraud Ernst (ed.), *Plural Medicine, Tradition and Modernity, 1800–2000* (London and New York: Routledge, 2002), p. 49.

[2] For a discussion on the scientific claims of homoeopathy in British Bengal, see Shinjini Das, 'Debating Scientific Medicine: Homoeopathy and Allopathy in Later Nineteenth-Century Medical Print in Bengal', *Medical History*, 56, 4 (2012), 463–80.

argued that 'although it costs a little to collect the plants and to prepare the drugs, yet so minute are the doses, each patient may be cured with as less as one paisa'.[3] Owing to the low prices both of drugs and homoeopathic manuals, it was reportedly 'as popular as almanacs in every Bengali home'.[4] Such impressions were so pervasive as to feed into the Bengal legislative assembly public health debates of the late 1930s.[5] Indeed, these provincial understandings eventually also reflected in the post-colonial national committees. Homoeopathy's cheapness and therefore its suitability for 'a poor agricultural country like India' was especially emphasised in the Homoeopathic Enquiry Committee's Report of 1948. This report formed the basis for the recommendations of the Constituent Assembly of 1948, which crucially shaped government policies on homoeopathy in post-colonial India.[6]

Its proponents in the province also claimed that the practice of homoeopathy did not necessarily require the intervention of an expert practitioner. Homoeopathy, it was argued, was intimately tied to the economic and corporeal needs and abilities of the people of Bengal, and therefore allowed literate householders to self-medicate. It was believed that once armed with relevant prescriptive medical manuals, and a box of different varieties of homoeopathic globules, literate Bengali householders could become self-reliant in protecting themselves from harmful diseases. This projected approachability of homoeopathy was bolstered further by the idea that homoeopathic pills suited Bengali taste. The sweetness of gentle sugar-coated homoeopathic drugs was contrasted with the tastelessness or the bitter taste of allopathic drugs.

Many authors in the Bengali medical print market suggested that certain core medical tenets of homoeopathy shared similarities with religious and philosophical notions prevalent in South Asia. The theory of minute doses was explained in terms of Indian philosophical thought about invisible immaterial spiritual forces such as Brahma or '*paramatma*'. Other essential homoeopathic tenets like 'vital force' were understood in relation to '*shakti*' or 'the cult of invisible female power', while Hahnemann himself was described as akin to figures such as Buddha and

[3] M. Chakrabarty, 'Homoeopahy Oushadh er Mulyo', *Hahnemann*, 5, 8 (1923), 419.

[4] ' Advertisement to the Fifth Edition', *Homoeopathic Paribarik Chikitsha (Homoeopathic Domestic Treatment)*, 5th edition (Calcutta: Mahesh Chandra Bhattacharya and Company, 1906).

[5] See *Bengal Legislative Assembly Proceedings*, Vol L. 1 (Number 3, 1937, Calcutta: Bengal Government Press), pp. 804–5 [WBSL]; and Shamshad Khan, 'Systems of Medicine and Nationalist Discourse in India: Towards "New Horizons" in Medical Anthropology and History', *Social Science and Medicine*, 62 (2006), 2791.

[6] Report of the Homoeopathic Enquiry Committee, *Ministry of Health*, Government of India (Delhi: Manager of Publications, 1949), pp. 2–3.

the Hindu Lord Siva. Homoeopathy was even conceptualised as '*amiya-patha*', a Sanskrit rendering of the name of the science as a potential route to immortality. These colonial associations of homoeopathy with South Asian spiritualism were so firmly entrenched that they often continued to have long afterlives deep into the twentieth century. The idea that Hahnemann was an incarnation of the monkey-god Hanumana features prominently in the encyclopaedic ode to Hanumana titled *Sri Sankat Mochan Hanuman Charit Manas* (*Life of Hanuman, Preventer of Crisis*), written on the model of the iconic sixteenth-century epic poem *Ramcharitmanas*, and published as late as in 1998.[7]

These varied claims of homoeopathy being an inexpensive, accessible, approachable, palatable and culturally amenable form of medicine converged to produce the notion that homoeopathy was, in fact, indigenous to South Asia. The preceding chapters have closely followed the *bhadralok* print discussions that discursively reshaped German homoeopathy as indigenous medicine over the late nineteenth to early twentieth centuries. Not only were similarities between homoeopathy and Indian philosophy elaborated upon, some authors went so far as to claim an ayurvedic origin for homoeopathy. It was argued that the main principle of homoeopathy was rooted in an ancient ayurvedic corpus which travelled west in the ancient times, and merely returned to India through British colonialism. Developments in Bengal's provincial politics in the 1930s and early 1940s also indicate a gradual bracketing of homoeopathy with the indigenous corpus through discussions of state legislation. Such a perception was further consolidated in national-level governmental discussions through the decades of the 1940s and 1950s. The major committees deliberating upon national health policies in post-colonial India (such as the Bhore and Chopra committees) identified ayurveda and unani as 'indigenous' or 'traditional' medicine, and often clubbed homoeopathy with them. The decisions taken on ayurveda and unani were made to bear on homoeopathy too. In its final summary recommendations the Bhore report stated, 'what we have said in regard to the indigenous systems applies to Homoeopathy also'.[8] The Dave Commission's report of 1956, which set out to regularise the education and teaching of indigenous medicine, also proclaimed, 'the present committee has been entrusted with the work of recommending the ways and methods and rules to bring about uniformity

[7] See Harvansh Lal Sundd, Sri Sankat Mochan Hanuman Charit Manas (Life of Hanuman, Preventer of Crisis) (Delhi: Aravali Books International, 1998), pp. 439–40.

[8] Dominik Wujastyk, 'The Evolution of Indian Government Policy on Ayurveda in the Twentieth Century' in Dagmar Wujastyck and Frederick Smith (eds.), *Modern and Global Ayurveda: Pluralism and Paradigms* (Albany: State University of New York Press, 2008), p. 57.

as regards legislation, medical education and practice of Vaidyas, Hakims and Homoeopaths'.[9] Even the Congress Health Minister Rajkumari Amrit Kaur's 1948 budget speech mentioned homoeopathy in the same breath as the other ostensibly indigenous or traditional practices. She held that '[t]he important thing for us to consider is in what condition the indigenous systems of medicine to-day are and what is necessary to make them a progressive scientific art ... Whatever in either the Ayurvedic or Unani systems of medicine or in homoeopathy stands the test of scientific scrutiny must and will be translated and synthesised in modern scientific medicine and added to the fund of world knowledge'.[10] In 1964, a composite Central Council Bill for ayurveda, unani and homoeopathy systems was introduced in parliament. It is therefore unsurprising that under Indira Gandhi in 1973, homoeopathy was proclaimed one of the national systems of medicine, and the Central Council of Homoeopathy was formed in 1974 around the same time as Central Councils were put together for regularising ayurveda and unani.[11] Today, along with ayurveda, unani, siddha, yoga and naturopathy, homoeopathy is considered to be one of the six forms of 'national medicine' governed by the Department of AYUSH (Ayurveda, Yoga and Naturopathy, Unani, Siddha and Homoeopathy). Experts commenting on policy developments in the post-colonial period, too, often regard homoeopathy as an 'Indian system of medicine'.[12]

Therefore, homoeopathy was constructed from the colonial period onwards in Bengal, if not in South Asia more generally, as simultaneously distant, abstract and exotic, on the one hand, and accessible, approachable and indigenous, on the other. These twin features of what I have described as 'familiar science' were not unique to colonial science and medicine. However, these features manifested with particular starkness in the colonial world, where medical genres established their dominance through multilingual, intercultural encounters occasioned by European imperial rule. Colonial science and medicine were, to a considerable extent, shaped by the incentives of the imperial rulers. However, recent scholarship has questioned the view that colonial science and medicine

[9] Ibid., p. 67.

[10] K. C. K. E. Raja, 'Developments in the Field of Health in India', *The British Medical Journal*, 1, 4650 (1950), 392.

[11] Ajoy Kumar Ghosh, 'A Short History of the Development of Homoeopathy in India', *Homeopathy*, 99, 2 (2010), 136; and Stefan Ecks, *Eating Drugs: Psychopharmaceutical Pluralism in India* (New York University Press, 2013), pp. 109–10.

[12] For instance, see the first footnote in Shamshad Khan, 'Systems of Medicine and Nationalist Discourse in India: Towards "New Horizons" in Medical Anthropology and History', p. 2787 and V. Sujatha, 'Medicine, State and Society', *Economic and Political Weekly*, 44, 16 (2009), 35–6.

were characterised by the unilateral imposition of imperial ideologies and interests on the colonised subjects. Rather, a distinct strand of research into colonial South Asia has examined the myriad negotiations undertaken by the colonised peoples themselves to come to terms with the advent of scientific modernity in the subcontinent. Gyan Prakash has dwelt on the idea that the domestication of 'western science' involved a process of historic translation through which the Indian peoples became familiarised with aspects of the sciences.[13] More recently, Projit Bihari Mukharji has illustrated the ways in which colonial state medicine was accessed, resisted and reconstituted in the emerging print culture in Bengal; while Ishita Pande's work has revealed the extent to which adaptation to western medicine was integral to shaping colonial modern subjectivities.[14] Srirupa Prasad has analysed how particular western biomedical notions such as 'hygiene' and 'contagion' were negotiated by the colonised peoples specifically in the realm of emotion and affect.[15]

The concept 'familiar science' extends this line of study by drawing attention in particular to the institution of family in histories of science and medicine. Indeed, the case of homoeopathy suggests that the concept of 'familiar science' should also open up, for more explicit analysis than these extant histories do, the role of familial institutions in the history of colonial medicine. I have closely tracked the interaction between homoeopathy and family between the 1860s and 1941 to explore the extent to which the two shaped one another. The concept of 'familiar science', therefore, inspires further investigations into the ways in which particular genres of medicine were deemed simultaneously familial and ubiquitous in the colonial context.

The use of the phrase 'familiar science' here is built especially upon recent scholarship that has attempted to foreground the role of family in histories of science and medicine. Deborah Coen's article 'The Common World: Histories of Science and Domestic Intimacy' reflects on the emerging historiographical literature at the intersection of the history of science and the history of family. Coen points out that at one level, historians of science have begun to consider the home as a key site for scientific research, during and even after what has been (somewhat controversially) termed the nineteenth-century laboratory

[13] Gyan Prakash, *Another Reason: Science and the Imagination of Modern India* (Princeton, NJ: Princeton University Press, 1999), pp. 6–7.
[14] Projit Bihari Mukharji, *Nationalising the Body: The Medical Market, Print and Daktari Medicine* (London and New York: Anthem Press, 2009); and I shita Pande, *Medicine, Race and Liberalism in British Bengal: Symptoms of Empire* (London and New York: Routledge, 2009).
[15] Srirupa Prasad, *Cultural Politics of Hygiene in India, 1890–1940: Contagions of Feeling* (New York: Palgrave Macmillan, 2015).

'revolution'.[16] But more importantly, she focuses on various other levels of conceptual enmesh between the two fields. She urges scholars to consider men of science as familial agents, and explores the imprint of familial ideologies and interests in their scholarly pursuits. Her work builds upon historians who have been evaluating the role of emotions and familial intimacies in the making of various scientific facts.[17] Likewise, Melanie Keene has recently focused on the importance of the two tropes of the 'familiar' (vocabularies and objects) and the 'familial' (the domestic space) in the popularisation of science in nineteenth-century Britain.[18] She proposes 'familiar science' as a corrective to the analytical category of 'popular science', which she states has become a 'disputed historical tool . . . yet few constructive new ways of mapping the landscape have been proposed'.[19] Of course, studies of 'popular science' have proliferated since the late 1980s, and have provided alternative models within the historiography of science and medicine for questioning the overwhelming scholarly emphasis on a few western expert discoverers and institutions.[20] Yet, the concept of 'popular science' itself has also come under critical scrutiny for being much too general and ambiguous as an analytical tool. It has been contended that the concept of 'popular' does not entirely do justice to the 'rich variety of activities, sites and experiences in the heterogeneous cultures of nineteenth-century sciences'.[21] Rather than being predicated on any simple professional-popular dyad, it is argued that newer histories of science should devise fresh vocabularies to specify the particular kinds and levels of social engagement with science or medicine. Keene's study brings together three interlocking components: the domestic space; the invocation of familiar language; and that of familiar objects, which helped create a new mass audience for science in the nineteenth century.[22] In his book-length study of medicine in post-colonial, post-Cold War Vietnam entitled *Familiar Medicine: Everyday Health Knowledge and Practice in Today's Vietnam*, David Craig too uses the framework of 'familiar medicine' to analyse everyday health regimen

[16] Deborah Coen, 'The Common World: Histories of Science and Domestic Intimacy', *Modern Intellectual History*, 11, 2 (2014), 420–1.
[17] Paul White, 'Darwin's Emotions: The Scientific Self and the Sentiment of Objectivity', *Isis*, 100, 4 (2009), 811–26, 812.
[18] Melanie Keene, 'Familiar Science in Nineteenth-Century Britain', *History of Science*, 52, 1 (2014), 53–71.
[19] Ibid., pp. 53–4.
[20] For a review of the historiography of popular science in history of science, see Bernard Lightman, *Victorian Popularisers of Science: Designing Nature for New Audiences* (Chicago: University of Chicago Press, 2007), pp. 13–16.
[21] Melanie Keene, 'Familiar Science in Nineteenth-Century Britain', pp. 54–5.
[22] Ibid., pp. 53–71.

and drug consumption in Vietnam.[23] He shows that with the opening up of markets and the free inflow of western drugs into contemporary Vietnam, household drug choice is being heavily guided by the notion of familiarity. Traditional and family-inherited knowledge about healing is being garnered to repackage the multitude of available western therapeutic options.

While several studies on colonial medicine have examined the multifaceted transaction of medico-scientific ideas between Europe and India, they have only rarely considered the fundamental location of families within these historical processes. My use of the expression 'familiar science' does not only encapsulate the processes through which colonised subjects in provincial India established intimacies with seemingly distant science and medicine. It also emphasises the significance of familial agency to the ways in which medical genres were translated and adapted in colonial India. Drawing on these insights, I have explored the entangled constructions of homoeopathic medicine, families and the everyday in colonial Bengal.

In developing this project, my work responds to recent calls to dismantle any notion of the family as a rigid or unchanging phenomenon. In an agenda-setting work, Indrani Chatterjee has pointed out that the most imminent task facing historians engaged in writing new histories of the South Asian family is to make the institution unfamiliar, 'to get rid of our all-too-known familiarity of the here-and-now'.[24] As I have discussed earlier in this book, several scholars have recently drawn our attention to the evolving and flexible nature of the family as an institution in South Asia throughout the colonial period. They have studied the colonial family from the vantage points of law, labour, sexuality, marriage and governance.[25] Some among them have focused on the production of family as an

[23] David Craig, *Familiar Medicine: Everyday Health Knowledge and Practice in Today's Vietnam* (Honolulu: University of Hawaii Press, 2002).

[24] Indrani Chatterjee, *Unfamiliar Relations: Family and History in South Asia* (New Brunswick: Rutgers University Press, 2004), pp. 5–7.

[25] Indrani Chatterjee, 'Gossip, Taboo and Writing Family History', in Indrani Chatterjee (ed.) *Unfamiliar Relations*, pp. 222–60; Durba Ghosh, *Sex and the Family in Colonial India: The Making of Empire* (Cambridge: Cambridge University Press, 2006); Swapna Banerjee, *Men, Women and Domestics: Articulating Middle-Class Identity in Colonial India* (Delhi and New York: *Oxford University Press*, 2006); Rachel Sturman, *Government of Social Life in Colonial India: Liberalism, Religious Law and Women's Rights* (Cambridge: Cambridge University Press, 2012); Eleanor Newbigin, *The Hindu Family and the Emergence of Modern India: Law, Citizenship and Community* (Cambridge: Cambridge University Press, 2013; and Leigh Denault, 'Partition and the Politics of the Joint Family in Nineteenth-Century North India', *Indian Economic and Social History Review*, 46, 1 (2009), 27–55.

economic unit.[26] Together they illustrate how the institution of family, rather than being an unchanging bedrock of values or emotions, is deeply implicated in histories of capitalism, patriarchy and political power.

Vernacular Medicine in Colonial India has examined the interactions between family and homoeopathy in various interrelated registers. The book has shown that the history of colonial homoeopathy in Bengal cannot be accounted for without engaging with the history of colonial family. Indeed, the history of Bengali homoeopathy was shaped considerably by physicians who claimed to represent families that practised homoeopathy over generations. Between fathers, sons and often grandchildren, these families continued to specialise in homoeopathy almost as a matter of cherished family lineage. Furthermore, these intergenerational kinship networks quite often organised themselves into family firms, business partnerships and enterprises. These family firms were the most significant producers of homoeopathic knowledge, publications and drugs in Bengal. This recurrent pattern chimes in with recent work in the history of science that contends that, during the nineteenth century, 'family partnerships became a model of organization not only for capitalist enterprises but also for newly emerging intellectual professions'.[27] Not only were these homoeopathic firms owned mostly by intergenerational physician-entrepreneurs, but their business operations were also predicated upon the rhetoric of family. Thus, along with filial and patrilineal business ownerships, an overwhelming rhetoric of familial paternalism thrived in the way these firms functioned. From caste and kinship-based recruitment patterns to envisioning the firm as an extended family, the idea of family animated the organisation of a range of homoeopathic firms both materially and metaphorically.

The processes of biography writing, translation and domestication, often initiated by family firms, made homoeopathy resonate with symbols and ideas that were ostensibly more recognisable to the Indians, such as the ayurvedic corpus, religio-spiritual motifs and regional languages. To that extent, familial ideologies, institutions, identities and metaphors shaped the ways in which homoeopathy familiarised itself in Bengal. Besides, Bengali homoeopathic discourse upheld an ideological mandate for making households self-sufficient in terms of health and economy by empowering the *grihasthas* (householders) and *grihinis* (lady of the house). An overwhelming number of health manuals contained words such as

[26] Ritu Birla, *Stages of Capital: Law, Culture and Market Governance in Late Colonial India* (Durham: Duke University Press, 2009).
[27] Deborah Coen, 'The Common World: Histories of Science and Domestic Intimacy', p. 420.

'garhasthya'/*'griha'* (household), 'domestic', 'home' and 'family' in their titles. This illustrates that families were the main target readership of these manuals, rather than individuals or the public at large. The manuals adopted specific pedagogic techniques for home-based medical education, invoking familial contexts and idioms.[28] The didactic dialogue form adopted in many manuals involved conversation between family members (especially between a mother-in-law and the daughter-in-law), or between the physician and the householder.[29] This often revealed tropes of a peculiarly home-centric medical education that addressed the everyday anxieties of colonial family. Besides, Bengali texts asserted homoeopathy's supposed indigenous character and affordability to recommend it as an instrument of national self-reliance. In this context, Bengali domesticity and families were idealised as the most appropriate site for the consumption (and even production) of homoeopathy. Homoeopathy was projected in these texts not just as a medical genre but also as an ethical way of living, befitting a healthy emergent nation. The homoeopathic disciplining of the Bengali home, with its insistence on indigenous consumption, self-reliance and economic frugality, exemplifies Gyan Prakash's observation on how, during the interwar period, nationalist politics 'subverted colonial governmentality and pursued its own programme of welfare of the population'.[30]

Vernacular Medicine in Colonial India has therefore argued that historicising the Bengali family is essential in order to analyse the reconfiguration of homoeopathy as a 'familiar science' in colonial Bengal. Seen through the lens of homoeopathy as a 'familiar science', the colonial Bengali family appears to be both a historical agent and a site of reform; a patrilineal unit of legitimate reproduction as well as a discursive product of nationalist ideological imagination; a site for the production of medical knowledge and pills, as well as a coveted market for a profit-making enterprise.

[28] Melanie Keene, 'Familiar Science in Nineteenth-Century Britain', p. 67.

[29] See, for example, Mahendranath Ghosh, *Soudaminir Dhatri Shikkha ebong Garbhini o Prashuti Chikitsha (Guidelines on Midwifery, Pregnancy and Reproductive Health Enunciated by Soudamini)* (Calcutta: Bharat Mihir Jontro, 1909). This text records a conversation between a fictional Calcutta-based female physician, Soudamini, and her maternal family members and some female neighbours in her native village. Also see Hemangini Ray Dastidar, *Grihinir Hitopodesh (Advice for the Wife)* (Srihatta: Karimganj Press, 1917), which is a text framed as a conversation between a newlywed wife and her mother-in-law.

[30] Gyan Prakash, *Another Reason*, pp. 156–8.

Bibliography

Unpublished Official Sources

West Bengal State Archives

Municipal Department, Medical Branch, September 1887–1913
Financial Department, Medical Branch, 1913–15
Local Self Government Department, Medical Branch Proceedings, Vol 1921–31

West Bengal Secretariat Library

Bengal Legislative Assembly Proceedings, Vol L. 1–L. VI (Alipur: Bengal Government Press, 1937–40).

Published Reports

Late Principle Bramley's Report, Report of the General Committee of Public Instruction of the Presidency of Fort William in Bengal for the year 1836 (Calcutta: Baptist Mission Press, 1837).

Report of the Homoeopathic Enquiry Committee, Ministry of Health, Government of India (Delhi: Manager of Publications, 1949).

Contemporary English Periodicals/Journals

Calcutta Journal of Medicine, 1868–1913
Calcutta Review, 1852
Home and Homoeopathy, 1931–38
Indian Homoeopathic Review, 1882–1912
Indian Medical Gazette, 1878–1910
The Hahnemannian Gleanings, 1930–42
The Lancet, 1861–88
The Medical Reporter, 1895–1900

Contemporary Bengali Periodicals/Journals

Antahpur, 1899–1904
Bangamahila, 1875–82
Banik, 1930
Bhishak Darpan, 1911
Bigyan, 1913
Chikitsha Sammilani, 1884–1900
Chikitsha Sammilani New Series, 1911–21
Chikitshak, 1923–26
Chikitshak o Samalochak, 1895
Grihastha, 1913–
Grihasthali, 1884–
Grihasthamangal, 1927–37
Hahnemann, 1883–1910?
Hahnemann, 1918–43
Homoeopathy Paricharak, 1927–28
Homoeopathy Pracharak, 1926–30
Krishak, 1910
Mahila, 1896–1905
Mashik Basumati, 1944–50
Svasthya, 1897–1900

Primary Sources in English

'An Address: Presented to Hon'ble Mr. Tamizuddin Khan, Minister Public Health, Bengal Government', *The Hahnemannian Gleanings*, 10 (May 1939), 213.

Anonymous Correspondent, 'India', *The Lancet*, 131, 3365 (25 February 1888), 399–400.

Anonymous, 'Homoeopathy and the University of Calcutta', *Indian Medical Gazette*, 13 (June 1878), 159.

Anonymous, 'Letter to the Editor, Correspondence: The Indian Systems of Medicine', *The Medical Reporter*, VI (16 August 1895), 125.

Anonymous, 'Letter to the Editor: Sir Benjamin Benjamin Brodie on Homoeopathy', *The Lancet*, 7, 1984 (7 September 1861), 238–9.

Bhattacharya, Benoytosh, *The Science of Tridosha* (Calcutta: Firma K. L. Mukhopadhyay, 1975 [1951]).

Borland, Douglas M., 'Homoeopathy and the Infant', *The Hahnemannian Gleanings*, 5 (1934), 80–1.

Choudhury, N. M., 'Organisation of Homoeopathy and Its Improvement', *Home and Homoeopathy* (May 1931), 445.

Choudhury, N. M., 'Second Andhra Homoeopathic Conference Presidential Address', *The Hahnemannian Gleanings*, 5 (February 1934), 42.

Chowdhury, J. N., 'Recognition, a Blessing or a Curse', *The Hahnemannian Gleanings*, 1, 5 (June 1930), 208–9.

Das, S. K., 'Editorial Notes and Comments', *The Hahnemannian Gleanings*, 5 (August 1934), 332–3.

Dutta, R. C., *The Economic History of British India* (London: Kegan Paul, 1902).

'Editorial: Calcutta Homoeopathic Hospital', *Indian Homoeopathic Review*, 19, 6 (June 1910), 102.

'Editorial: Calcutta Homoeopathic Society', *Indian Homoeopathic Review*, 19, 11 (November 1910), 321–2.

'Editorial: Dr. A. N. Mukherjee M. D. and Ourselves', *The Hahnemannian Gleanings*, 3 (June 1932), 235.

'Editorial: Fate of the Homoeopathic Faculty Bill', *The Hahnemannian Gleanings*, 9 (October 1938), 502–3.

'Editorial', *Homeopathy Paricharak*, 1, 4 (July 1927), 226–7.

'Editorial', *Indian Homoeopathic Review*, 15, 1 (January 1906), 1.

'Editorial: New Year's Retrospection and Introspection', *The Hahnemannian Gleanings*, 4, 1 (February 1933), 4–11.

'Editorial: News about the Advisory Committee of the State Homoeopathic Faculty of Bengal', *The Hahnemannian Gleanings*, 11 (July 1940), 334.

'Editorial Notes and Comments', *The Hahnemannian Gleanings*, 3, 6 (June 1932), 236.

'Editorial Notes and Comments', *The Hahnemannian Gleanings*, 5 (March 1934), 91–2.

'Editorial Notes and News: Reminiscences of Old Torch-bearers of Homoeopathy in India', *The Hahnemannian Gleanings*, 9 (June 1939), 266–7.

'Editorial: Our Creed', *Calcutta Journal of Medicine*, 1, 1 (1868), 190–1.

'Editorial: Reception of the Hon'ble Mr. A. K. Fazlul Huq Chief Minister of Bengal by the Members of the South Calcutta Homoeopathic Association', *The Hahnemannian Gleanings*, 10 (May 1939), 217–23.

Freebome, J. H., 'Talks about Homoeopathy', *The Hahnemannian Gleanings*, 3 (December 1932), 515.

Gangadin, *European Guide and Medical Companion to India* (Westminster: Roxburghe Press, 1895).

'General Council and State Faculty of Homoeopathic Medicine in Bengal: Government Announcement', *The Hahnemannian Gleanings*, 12, 7 (August 1941), 237.

Ghatak, N., 'Homoeopathy – Past and Present – in India', *The Hahnemannian Gleanings*, 8 (December 1937), 506.

Ghatak, Nilmani, 'School of Medicine in India', *The Hahnemannian Gleanings*, 1, 8 (September 1930), 340.

Ghose, S. C., 'Homoeopathy and Its First Missionary in India', *The Hahnemannian Gleanings*, 3, 7 (August 1932), 289.

Ghose, S. C., 'Homoeopathy and Its First Missionary in India', *The Hahnemannian Gleanings*, 3, 8 (September 1932), 337.

Ghose, S. C., 'Homoeopathy and Its First Missionary in India', *The Hahnemannian Gleanings*, 3, 10 (November 1932), 449–450.

Ghose, S. C., *Life of Mahendralal Sircar*, 1st edition (Calcutta: Oriental Publishing Company, 1909).
Ghose S. C., *Life of Mahendralal Sircar*, 2nd edition (Calcutta: Hahnemann Publishing Company, 1935).
Ghosh, Sarat Chandra, 'An Open Reply to the Letter Published by One Dr. H. Guha of Dacca on the Homoeopathic Bulletin of July 1932', *The Hahnemannian Gleanings*, 3 (September 1932), 365–77.
Ghosh, Sarat Chandra, *History of Homoeopathy in India* (Calcutta: International Institute of History of Homoeopathy, 1997 [1906]).
Goswami, S., 'Common Ailments of Women in Bengal and Their Causes', *Indian Homoeopathic Review*, 20, 1, (January 1911), 12.
Green, Julia Minnewa, 'Homoeopathy in the United States', *The Hahnemannian Gleanings*, 7, 10 (November 1936), 437–43.
'Homoeopathic News: A. N. Mukherjee and Calcutta Homoeopathic Hospital Society', *The Hahnemannian Gleanings*, 8 (February 1937), 49.
Hughes, Richard, 'On Translations of Hahnemannian Pathogenesis: With a Plea for a New English Version', *Calcutta Journal of Medicine*, 8, 5 and 6 (1876–77), 311–15.
Majumdar, Jitendranath, 'The International Homoeopathy Congress', *The Indian Homoeopathic Review*, 20, 9 (September 1911), 257–63.
Majumdar, J. N., 'State Recognition of Homoeopathy and Status of Homoeopaths in India', *The Hahnemannian Gleanings*, 7 (May 1936), 178.
Majumdar, J. N., 'The Sixth All India Homoeopathic Medical Conference', *The Hahnemannian Gleanings*, 9 (February 1938), 49–50.
Majumdar, J. N., 'The Sixth All India Homoeopathic Medical Conference', *The Hahnemannian Gleanings*, 9 (February 1938), 51.
McLeod, Kenneth, 'Medical Practice in Calcutta', *Indian Medical Gazette*, 17 (August 1882), 213–17.
Mitra, Rajendralal, *A Scheme for the Rendering of European Scientific Terms in India* (Calcutta: Thacker, Spink and Company, 1877).
Mukherjee, A. N., 'Hahnemann's Birthday Celebration', *The Hahnemannian Gleanings*, 7 (May 1936), 191.
Mukherjee, A. N., 'Progress of Homoeopathy in India', *The Hahnemannian Gleanings*, 8 (January 1937), 560.
Raja, K. C. K. E., 'Developments in the Field of Health in India', *The British Medical Journal*, 1, 4650 (1950), 392.
'Resolution Re Introduction of Homoeopathic Treatment in Government Hospitals and Recognition of Homoeopathic Colleges in India', *The Hahnemannian Gleanings*, 8 (August 1937), 301–11.
Robson, W., *Homoeopathy Expounded and Exposed: A Lecture Delivered in the Theatre of the Medical College, Calcutta March 20th, 1867* (Calcutta: Wyman Bros, 1867).
Roy, C., 'The Spiritual Power of Medicine Does Not Accomplish Its Object by Means of Quantity But by Potentiality and Quality', *The Hahnemannian Gleanings*, 1, 1 (February 1930), 59.
Roy, C., 'Etiology in Homoeopathy', *The Hahnemannian Gleanings*, 1, 1 (1930), 53–4.

Royal, George, 'World Progress in Homoeopathy', *The Hahnemannian Gleanings*, 3, 6 (June 1932), 213–18.

Salzer, Leopold, 'On the Necessity of Drug Proving in India', *Calcutta Journal of Medicine*, 2, 5 and 6 (May-June 1869), 177–8.

Salzer, Leopold, *Rational Practice of Medicine: A Lecture Delivered at the School of Arts, Jeypore* (Calcutta: Thacker and Spink, 1871).

Sircar, Amritalal, 'The Late Dr. Mahendralal Sircar, CIE, MD, DL', *Calcutta Journal of Medicine*, 23, 2 (February 1904), 45–66.

Sircar, Amritalal, *Obituary Notice of Dr. Mahendralal Sircar* (Kolkata: Anglo Sanskrit Press, 1905).

Sircar, Mahendralal, 'British Homoeopathic Congress of 1874', *Calcutta Journal of Medicine*, 7 (June–July 1874), 241.

Sircar, Mahendralal, 'Public Conference upon Homoeopathy: On the Reform of Hahnemann as the Basis of Positive Therapeutics', *Calcutta Journal of Medicine*, 1, 1 (January 1868), 14–15.

Sircar, Mahendralal 'Outdoor Homoeopathic Dispensary', *Calcutta Journal of Medicine*, 7, 1 and 2 (1874), 47–52.

Sircar, Mahendralal, 'Further Considerations on the Necessity for a Homoeopathic Hospital and Dispensary in Calcutta', *Calcutta Journal of Medicine*, 8, 2 (1876), 57–62.

Sircar, Mahendralal, 'Hahnemann and His Work', *Calcutta Journal of Medicine*, 12, 10 (May 1887), 391–416.

Sircar, Mahendralal, 'The Story of Dr. Sircar's Conversion to Homoeopathy', *Calcutta Journal of Medicine*, 21 (1902), 276.

Sircar, Amritalal, *Therapeutics of Plague*, 4th edition (Calcutta: Anglo-Sanskrit Press, 1913).

Sircar, Mahendralal, *On the Supposed Uncertainty in Medical Science and on the Relation between Diseases and Their Remedial Agents* (Calcutta: Anglo-Sanskrit Press, 1903 [1867]).

Skipwith, F. C., 'Homoeopathy and Its Introduction into India', *Calcutta Review*, 17 (1852), 19.

Sundd, Harvash Laal, *Sri Sankat Mochan Hanuman Charit Manas (Life of Hanuman, Preventer of Crisis)* (Delhi: Aravali Books International, 1998).

'The Bengal Homoeopathic Pharmacist's Association', *The Hahnemannian Gleanings*, 12 (October 1941), 454.

Wood, James C., 'Value and Limitations of Homoeopathy', *The Hahnemannian Gleanings*, 3 (December 1932), 501.

Primary Sources in Bengali

Abiar, Bidyabati Saraswati (ed.), *Griha Dharma* (*Religion of Domesticity*), 2nd edition (Calcutta: Hitabadi Press, 1910).

Anonymous (Translated from the English of Herbert A. Roberts), 'Jeebani Shakti' ('Vital Force'), *Hahnemann*, 20, 7 (1937), 362.

Anonymous Hindu Female, 'Mahilar Svasthya' ('Health of Women'), *Antahpur*, 6, 3, (1903), 57–61.

Anonymous, 'Amader Atmakahini' ('Our Autobiography'), *Hahnemann*, 9, 7 (1926), 370–6.
Anonymous, 'Atma Nirbharata' ('Self-Sufficiency'), *Svasthya*, 3, 7 (1899), 204–5.
Anonymous, 'Bange Ekannabarti Paribar' ('Joint Family in Bengal'), *Grihasthali*, 1, 4 (1884), 94–6.
Anonymous, 'Bharat Mahilar Svasthya' ('Health of Women in India'), *Antahpur*, 4, 7 (1901), 149–51.
Anonymous, 'Bhishak Kalima Udghaton' ('Exposing a Fraud Physician'), *Hahnemann*, 8, 7 (1925), 359.
Anonymous, 'Deshiya Dhatri' ('Indigenous Midwife'), *Hahnemann*, 2, 9 (1884), 161–3.
Anonymous, 'Homoeopathy Chikitshak' ('Homoeopathic Physician'), *Hahnemann*, 9, 6 (1926), 318.
Anonymous, 'Jvar Tattva O Shishur Akal Mrittyu' ('Theories of Fever and Untimely Deaths of Children'), *Hahnemann*, 4, 5 (1921), 161–213.
Anonymous, 'Letter to the Editor: Alochona' ('Discussion'), *Hahnemann*, 8, 5 (1925), 234–8.
Anonymous, 'Letter to the Editor', *Chikitsha Sammilani*, 5 (1888), 98.
Anonymous, 'Letter to the Editor', *Svasthya*, 4, 8 (1900), 238.
Anonymous, 'Madyapan Jonito Rog' ('Diseases Relating to Drinking Alcohol'), *Chikitsha Sammilani*, 4 (1887), 26–8.
Anonymous, 'Paralok e Dr. Baridbaran Mukhopadhyay' ('Late Dr. Baridbaran Mukhopadhyay'), *Hahnemann*, 23, 7 (1940), 428.
Anonymous, 'Presidential Address at the Annual Meeting of the Midnapore Hahnemann Association', *Hahnemann*, 10, 2 (1927), 65–6.
Anonymous, 'Shok- Sangbad' ('Sad News'), *Hahnemann*, 5, 7 (1922), 383.
Anonymous, 'Stree Chikitshak' ('Women Physician'), *Hahnemann*, 1, 4 (1883), 49–52.
Anonymous, 'Sukhi Paribar' ('Happy Family'), *Mahila*, 9, 8 (March 1907), 207.
Anonymous, 'Upodangsho o Bibaho' ('Syphilis and Marriage'), *Hahnemann*, 3, 1 (1885), 26.
Anonymous, *Daktarbabu (The Physician)* (Calcutta: Jogendra Ghosh, 1875).
Anonymous, *Homoeopathic Paribarik Chikitsha (Homoeopathic Domestic Treatment)*, 5th edition (Calcutta: M. Bhattacharya and Company, 1906).
Anonymous, *Homoeopathy Mowt e Adorsho Griha Chikitsha (The Ideal Domestic Treatment according to the Homoeopathic Method)* (Calcutta: The Standard Homoeopathic Pharmacy, 1914).
Bandopadhyay, Bhupendranath, 'Smriti Sabha' ('Memorial Meeting'), *Hahnemann*, 9, 1 (1926), 34.
Bandopadhyay, Chintaharan, 'Homoeopathy Shebir Asha o Nirasha' ('The Anxieties of a Servant of Homoeopathy'), *Homoeopathy Paricharak*, 2, 8 (November 1928), 296–303.
Bandopadhyay, Raimohan, *Homoeopathic Griha Chikitshak (Homoeopathic Family Physician)* (Calcutta: Gurudas Chattopadhyay and Sons, 1926).
Bandopadhyay, Saradindu, '*Satvanneshi*' *(The Searcher of Truth)*, Byomkesh *Omnibus*, Vol I (Calcutta: Ananda Publishers, 1932/2000), pp. 13–32.

Bandopadhyay, Tarashankar, 'Srinath Daktar', *Tarashankar er Galpaguchha* (Kolkata: Sahitya Samsad, 1934/1990), pp. 373–83.

Banerjee, J. C., 'Howrah Zilla Homoeopathy Sammelan ('Homoeopathy Conference for the District of Howrah'), *Hahnemann*, 23, 4 (1940), 363.

Basu, Amritalal, *Amrita Madira (The Intoxicating Elixir)* (Calcutta, 1903).

Basu, Bijoya Kumar, 'Jouna Samasya Samadhan er Ingit' ('Hint towards Solving Sexual Problems'), *Hahnemann*, 22, 1 (1939), 26.

Basu, K. N., 'Homoeopathic Upadhi Samasya' ('Problem of Homoeopathic Degrees'), *Hahnemann*, 9, 10 (1926), 547.

Basu, Khagendranath, 'Palligram e Homoeopathy O Tar Durobastha' ('Deplorable Condition of Homoeopathy in the Villages'), *Homoeopathy Paricharak*, 1, 3 (June 1927), 164–6.

Basu, Narayan Chandra, *Shishu Rog Samhita (Compendium of Children's Disease)* (Calcutta: Sadhana Library, 1922).

Benimadhab Dey and Company Almanac (Calcutta: Benimadhab Dey and Company, 1896–97).

Bhaduri, Biharilal, *Homoeopathic Bhaishajjya Tattwa (Homoeopathic Materia Medica)* (Calcutta: Harachandra Das, 1878).

Bhaduri, Biharilal, *Homoeopathic Chikitsha Bigyan (Homoeopathic Medical Science)* (Calcutta: Saraswat Jantra, 1874).

Bhattacharjee, M. N., *Contributions towards a Knowledge of the Peculiarities of all Homoeopathic Medicines* (Hooghli: Mahendranath Bhattacharya, 1921).

Bhattacharya, Kalikumar, 'Ashar Alok' ('Light of Hope') *Hahnemann*, 7, 2 (1924), 80.

Bhattacharya, Kalikumar, 'Atista Indica Proving er Itibritta' ('Account of Proving Atista Indica'), *Hahnemann*, 4, 9 (1921), 323.

Bhattacharya, Kalikumar, 'Bacteriar Shohit Rog er Ki Sombondho' ('What Is the Relation between Bacteria and Disease'), *Homoeopathy Paricharak*, 2, 12 (March 1929), 463–9.

Bhattacharya, Kalikumar, 'Letter to the Editor: Alochonar Prattyuttor' ('Reply to Discussion'), *Hahnemann*, 8, 5 (1925), 239–48.

Bhattacharya, Kalikumar, 'Prabhu Hahnemann er Proti' ('To Hahnemann, the Divine'), *Hahnemann*, 8, 5 (1925), 1.

Bhattacharya, Kalikumar, 'Samasya o Pratikar' ('Problem and Its Solution'), *Hahnemann*, 7, 1 (1924), 51.

Bhattacharya, Kamal Krishna, 'Homoeopathy Bonam Allopathy O Onyanyo Chikitsha Pronali' ('Homoeopathy vs. Allopathy and Other Medical Systems'), *Hahnemann*, 23, 6 (1940), 345.

Bhattacharya, Krishnahari, *Homoeopaty Mowt e Stree Rog Chikithsa (Treatment of Female Diseases According to Homoeopathy)* (Calcutta: Medical Library, 1886).

Bhattacharya, Mahesh Chandra, *Atmacharit (My Life)*, 4th edition (Calcutta: Economic Press, 1957).

Bhattacharya, Mahesh Chandra, *Bheshaja Bidhan (Pharmaceutical Prescription)*, 5th edition (Calcutta: M. Bhattacharya and Company, 1920).

Bhattacharya, Mahesh Chandra, *Byabshayee (Businessman)*, 1st edition (Calcutta: M. Bhattacharya and Company, 1905 [4th edition, 1921]).

Biswas, Pramada Prasanna, 'Deshiya Oushadh Sambondhe Aboshyokiyo Kotoguli Kotha' ('A Few Useful Words on the Indigenous Drugs'), *Hahnemann*, 8, 7 (1925), 372.

Biswas, Pramada Prasanna, 'Homeopathic Bhaishajya Tattwer Bishesattva o Sustho Manob Dehe Oushadh er Porikkha' ('Peculiarity of the Homoeopathic Materia Medica and Proving Drugs on Healthy Human Bodies'), *Hahnemann*, 6, 10 (1923), 100.

Biswas, Pramada Prasanna, 'Letter to the Editor', *Hahnemann*, 7, 7 (1924), 332.

Biswas, Pramada Prasanna, *Bharat Bhaishajya Tattva: Materia Medica of Indian Drugs* (Pabna: Hahnemann Medical Mission, 1924).

Biswas, R., 'Homoeopathy Balika School' ('Homoeopathic Girls' School'), *Hahnemann*, 22, 7 (1939), 414–15.

Biswas, R., 'Homoeopathy Mowt e Jounabyadhi Chikitshar Ingit' ('Hints towards Curing Sexual Ills with Homoeopathy'), *Hahnemann*, 21, 10 (1938), 613.

Biswas, Radharaman, 'Deboddeshe' ('To the Almighty'), *Hahnemann*, 23, 1 (1940), 19.

Boral, Sripati Chandra, 'Protibaad' ('Protest'), *Hahnemann*, 3, 4 (1920), 169–73.

Chakrabarti, Hariprasad, *Homoeopathic Bhaishajya Tattwa Chikitsha Pradarshika (Guide to the Materia Medica of Homoeopathic Treatment)* (Calcutta: Chikitsha Tattwa Jontro, 1902).

Chakrabarti, Lalmohan, *Paribarik Chikitshay Grihini (Role of the Wife in Domestic Treatment)* (India: Dhaka Shakti Press, 1925).

Chakrabarti, M., 'Rog o Pashchatya Sabhyata' ('Disease and Western Civilisation'), *Hahnemann*, 3, 6 (1920), 217.

Chakrabarti, Manmathanath, *Thakurma (Grandmother)* (Calcutta: Indian Art School, 1912).

Chakrabarty, M., 'Homoeopahy Oushadh er Mulyo' ('Price of Homoeopathic Drugs'), *Hahnemann*, 5, 8 (1923), 419.

Chakrabarty, Tarak Das, 'Homoeopathy aj Kon poth e?' ('What Is the Future of Homoeopathy'), *Hahnemann*, 23, 11 (1940), 692.

Chandra, Amulya Kumar, 'Government O Homoeopathy', *Hahnemann*, 7, 3 (1924), 142.

Chandra, Amulya Kumar, 'Patra' ('Letter'), *Hahnemann*, 9, 10 (1926), 543–5.

Chatterjee, Haricharan, *Oushudh Nirbachan Bigyan: The Practical Materia Medica of Homoeopathic Treatment* (Dacca: Popular Library Patuatoli, 1911).

Chatterjee, K., 'Bharate Kromo Somosya' ('The Problem of Potency in India'), *Hahnemann*, 8, 5 (1925), 406.

Chatterjee, Prabal Chandra, 'Gharer Dheki' ('Internal Problems'), *Hahnemann*, 6, 3 (1923), 121.

Chattopadhyay, Abhaypada, 'Chikitsha Jogote Homoeopathy' ('Homoeopathy in the Medical World'), *Chikitshak*, 4 (1926), 38–9.

Chattopadhyay, Khetranath, *Homoeopathic Griha Chikitsha (Homoeopathic Domestic Treatment)*, 1st edition (Calcutta: People's Press, 1887).

Chattopadhyay, Sarat Chandra, 'Bamun er Meye' ('Daughter of Brahmin'), *Sarat Sahitya Samagra*, Vol I (Kolkata: Ananda Publishers, 1920/1986), pp. 979–1013.

Chattopadhyay, Sashi Bhushan, 'Prokrito o Adorsho Homoeopath o Homoeopathy' ('Real and Ideal Homoeopaths and Homoeopathy'), *Homoeopathy Paricharak*, 2, 6 (September 1928), 243–4.

Choudhury, Basanta Kumar, 'Baje Kharach' ('Bad Expenditure'), *Grihasthamangal*, 5, 2–3 (1931), 35.

Das, Dharmadas, 'Jigashya' ('Question'), *Hahnemann*, 21, 10 (1938), 545.

Dasgupta, Bipin Bihari, *Homoeopathy Mowt e Manashik Rog Chikitsha (Homoeopathic Treatment of Mental Illness)* (Murshidabad: Kanika Press, 1904).

Dasgupta, Surajit, *Rog o Arogyo (Disease and Recovery)* (Mymensingh: Surajit Dasgupta, 1925).

Datta, Basanta Kumar, 'Homoeopathic Bangla Sahitya' ('Homoeopathic Bengali Literature'), *Hahnemann*, 2, 10 (1884), 181–3.

Datta, Basanta Kumar, 'Homoeopathic Bangla Sahitya', ('Homoeopathic Bengali Literature') *Hahnemann*, 2, 11 (1884), 202.

Datta, Basanta Kumar, 'Homoeopathic Bangla Sahitya' ('Homoeopathic Bengali Literature'), *Hahnemann*, 2, 12 (1884), 222.

De, Ajit Shankar, 'Shantir Shandhan' ('In Search of Peace'), *Homoeopathy Pracharak*, 2, 1 (April 1928), 42–5.

Devi, Nirupama, 'Ekannabhukta Paribar er Ashanti Nibaran er Upay Ki?' ('What Are the Ways to Pacify the Problems in a Joint Family?'), *Antahpur*, 6, 9 (January 1904), 197.

Dey, Keshablal, 'Protibaad' ('Protest'), *Hahnemann*, 5, 10 (1922), 514–15.

Dey, Manomohan, 'Patra' ('Letter'), *Hahnemann*, 8, 11 (1925), 601–4.

Dey, S. C., 'Homoeopathy Mowt e Oushadh Porikkha' ('Drug Testing According to Homoeopathy'), *Hahnemann*, 21, 5 (1938), 272.

Dirghangi, G., 'Bharatbarshe Homeopathy' ('Homoeopathy in India'), *Hahnemann*, 3, 11 (1920), 401.

Dirghangi, G., 'Homoeopathic College', *Hahnemann*, 1, 10 (1918), 308.

Dirghangi, G., 'Homoeopathy Parikkha Samiti' ('Homoeopathic Examination Committee'), *Hahnemann*, 4, 12 (1921), 451–9.

Dirghangi, G., 'Oushadh er Shakti Tattva' ('Theories Relating to the Potency of Drugs'), *Hahnemann*, 3, 8 (1920), 297.

Dirghangi, G., 'Upadhir Byabsha' ('Degree Trade'), *Hahnemann*, 5, 11 (1922), 553–4.

Dutta, Basanta Kumar (ed.), *Datta's Homoeopathic Series in Bengalee*, 1876 (monthly publication).

Dutta, Sarat Chandra, *Primary Guide to Homoeopathy or Companion to the Family Medical Chest* (Calcutta: Homoeopathic Medical Hall, 1899).

'Editorial: Hahnemann er Borsho Bridhhi' ('Growth of Hahnemann over the Years'), *Hahnemann*, 3, 1 (Baishakh 1885), 4.

'Editorial', *Hahenmann*, 6, 7 (1923), 290.

'Editorial: Homoeopathy Chikitshak er Shasti' ('Punishment of a Homoeopathic Physician'), *Homoeopathy Paricharak*, 2, 5 (August 1928), 185.

'Editorial: 'Homoeopathy r Dheki' ('Problems of Homoeopathy'), *Homoeopathy Pracharak*, 3, 9 (December 1929), 316–21.

'Editorial: Bharat Government Homoeopathic Chikitsha Podhhoti Sombandhe Onumodan' ('Government Acknowledges the Homoeopathic Mode of Treatment'), *Hahnemann*, 20, 1 (1937), 3–4.
'Editorial: Homoeopathic Faculty Bill, 1937', *Hahnemann*, 20, 4 (1937), 210.
'Editorial: Homoeopathic Faculty Bill, 1937', *Hahnemann*, 20, 5 (1937), 269.
'Editorial: Bangiya Byabastha Parishad e Homoeopathy Faculty Bill Prabartan er Sothik Sangbad' ('The Accurate Account of the Introduction of the Homoeopathic Faculty Bill at the Bengal Assembly'), *Hahnemann*, 20, 6 (1937), 320.
'Editorial: Nikhil Bharat Homoeopathy Sammelan' ('All India Homoeopathic Conference'), *Hahnemann*, 20, 10 (1937), 537.
'Editorial: Khulna Jela Homoeopathic Sammelan' ('Homoeopathic Conference at the Distirict of Khulna'), *Hahnemann*, 20, 12 (1937), 661.
'Editorial: Manoniyo Pradhan Mantri Fazlul Haq er Sambardhana' ('Felicitation of Fazlul Haq, the Honourable Chief Minister'), *Hahnemann*, 22, 1 (1939), 3–5.
'Editorial: Bengal Homoeopathic Faculty Sombondhe Sothik Sangbad' ('The Accurate Account of the Introduction of the Homoeopathic Faculty Bill at the Bengal Assembly'), *Hahnemann*, 23, 2 (1939), 113.
'Editorial: Daktar Rajendralal Dutta Sambandhe Homoeopathic Samachar er Uktir Uttor' ('Reply to the Remark on Dr. Rajendralal Dutta by Homoeopathic Samachar'), *Hahnemann*, 22, 3 (1939), 181–3.
'Editorial: Homoeopathic State Faculty Songothon' ('Formation of the Homoeopathic State Faculty'), *Hahnemann*, 23, 9 (1939).
'Editorial: Rog, Doridrota o Oshikkhar Birudhhe Bengal Government er Procheshta' ('The Efforts of Bengal Government in Combating Disease, Poverty and Illiteracy'), *Hahnemann*, 22, 9 (1939), 563.
'Editorial', *Hahnemann*, 21, 7 (1938), 422–23.
Editors, 'Mantabya' ('Comment'), *Hahnemann*, 3, 4 (1920), 173–7.
'Sangbad' ('News'), *Hahnemann*, 20, 1 (1937), 36–7.
Gangopadhyay, Manmatha Nath, 'Bisadrisa Chikitshay Sadrisa ba homoeo shabder Obantor proyog' ('Irrelevant Use of the Word Homoeo in Treatment of Dissimilars'), *Homoeopathy Paricharak*, 1, 1 (April 1927), 60–2.
Gangopadhyay, Yaminikanta, *Hahnemann's Nature of Chronic Diseases* (Dacca: Baikunthanath Press, 1933).
Ghatak, Nilmani, 'Allopathy r Moho' ('The Allure of Allopathy'), *Homoeopathy Paricharak*, 2, 5 (August 1928), 165–8.
Ghatak, Nilmani, 'Lok Shikkha' ('Lessons for People'), *Hahnemann*, 10, 6 (1927), 285.
Ghatak, Nilmani, 'Nijeder Kotha' ('Our Words'), *Hahnemann*, 5, 4 (1922), 184–8.
Ghatak, Nilmani, *Prachin Peerar Karon o Tahar Chikitsha (The Etiology and Treatment of Chronic Diseases)*, 10th edition (Calcutta: Sasadhar Printing works, 1927/1967).
Ghosh, Anilchandra, *Bigyane Bangali (Science and the Bengalis)* (Calcutta: Presidency Library, 1931).

Ghosh, Himangshushekhar, 'Hahnemann O Adhunik Bigyan' ('Hahnemann and Modern Science'), *Hahnemann*, 23, 1 (1940), 22–3.

Ghosh, Mahendranath, *Soudaminir Dhatri Shikkha ebong Garbhini o Prashuti Chikitsha (Guidelines on Midwifery, Pregnancy and Reproductive Health Enunciated by Soudamini)* (Calcutta: Bharat Mihir Jontro, 1909).

Ghosh, N. C., 'Homoeopathy Sombondhe Du ekti Kotha' ('A Few Words on Homoeopathy'), *Hahnemann*, 21, 7 (1938), 508.

Ghosh, N. C., 'Sahar o Mofussil Bashi der Pakkha hoite Homoeopathy o Ashikhita ba Ardha Shikhita Homoeopath Sombondhe Du ekti Kotha' ('From the Inhabitants of Towns and Mofussil a Few Words on the Illiterate or the Semi-Literate Homoeopaths'), *Hahnemann*, 21, 2 (1938), 75.

Ghosh, R. R., 'Organon ba Homoeopathy Bigyan' ('Organon or the Science of Homoeopathy'), *Hahnemann*, 1, 1 (1918), 11.

Ghosh, Sarat Chandra, 'Bharatbarshe Homoeopathic Chikitshar Sorboprothom Pothoprodorshok o Pracharak Dr. Rajendralal Dutta' ('The Pioneer Physician and Perpetrator of Homoeopathy in India'), *Hahnemann*, 22, 1 (1939), 14–23.

Ghosh, Sarat Chandra, 'Daktar Lokenath Maitra', *Hahenmann*, 22, 12 (1939), 309.

Ghosh, Sarat Chandra, 'Daktar Lokenath Maitra', *Hahnemann*, 22, 12 (1939), 708–10.

Ghosh, Sarat Chandra, 'Daktar Mahendralal Sircar er Jibon-katha', *Hahnemann*, 22, 2 (1939), 67, 77–9.

Ghosh, Sarat Chandra, 'Daktar Mahendralal Sircar er Jibon-katha', ('Life of Dr Mahendralal Sircar'), *Hahnemann*, 22, 3 (1939), 137–43.

Ghosh, Sarat Chandra, 'Dr. Akshay Kumar Datta L. M. S', *Hahnemann*, 23, 4 (1940), 199.

Ghosh, Sarat Chandra, 'Dr. Bamacharan Das L. M. S', *Hahnemann*, 23, 10 (1940), 580–1.

Ghosh, Sarat Chandra, 'Dr. Brajendranath Bandopadhyay M. D.', *Hahnemann*, 23, 3 (1940), 133.

Ghosh, Sarat Chandra, 'Kishorimohan Bandopadhyay', *Hahnemann*, 23, 12 (1940), 728–9.

Ghosh, Sarat Chandra, 'Dr. L. Salzer M. D', *Hahnemann*, 22, 6 (1939), 326–7.

Ghosh, Sarat Chandra, 'Dr. T. Berigny', *Hahnemann*, 22, 4 (1939), 198.

Ghosh, Surendra Mohan, *Susrut o Hahnemann (Susrut and Hahnemann)* (Calcutta: Bengal Medical Library, 1906).

Guha, S. N., 'Kaj er Kotha' ('Useful Words'), *Hahnemann*, 6, 10 (1923), 437.

Hui, Nilambar, 'Our Letter to the Publisher' in *Sadrisa Bigyan Sutra (Principles for the Science of Similars)* (Calcutta: Sanyal and Company, 1896).

Kali, C. S., *Homoeopathic Chikitsha Bidhan (Prescriptions of Homoeopathic Treatment)*, 13th edition (Calcutta: S. Kyle and Company, Vol II, 1928).

Kali, Chandra Shekhar, *Homoeopathic Practice of Medicine* (Calcutta: L. V. Mitra and Company, 1890).

Kali, Chandra Shekhar., *Brihat Olautha Samhita (Enlarged Compendium of Treatment of Cholera)*, 12th edition (Calcutta: C. Kylye and Company, 1926).

Kanjilal, Amaresh, *Byaktigata Arthaneeti (Personal Economics)* (Calcutta: Samyo Press, 1921).

Khatun, M. M., 'Homoeopathy r Abyartho Sandhan' ('The Guaranteed Cure of Homoeopathy'), *Hahnemann*, 20, 3 (1937), 158–60.

Laha, Satyacharan, *Homoeopathic Griha Chikitsha (Homoeopathic Domestic Treatment)* (Calcutta: Akhil Chandra Shil, 1914).

Lahiri, Jagadish Chandra, *Homoeopathy r Bipokkhe Apatti Khandan (Denouncing the Arguments Made Against Homoeopathy)* (Calcutta: Lahiri and Company, 1907).

Maitra, Bipin Bihari, *Diseases of Children and Its Homoeopathic Treatment* (Calcutta: Maitra and Company, 1887).

Maitra, Jnanendra Kumar, *Sachitra Rati Jantradi r Peera: Sexual and Venereal Ills and Evils* (Calcutta: Maitra and Sons, 1923 [Vols I and II bound together]).

Maity, H. P., 'Deshiya Beshaja o Tahar Shakti' ('Indigenous Vegetation and Its Power'), *Hahnemann*, 7, 4 (1924), 174.

Majumdar, P. C., *Oushadh Guna Sangraha: Outlines of Materia Medica and Therapeutics*, 6th edition (Calcutta: Indian Press, 1911).

Majumdar, J. N., 'Dr. Pratap Chandra Majumdar MD', *Hahnemann*, 23, 5 (1940), 261–7.

Majumdar, J. N., 'Dr. Pratap Chandra Majumdar MD', *Hahnemann*, 23, 6 (1940), 324–5.

Majumdar, J. N., 'Dr. Pratap Chandra Majumdar MD', *Hahnemann*, 23, 7 (1940), 453.

Majumdar, J. N., 'Dr. Pratap Chandra Majumdar MD', *Hahnemann*, 23, 8 (1940), 451–5.

Majumdar, Jitendranath, 'Dr. Pratapchandra Majumdar', *Hahnemann*, 22, 5 (1939), 260–7.

Majumdar, Jitendranath, *Arther Sandhan (Pursuit of Wealth)* (Calcutta: Sisir Publishing House, 1932).

Majumdar, Nalininath, 'Amiya Samhita' ('Collection of Principles Ensuring Immortality'), *Hahnemann*, 8, 4 (1925), 192–6. (Note: this article was published serially in *Hahnemann* through 1925 and 1926).

Majumdar, Nalininath, 'Baro Daktar Rahasya' ('Mystery about Big Doctors'), *Hahnemann*, 8 (1925), 427.

Majumdar, Nalininath, 'Homoeopathy r Bartaman Durabastha' ('The Present Predicament of Homoeopathy'), *Hahnemann*, 8, 12 (1925), 663.

Majumdar, Rajanikanta, 'Bheshaja Shatak' ('Compendium of Hundred Drugs'), *Grihasthamangal*, 1, [Ben: Baisakh-Chaitra] (1927), 17.

Mallik, Harikrishna, *Berigny and Company's Bengali Homoeopathic Series V: Sadrisa Byabostha Bajhyik Proyog (Drugs for External Use According to the System of Similars)* (Calcutta: Berigny and Company, 1870).

Mallik, Harikrishna, *Berigny and Company's Bengali Homoeopathic Series Number III: Sadrisa Byabastha Chiktsha Dipika (Glossary for Treatment According to the System of Similars)* (Calcutta: Berigny and Company, 1870).

Mallik, Harikrishna, *Berigny and Company's Bengali Homoeopathic Series Number II: Sadrisa Byabastha Jvar Chikitsha (Treatment of Fever According to the System of Similars)* (Calcutta: J. G. Chatterjee and Co's Press, 1871).

Mallik, Harikrishna, *Berigny and Company's Bengali Homoeopathic Series Number IV: Sadrisa Byabastha Chikitsha Dipika (Glossary for Treatment According to the System of Similars)* (Calcutta: Berigny and Company, 1870).

Mandal, Dharmadas, 'Homoeopath er Dak e Saara' ('Response to the Calls of a Homoeopath'), *Hahnemann*, 23, 5 (1940), 289.

Mukhati, H. N., *Pothyo Nirbachan (Selection of Diet)* (Dacca: 1925).

Mukhopadhyay, Rashbehari, 'Shworgiyo Raysaheb Dinabandhu Mukhopadhyay er Jiboni', *Hahnemann*, 4, 8 (1921), 276.

Mukhopadhyay, Bhudeb, *Paribarik Prabandha (Essays on Family)*, 3rd edition (Hooghly: Budhoday Jantra, 1889).

Mukhopadhyay, Gopal Chandra, *Sadhu Batakrishna Pal (The Saintly Batakrishna Pal)* (Calcutta: Batakrishna Pal, 1919 [Vols I and II bound together]).

Mukhopadhyay, Harendra Nath, 'Homoeopathic Chhatragan er Proti' ('To the Students of Homoeopathy'), *Hahnemann*, 21, 6 (1938), 347.

Mukhopadhyay, Piyari Mohan, 'Amar Deeghayu Labh er Karon' ('How I Attained my Long Life'), *Hahnemann*, 21, 7 (1938), 411–13.

Mukhopadhyay, Purnachandra, *Grihastha Darpan (Mirror of Domesticity)* (Calcutta: Basumati Sahityo Mandir, 1932).

Mukhopadhyay, Radhakamal, 'Madhyabitta Srenir Durobostha' ('Wretched Condition of the Middle Class') *Grihastha* [Ben: Ashadh] (1913), 573.

Mukhopadhyay, Rashbehari, 'Shworgiyo Raysaheb Dinabandhu Mukhopadhyay er Jiboni' ('Life of Late Honourable Rashbehari Mukhopadhyay'), *Hahnemann*, 4, 7 (1921), 147.

Mukhopadhyay, Rashbehari, 'Shworgiyo Raysaheb Dinabandhu Mukhopadhyay er Jiboni' ('Life of Late Honourable Rashbehari Mukhopadhyay'), *Hahnemann*, 4, 8 (1921), 293.

Mukhopadhyay, Shashibhushan, 'Baidya Chikitshak er Ashumparnata' ('Inadequacies of the Kavirajes'), *Chikitsha Sammilani*, 8 (1891), 269–72.

Nandi, Srish Chandra, *Monpyathy* (Kasimbazar: Publisher not cited, 1931).

Pal, Batakrishna, *Homoeopathic Mowt e Saral Griha Chikitsha (Simple Domestic Treatment According to Homoeopathy)*, 7th edition (Calcutta: Great Homoeopathic Hall, 1926).

Pal, LM, *Infantile Liver* (Calcutta: Hahnemann Publishing Company, 1935).

Pan, Gyanendra Mohan, 'Edesh e Homoeopathy Chikitshar Unnotir Ontoray Ki?' ('What Are the Hindrances to the Development of Homoeopathy in India?'), *Hahnemann*, 21, 10 (1938), 583–5.

Rakshita, Ambikacharan, *Homoeopathic Oushadh Shorashak (Sixteen Rules for Homoeopathic Drugs)* (Calcutta, 1909).

Ray, Akhil Chandra, 'Jouna Samasya Samadhan Sambandhe Du Ekti Kotha' ('One or Two Words on the Treatment of Venereal Diseases'), *Hahnemann*, 23, 7 (1940), 29–32.

Ray, D. N., *Daktar D. N. Ray er Atmakatha (Autobiography of D. N. Ray)* (Publisher not cited, 1929).

Ray Dastidar, Hemangini, *Grihinir Hitopodesh (Advice for the Wife)* (Srihatta: Karimganj Press, 1917).

Ray, Dwijendralal, *Trhyasparsha ba Sukhi Paribar (The Triangular Impact or Happy Family)*, 2nd edition (Calcutta: Surdham, 1915).

Ray, Haranath, 'Homoeopathic Mowt e Jvar Chikitsha' ('Homoeopathic Treatment of Fever'), *Chikitsha Sammilani*, 4 (1887), 122–6.
Ray, Haranath, 'Homoeopathy Mowt e Jvar Chikitsha ('Homoeopathic Treatment of Fever'), *Chikitsha Sammilani*, 3 (1886), 222.
Ray, K. K., 'Editorial: Prodorshoni te Deshiya Homeo Oushadh'('Indigenous Homoeopathic Drugs at Exhibition') *Homeopathy Pracharak*, 2, 9 (December 1928), 366.
Ray, Mahendranath, *Homoeopathy Abishkorta Samuel Hahnemann er Jiboni (Life of Samuel Hahnemann the Inventor of Homoeopathy)* (Taligunj: Kasi Kharda Press, 1881).
Ray, Satyendranath, *Asia r Hahnemann: Dr. Mahendralal Sircar (Dr. Mahendralal Sircar, the Hahnemann of Asia)* (Calcutta: Institute of History of Homoeopathy, year not cited).
Raya, Jagachandra, *Garhasthya Svasthya ebong Homoeopathic Chikitsha Bigyan (Domestic Health and Homoeopathic Medical Science)* (Calcutta: Harendranath Roy, 1917).
Roy, Akhilchandra, 'Homoeopathy'r Mul Tattva Sombondhe Du Ekti Kotha' ('A Few Words on the Fundamental Principle of Homoeopathy'), *Hahnemann*, 22, 11 (1939), 661.
Roy, Madhusudan, 'Abadhoutik ba Sadrisa Chikitsha' ('Abadhoutik or Homoeopathic treatment'), *Chikitsha Sammilani*, 2 (1885), 146–61.
Roy, SN, 'Rog Kahake Bole' ('What Is Disease'), *Hahnemann*, 6, 12 (1923), 555.
Sadhukhan, Ramcharan, 'Patra' ('Letter'), *Hahnemann*, 9, 10 (1926), 435–6.
Saha, Harendra Kumar, *Bartaman Chikitsha Rahasya O Akal Mrityur Baan (Mysteries of Modern Medicine and Increase in Untimely Deaths)* (Faridpur: Bijoy Chandra Roy, 1922).
Sanyal, Pulin Chandra, 'Ini Abar Ki Bolen' ('What Does He Say'), *Chikitsha Sammilani*, 4 (1887), 304–8.
Sen, Kunjalal, 'Abishvashir Homoeo Mantre Deekha' ('Conversion of an Unbeliever to Homoeopathy'), *Hahnemann*, 10, 6 (1927), 295–300.
Shastri, Shivnath, *Atmacharit (My Life)* (Calcutta: Prabasi Karjalay, 1918; Reprint Dey's, 2003).
Talapatra, Srish Chandra, *Mahesh Chandra Charitkatha (Life of Mahesh Chandra)* (Calcutta: Economic Press, 1946).
Thakur, S. C., 'Homoeopathic Philosophy', *Hahnemann*, 3, 8 (1919), 284–9.

Bengali Secondary Readings

Bhadra, Gautam, *Nyara Battalay Jay Kawbar?* (Kolkata: Chhatim Books, 2011).
Harun-ar-Rashid, Mohammad, 'Homoeopathy Chikitsha Bigyane Rabindranath', *Bangla Academy Patrika* [Bengali 1401] (1994), 113–45.
Sripantha, *Battala* (Calcutta: Ananda, 1997).

English Secondary Readings

Adams, Vincanne, 'Randomised Control Crime, Postcolonial Sciences in Alternative Medicine Research', *Social Studies of Science*, 32, 5/6 (2002), 659–90.

Adams, Vincanne, 'The Sacred in the Scientific: Ambiguous Practices of Science in Tibetan Medicine', *Cultural Anthropology*, 16, 1 (2001), 542–75.

Ahluwalia, Sanjam, *Reproductive Restraints: Birth Control in India, 1877–1947* (New Delhi: Permanent Black, 2008).

AHR Roundtable Special Issues, 'Historians and Biography', *American Historical Review*, 114, 3 (June 2009).

Alavi, Seema, *Islam and Healing: Loss and Recovery of an Indo-Muslim Medical Tradition 1600–1900* (Basingstoke: Palgrave Macmillan, 2008).

Ali, Daud (ed.), *Invoking the Past: The Uses of History in South Asia* (Delhi: Oxford University Press, 2002).

Alter, Joseph, 'Celibacy, Sexuality and the Transformation of Gender into Nationalism in North India', *Journal of Asian Studies*, 53, 1 (1994), 45–66.

Alter, Joseph, *Gandhi's Body: Sex, Diet and the Politics of Nationalism* (Pennsylvania: University of Pennsylvania Press, 2000).

Althusser, Louis, 'Ideology and Ideological State Apparatuses', *Lenin and Philosophy, and Other Essays*, Trans. Ben Brewster (London: New Left Books, 1971), pp. 121–76.

Anderson, Clare, *Subaltern Lives: Biographies of Colonialism in the Indian Ocean World, 1790–1920* (Cambridge: Cambridge University Press, 2012.

Appadurai, Arjun, 'Archive and Aspiration' in Joke Brouwer and Arjen Mulder (eds.), *Information Is Alive* (Rotterdam: V2_Publishing/NAI Publishers, 2003), pp. 14–25.

Aquil, Raziuddin and Partha Chatterjee (eds.), *History in the Vernacular* (Ranikhet: Permanent Black, 2008).

Arnold, David and Stuart Blackburn (eds.), *Telling Lives in India: Biography, Autobiography and Life History* (New Delhi: Permanent Black, 2004).

Arnold, David and Sumit Sarkar, 'In Search of Rational Remedies: Homoeopathy in Nineteenth-century Bengal' in Waltraud Ernst (ed.), *Plural Medicine, Tradition and Modernity, 1800–2000* (London and New York: Routledge, 2002), pp. 40–54.

Arnold, David, 'Touching the Body: Perspectives on the Indian Plague, 1896–1900', Ranajit Guha (ed.) *Subaltern Studies V* (Delhi: Oxford University Press, 1987), pp. 55–90.

Arnold, David, *Colonising the Body: State Medicine and Epidemic Disease in Nineteenth Century India* (Berkeley: University of California Press, 1993).

Arnold, David, *Everyday Technology: Machines and the Making of India's Modernity* (Chicago and London: University of Chicago Press, 2013).

Arnold, David, *Imperial Medicine and Indigenous Societies* (Manchester: Manchester University Press, 1988).

Arnold, David, *Science, Technology and Medicine in Colonial India* (New Cambridge History of India III: 5) (Cambridge, Cambridge University Press, 2000).

Arnold, David, *Tropics and the Travelling Gaze: India, Landscape and Science, 1800–1856* (Seattle: Washington University Press, 2006).

Arondekar, Anjali, *For the Record: On Sexuality and the Colonial Archive in India* (Durham, NC: Duke University Press, 2009).

Attewell, Guy, *Refiguring Unani Tibb: Plural Healing in Late Colonial India* (New Delhi: Orient Longman, 2007).

Bagchi, Amiya Kumar, 'European and Indian Entrepreneurship in India, 1900–1930' in Rajat K Ray (ed.), *Entrepreneurship and Industry in India: 1800–1947* (Delhi: Oxford University Press, 1992), 169–81.

Bagchi, Amiya Kumar, *Private Investment in India 1900–1939* (Cambridge: Cambridge University Press, 1972).

Bagchi, Ashok K., *Rabindranath Tagore and His Medical World* (Delhi: Konark Publishers, 2000).

Bandopadhyay, Shekhar (ed.), *Bengal: Rethinking History: Essays in Historiography* (Delhi: Manohar Publishers, 2001).

Banerjee, Madhulika, 'Public Policy and Ayurveda: Modernising a Great Tradition', *Economic and Political Weekly*, 37, 12 (2002), 1136–46.

Banerjee, Madhulika, *Power, Knowledge, Medicine: Ayurvedic Pharmaceuticals at Home and in the World* (Hyderabad: Orient Blackswan, 2009).

Banerjee, Prathama, *Politics of Time: 'Primitives' and History Writing in a Colonial Society* (New Delhi: Oxford Universoty Press, 2006).

Banerjee, Sumanta, *Dangerous Outcaste: Prostitutes in Nineteenth Century Bengal* (Calcutta: Seagull, 1998).

Banerjee, Swapna M., *Men, Women and Domestics: Articulating Middle Class Identity in Colonial Bengal* (New Delhi: Oxford University Press, 2004).

Basu, Amitranjan, 'Emergence of a Marginal Science in a Colonial City: Reading Psychiatry in Bengali Periodicals', *Indian Economic and Social History Review*, 41, 2 (2004), pp. 103–41.

Bates, Donald G., 'Why Not Call Modern Medicine "Alternative"', *Perspectives in Biology and Medicine*, 43, 4 (2000), 502–18.

Bayly, Christopher, 'The Origins of Swadeshi: Cloth and Indian Society' in Arjun Appadurai (ed.), *The Social Life of Things* (Cambridge: Cambridge University Press, 1986), pp. 285–321.

Bayly, Christopher, *Rulers, Townsmen and Bazaars: North Indian Society in the Age of British Expansion, 1770–1870* (Cambridge: Cambridge University Press, 1983).

Bean, Susan S., 'Gandhi and Khadi: The Fabric of Indian Nationalism' in Annette B. Weiner and Jane Schneider (eds.), *Cloth and Human Experience* (Washington: Smithsonian Institution Press, 1989), pp. 355–76.

Berger, Rachel, 'Ayurveda and the Making of the Urban Middle Class in North India 1900–1945' in Dagmar Wujastyk and Frederick Smith (eds.), *Modern and Global Ayurveda: Pluralism and Paradigms* (Albany: State University of New York Press, 2008), pp. 101–16.

Berger, Rachel, *Ayurveda Made Modern: Political Histories of Indigenous Medicine, 1900–1955* (Basingstoke: Palgrave Macmillan, 2013).

Bhadra, Gautam, 'Four Rebels of Eighteen Fifty-Seven' in Ranajit Guha and Gayatri Spivak (eds.), *Selected Subaltern Studies* (Delhi: Oxford University Press, 1988), pp. 129–78.

Bhardwaj, Surinder M., 'Homoeopathy in India' in Giri Raj Gupta (ed.), *The Social and Cultural Context of Medicine in India* (Delhi: Vikas, 1981), pp. 31–54.

Bhattacharya, Nandini, 'Between the Bazaar and the Bench: Making of the Drug Trade in Colonial India, ca. 1900–1930', *Bulletin of the History of Medicine*, 90, 1 (April 2016), 61–91.

Bhattacharya, Sabyasachi, 'Cotton Mills and Spinning Wheels: Swadeshi and the Indian Capitalist Class, 1920–22', *Economic and Political Weekly*, 11, 47 (1976), 1828–34.

Bhattacharya, Tithi, *Sentinels of Culture: Class, Education and the Colonial Intellectual in Bengal* (New York: Oxford University Press, 2005).

'Biography and History: Inextricably Interwoven', Special Issue, *Journal of Interdisciplinary History*, 40, 3 (Winter 2010).

Birla, Ritu, *Stages of Capital: Law, Culture and Market Governance in Late Colonial India* (Durham: Duke University Press, 2009).

Biswas, Arun Kumar (ed.), *Gleanings of the Past and the Science Movement: In the Diaries of Drs. Mahendralal and Amritalal Sircar* (Kolkata: Asiatic Society, 2000.

Biswas, Arun Kumar, *Collected Works of Mahendralal Sircar, Eugene Lafont and the Science Movement, 1860–1910* (Kolkata: Asiatic Society, 2003).

Bivins, Roberta, *Alternative Medicine? A History* (Oxford and New York: Oxford University Press, 2007).

Bivins, Roberta, 'Histories of Heterodoxies' in Mark Jackson (ed.), *The Oxford Handbook of Medicine* (Oxford University Press, 2011), 576–97.

Bode, Maarten, *Taking Traditional Knowledge to Market: The Modern Image of the Ayurvedic and Unani Industry, 1980–2000* (Hyderabad: Orient Longman, 2008).

Bose, Pradip, 'Sons of the Nation: Child Rearing in the New Family' in Partha Chatterjee (ed.), *Texts of Power: Emerging Discipline in Colonial Bengal* (Minneapolis: University of Minnesota Press, 1995), pp. 118–44.

Bose, Sugata, and Kris Manjapra (eds.), *Cosmopolitan Thought Zones: South Asia and the Global Circulation of Ideas* (Basingstoke: Palgrave Macmillan, 2010).

Bose, Sugata, *His Majesty's Opponents: Subhas Chandra Bose and India's Struggle Against Empire* (Cambridge: Harvard University Press, 2011).

Bradley, James, 'Medicine on the Margins: Hydropathy and Orthodoxy in Britain, 1840–1860' in Waltraud Ernst (ed.), *Plural Medicine, Tradition and Modernity, 1800–2000* (London and New York: Routledge, 2002).

Brown, Judith M., *Jawaharlal Nehru: A Political Life* (New Haven: Yale University Press, 2003).

Buchanan, Ian, and Adrian Parr (eds.), *Deleuze and the Contemporary World* (Edinburgh: Edinburgh University Press, 2006).

Buettner, Elizabeth, *Empire Families: Britons and Late Imperial India* (New York: Oxford University Press, 2004).

Bynum, W. F., and Roy Porter (eds.), *Medical Fringe and Medical Orthodoxy 1750–1850* (London and Wolfeboro: Croom Helm, 1987).

Cabrita, Joel, 'People of Adam: Divine Healing and Racial Cosmopolitanism in the Early Twentieth Century Transvaal', *Comparative Studies in Society and History*, 57, 2 (2015), 1–36.

Callewaert, Wianad and Rupert Snell (eds.), *According to Tradition: Hagiographical Writing in India* (Wiesbaden: Harrasowitz Verlag, 1994).

Cantor, Geoffrey, et al. (eds.), *Science in the Nineteenth-Century Periodical: Reading the Magazine of Nature* (Cambridge: Cambridge University Press, 2004).

Chakrabarti, Pratik, 'Medical Marketplaces beyond the West: Bazaar medicine, Trade and the English Establishment in Eighteenth Century India' in Mark Jenner and Patrick Wallis (eds.), *Medicine and the Market in England and Its Colonies, c. 1450–c. 1850* (Basingstoke: Palgrave Macmillan, 2007), pp. 196–215.

Chakrabarti, Pratik, 'Science and Swadeshi: The Establishment and Growth of the Bengal Chemical and Pharmaceutical Works' in Uma Dasgupta (ed.), *Science and Modern India: An Institutional History, 1784–1947* (Delhi: Pearson Education, 2010), pp. 117–42.

Chakrabarti, Pratik, 'Science, Morality, and Nationalism: The Multifaceted Project of Mahendra Lal Sircar', *Studies in History*, 17, 2 (2001), 245–74.

Chakrabarti, Pratik, *Western Science in Colonial India: Metropoitan Methods, Colonial Practices* (Delhi: Permanent Black, 2004).

Chakrabarty Dipesh, 'The Public Life of History: An Argument Out of India', *Public Culture*, 20, 1 (2008), 143–49.

Chakrabarty, Dipesh, 'Bourgeois Categories Made Global: Utopian and Actual Lives of Historical Documents in India', *Economic and Political Weekly*, 25 (June 2009), 69–75.

Chakrabarty, Dipesh, '*Family Fraternity, Salaried Labor' in Provincializing Europe: Postcolonial Thought and Historical Difference* (Princeton, NJ: Princeton University Press, 2000), pp. 214–236.

Chakrabarty, Dipesh, 'The Birth of Academic Historical Writing in India' in Stuart Macintyre et al. (eds.) *The Oxford History of Historical Writing, Vol 4: 1800–1945* (Oxford: Oxford University Press, 2011).

Chakrabarty, Dipesh, 'The Difference: Deferral of (A) Colonial Modernity: Public Debates on Domesticity in Colonial Bengal', *History Workshop*, 36 (1993), 1–36.

Chakrabarty, Dipesh, *Provincializing Europe: Postcolonial Thought and Historical Difference* (Princeton, NJ: Princeton University Press, 2000).

Chatterjee, Kumkum, 'The King of Controversy: History and Nation Making in Late Colonial India', *American Historical Review*, 110, 5 (2005), 1454–75.

Chatterjee, Kumkum, 'History and Nation-Making in Late Colonial India' in Partha Chatterjee and Raziuddin Aquil (eds.). *History in the Vernacular* (Delhi: Permanent Black, 2008), pp. 107–32.

Chatterjee, Indrani (ed.), *Unfamiliar Relations: Family and History in South Asia* (Delhi: Permanent Black, 2004).

Chatterjee, Indrani, 'Gossip, Taboo and Writing Family History' in Indrani Chatterjee (ed.), *Unfamiliar Relations: Family and History in South Asia* (Delhi: Permanent Black, 2004), pp. 222–60.

Chatterjee, Partha, 'Nationalist Resolution of the women's question' in Kumkum Sangari and Sudesh Vaid (eds.), *Recasting Woman: Essays in Indian Colonial History* (New Brunswick: Rutgers University Press, 1989), pp. 233–53.

Chatterjee, Partha, 'The Disciplines of Colonial Bengal' in Partha Chatterjee (ed.), *Texts of Power: Emerging Disciplines in Colonial Bengal* (Minneapolis: University of Minnesota Press, 1995).

Chatterjee, Partha, *The Nation and Its Fragments: Colonial and Postcolonial Histories* (Princeton, NJ: Princeton University Press, 1993).

Chatterji, Joya, *Bengal Divided: Hindu Communalism and Partition, 1932–1947* (Cambridge: Cambridge University Press, 1994).

Cleall, Esme, Laura Ishiguro and Emily Manktelow (eds.), 'Imperial Relations: Histories of Family in the British Empire', *Journal of Colonialism and Colonial History*, 14, 1 (2013), www.muse.jhu.edu/article/503247 (last accessed 11 August 2018).

Codell, Julie F., 'Constructing the Victorian Artist: National Identity, the Political Economy of Art and Biographical Mania in the Periodical Press', *Victorian Periodicals Review*, 33, 3 (2000), 283–316.

Codell, Julie F., 'Serialised Artist's Biographies: Culture Industry in Late Victorian Britain', *Book History*, 3 (2000), 94–124.

Codell, Julie F., *The Victorian Artist: Artists' Lifewriting in Britain c. 1870–1910* (Cambridge: Cambridge University Press, 2003).

Coen, Deborah, 'The Common World: Histories of Science and Domestic Intimacy', *Modern Intellectual History*, 11, 2 (2014), 417–38.

Cohn, Bernard and Nicholas B. Dirks, 'Beyond the Fringe: The Nation State, Colonialism, and the Technologies of Power', *Journal of Historical Sociology*, 1, 2 (June 1988), 224–9.

Cohn, Bernard S., *Colonialism and Its Forms of Knowledge: The British in India* (Princeton, NJ: Princeton University Press, 1996).

Cohn, Bernard S., 'Command of Language and Language of Command' in *Colonialism and Its Forms of Knowledge: The British in India* (Princeton, NJ: Princeton University Press, 1997).

Cook, Harold, *The Decline of the Old Medical Regime in Stuart London* (Ithaca: Cornell University Press, 1986).

Cooter, Roger (ed.), *Studies in the History of Alternative Medicine* (New York: St Martin's Press, 1988).

Coulter, H. L., *Divided Legacy Vol III: The Conflict between Homoeopathy and the American Medical Association: Science and Ethics in American Medicine: 1800–1900* (Berkeley: North Atlantic Books, 1982).

Coulter, H. L., *Homoeopathic Science and Modern Medicine: The Physics of Healing with Microdoses* (Berkeley: North Atlantic Books, 1981).

Craig, David, *Familiar Medicine: Everyday Health Knowledge and Practice in Today's Vietnam* (Honolulu: University of Hawaii Press, 2002).

Curley, David, *Poetry and History: Bengali Mangal Kabya and Social Change in Precolonial Bengal* (Delhi: Chronicle Books, 2008).
Darnton, Robert, *The Business of Enlightenment: A Publishing History of the Encyclopaedia, 1775–1800* (Cambridge: Harvard University Press, 1987).
Das, Shinjini, 'Biography and Homoeopathy in Bengal: Colonial Lives of a European Heterodoxy', *Modern Asian Studies*, 49, 6 (2015), 1732–71.
Das, Shinjini, 'Debating Scientific Medicine: Homoeopathy and Allopathy in Later Nineteenth-Century Medical Print in Bengal', *Medical History*, 56, 4 (2012), 463–80.
Deb Roy, Rohan, 'Debility, Diet, Desire: Food in Nineteenth and Early Twentieth Century Bengali Manuals' in Supriya Chaudhari and Rimi B. Chatterjee (eds.), *The Writer's Feast: Food and the Cultures of Representation* (Hyderabad: Orient Blackswan, 2011), pp. 179–205.
Denault, Leigh, 'Partition and the Politics of the Joint Family in Nineteenth Century North India', *Indian Economic and Social History Review*, 46, 1 (2009), 27–55.
Dinges, Martin (ed.), *Patient's Perspective in the History of Homoeopathy*, Network Series Number 5 (Sheffield, UK, European Association for the History of Medicine and Health, 2002).
Dodson, Michael, *Orientalism, Empire, National Culture, India 1770–1880* (Basingstoke: Palgrave Macmillan, 2007).
Dube, Saurabh, 'Colonial Registers of a Vernacular Christianity: Conversion to Translation', *Economic and Political Weekly*, 39, 1 (2004), 161–71.
Eaton, Richard, *Social History of Deccan, 1300–1761: Eight Indian Lives* (Cambridge: Cambridge University Press, 2005).
Ecks, Stefan, *Eating Drugs: Psychopharmaceutical Pluralism in India* (New York: New York University Press, 2013).
Elshakry, Marwa, 'Knowledge in Motion: The Cultural Politics of Modern Science Translation in Arabic', *Isis*, 99, 4 (2008), 701–30.
Elshakry, Marwa, *Reading Darwin in Arabic, 1860–1950* (Chicago and London: University of Chicago Press, 2013).
Ernst, Waltraud, 'Colonial Psychiatry, Magic and Religion: The Case of Mesmerism in British India', *History of Psychiatry*, 15, 1 (2004), 57–68.
Fissell, Mary E., *Vernacular Bodies: The Politics of Reproduction in Early Modern England* (New York: Oxford University Press, 2004).
Forbes, Geraldine, *Women in Colonial India: Politics, Medicine and Historiography* (Delhi: Chronicle Books, 2005).
Foucault, Michel, 'Governmentality' in Graham Burchell, Colin Gordon and Peter Miller (eds.) *The Foucault Effect: Studies in Governmentality* (Chicago: University of Chicago Press, 1991), pp. 87–104.
Foucault, Michel, *Power/Knowledge: Selected Interviews and Other Writings, 1972–1977*, Colin Gordon (ed.) (New York: Pantheon, 1980).
Ghosh, Ajoy Kumar, 'A Short History of the Development of Homoeopathy in India', *Homeopathy*, 99, 2 (2010), 130–6.
Ghosh, Anindita, 'Revisiting the "Bengal Renaissance": Literary Bengali and Low Life Print in Colonial Calcutta', *Economic and Political Weekly*, 37, 42 (2002), 4329–38.

Ghosh, Anindita, *Power in Print: Popular Publishing and Politics of Language and Culture in a colonial Society, 1778–1905* (Delhi: Oxford University Press, 2006).

Ghosh, Atig, 'The Mofussil and the Modern: The Discreet Charms of Kangal Harinath', *Modern Makeovers: Handbook of Modernity in South Asia* (Delhi: Oxford University Press, 2011), pp. 76–90.

Ghosh, Durba, *Sex and the Family in Colonial India: The Making of Empire* (Cambridge: Cambridge University Press, 2006).

Gijswijt-Hofstra, Marijke, 'Homeopathy and Its Concern for Purity: the Dutch Case in the Early 20th Century' in M. Gijswijt-Hofstra, G. M. Van Heteren and E. M. Tansey (eds.), *Biographies of Remedies: Drugs, Medicines and Contraceptives in Dutch and Anglo-American Healing Cultures* (Amsterdam: Rodopi, 2002), pp. 99–121.

Gold, Peter W., S. Novella, R. Roy, D. Marcus, I. Bell, N. Davidovitch and A. Saine, 'Homoeopathy – Quackery or a Key to the Future of Medicine?', *Homoeopathy*, 97 (2008), 28–33.

Goswami, Manu, *Producing India: From Colonial Economy to National Space* (Chicago: Chicago University Press, 2004).

Goswami, Manu, 'From Swadeshi to Swaraj: Nation, Economy, and Territory in Colonial South Asia, 1870 to 1907', *Comparative Studies in Society and History*, 40, 4 (1998), 609–36.

Goswami, Omkar, 'Sahibs, Babus and Banias: Changes in Industrial Control in Eastern India', *Journal of Asian Studies*, 48, 2 (1989), 289–309.

Greene, Mott, 'Writing Scientific Biography', *Journal of the History of Biology*, 40, 4 (2007), 727–59.

Greenough, Paul R., *Prosperity and Misery in Modern Bengal: The Famine of 1943–1944* (New York and Oxford: Oxford University Press, 1982).

Guha, Supriya, 'The Best Swadeshi: Reproductive Health in Bengal' in Sarah Hodges (ed.), *Reproductive Health in Colonial India: History, Politics, Controversies* (Hyderabad: Orient Longman, 2006), pp. 139–63.

Gupta, Charu, 'Procreation and Pleasure: Writings of a Woman Ayurvedic Practitioner in Colonial North India', *Studies in History*, 21, 1 (2005), 17–44.

Gupta, Charu, *Sexuality, Obscenity, and Community: Women, Muslims and the Hindu Public in Colonial India* (Delhi: Permanent Black, 2001).

Hall, Catherine and Leonore Davidoff, *Family Fortunes: Men and Women of the English Middle Class, 1780–1850* (Chicago: University of Chicago Press, 1987).

Hancock, Mary, 'Gendering the Modern: Woman and Home Science in British India' in Antoinette Burton (ed.), *Gender, Sexuality and Colonial Modernities* (London and New York: Routledge, 1999), pp. 149–62.

Hardiman, David, 'A Subaltern Christianity: Faith Healing in Southern Gujrat' in David Hardiman and Projit Mukharji (eds.), *Medical Marginality in South Asia: Situating Subaltern Therapeutics* (New York: Routledge, 2012).

Harrison, Mark and Biswamoy Pati (eds.), *Health, Medicine and Empire: Perspectives on Colonial India* (New Delhi: Orient Longman, 2001).

Harrison, Mark and Biswamoy Pati (eds.), *Social History of Health and Medicine in Colonial India* (New York: Routledge, 2009).

Harrison, Mark, 'Science and the British Empire', *Isis*, 96, 1 (2005), 56–63.
Harrison, Mark, *Climates and Constitutions, Health, Race, Environment and British Imperialism in India, 1600–1850* (Oxford: Oxford University Press, 1999).
Harrison, Mark, *Public Health in British India: Anglo India Preventive Medicine 1859–1914* (Cambridge: Cambridge University Press, 1994).
Hausman, Gary S., 'Making Medicine Indigenous: Homoeopathy in South India', *Social History of Medicine*, 15, 2 (2002), 303–22.
Hibbard, Allen, 'Biographer and Subject: A Tale of Two Narratives', *South Central Review*, 23, 3 (2006), 25–32.
Hobsbawm, Eric J., and Terence O. Ranger (eds.), *The Invention of Tradition* (Cambridge: Cambridge University Press, 1992).
Hodges, Sarah, *Reproductive Health in India: History, Politics, Controversies* (Hyderabad: Orient Longman, 2006).
Holmes, Richard, 'A Proper Study?' in William St Claire (ed.), *Mapping Lives: The Uses of Biography* (Oxford: *Oxford University Press*, 2002).
Howland, Douglas, 'Predicament of Ideas in Culture: Translation and Historiography', *History and Theory*, 42, 1 (2003), 45–60.
Ito, Akito, 'How Electricity Energizes the Body: Electrotherapeutics and Its Analogy of Life in Japanese Medical Context' in Dhruv Raina and Feza Gunergun (eds.), *Science between Europe and Asia, Historical Studies on the Transmission, Adoption and Adaptation of Knowledge* (Netherlands: Springer, 2011), pp. 245–58.
Jain, Kajri, *Gods in the Bazaar: Economies of Indian Calendar Art* (Durham: Duke University Press, 2007).
Jenner, Mark and Patrick Wallis, *Medicine and the Market in England and Its Colonies, c. 1450–c. 1850* (Basingstoke: Palgrave Macmillan, 2007).
Jodhka, Surinder S., 'Nation and Village: Images of Rural India in Gandhi, Nehru and Ambedkar', *Economic and Political Weekly*, 37, 32 (2002), 3343–53.
Jutte, Robert, Guenter Risse and John Woodward (eds.), *Culture, Knowledge and Healing: Historical Perspective of Homoeopathic Medicine in Europe and North America* (Sheffield: European Association for the History of Medicine and Health Publications, 1998).
Kapila, Shruti, 'The Enchantment of Science in India', *Isis*, 101, 1 (2010), 120–32.
Kar, Bodhisattva, 'Can the Postcolonial Begin? Deprovincializing Assam' in Saurabh Dube (ed.), *Modern Makeovers: Handbook of Modernity in South Asia* (Delhi: Oxford University Press, 2011), pp. 43–58.
Kasturi, Malavika, *Embattled Identities: Rajput Lineages and the Colonial State in Nineteenth Century North India* (Delhi: Oxford University Press, 2002).
Kaur, Raminder, *Performative Politics and the Cultures of Hinduism: Public Uses of Religion in Western India* (London: Anthem Press, 2005).
Kaviraj, Sudipta, 'Laughter and Subjectivity: The Self-Ironical Tradition in Bengali Literature', *Modern Asian Studies*, 34, 2 (May 2000), 379–406.
Kaviraj, Sudipta, 'The Invention of Private Life' in David Arnold and Stuart Blackburn (eds.), *Telling Lives in India: Biography, Autobiography and Life History* (Bloomington: Indiana University Press, 2004), pp. 83–115.

Keene, Melanie, 'Familiar Science in Nineteenth-Century Britain', *History of Science*, 52, 1 (2014), 53–71.

Khaleeli, Zhaleh, 'Harmony or Hegemony? Rise and Fall of the Native Medical Institution in Calcutta, 1822–1835', *South Asia Research*, 21, 1 (2001), 77–102.

Khan, Shamshad, 'Systems of Medicine and Nationalist Discourse in India: Towards "New Horizons" in Medical Anthropology and History', *Social Science and Medicine*, 62 (2006), 2786–97.

Kishore, Jugal, 'About Entry of Homoeopathy in India', *Bulletin of the Institution of History of Medicine*, 2, 2 (1973), 76–8.

Kopf, David, *Brahmo Samaj and the Shaping of the Modern Indian Mind* (Princeton, NJ: Princeton University Press, 1979).

Kucich, John, *Ghostly Communion: Cross-cultural Spiritualism in the Nineteenth Century* (New Hampshire: UPNE, 2004), pp. 36–58.

Kumar, Anil, *Medicine and the Raj: British Medical Policy in India 1935–1911* (New Delhi: Sage Publications, 1998).

Kumar, Udaya, 'Writing the Life of the Guru: Chattampi Swamikal, Sree Narayan Guru and the Modes of Biographical Construction' in Vijaya Ramaswamy and Yogesh Sharma (eds.), *Biography as History: Indian Perspectives* (Hyderabad: Orient BlackSwan, 2009), pp. 53–87.

Lal, Maneesha, 'Purdah as Pathology: Gender and the Circulation of Medical Knowledge in Late Colonial India' in Sarah Hodges (ed.), *Reproductive Health in India: History, Politics, Controversies* (New Delhi: Orient Longman, 2006), pp. 85–114.

Lal, Maneesha, 'The Politics of Gender and Medicine in Colonial India: The Countess of Dufferin's Fund, 1885–1888', *Bulletin of the History of Medicine*, 68, 1 (1994), 29–66.

Laurie, Timothy and Hannah Stark, 'Reconsidering Kinship: Beyond the Nuclear Family with Deleuze and Guattari', *Cultural Studies Review*, 18, 1 (2012), 19–39.

Lepore, Jill, 'Historians Who Love Too Much: Reflections on Microhistory and Biography', *Journal of American History*, 88, 1 (2001), 129–44.

Lightman, Bernard and Aileen Fyfe (eds.), *Science in the Marketplace: Nineteenth Century Sites and Experiences* (Chicago: University of Chicago Press, 2007).

Lightman, Bernard, *Victorian Popularisers of Science: Designing Nature for New Audiences* (Chicago: University of Chicago Press, 2007).

Liu, Lydia (ed.), *Tokens of Exchange: The Problem of Translation in Global Circulations* (Durham: Duke University Press, 2000).

Liu, Lydia, *Translingual Practice: Literature, National Culture and Translated Modernity: China 1900–1937* (Palo Alto: Stanford University Press, 1995).

Livingstone, David and Charles Withers (eds.), *Geographies of Nineteenth Century Science* (Chicago: University of Chicago Press, 2011).

Lubenow, William, 'Intimacy, Imagination, and the Inner Dialectics of Knowledge Communities: The Synthetic Society, 1896–1908' in Martin Daunton (ed.), *The Organisation of Knowledge in Victorian Britain* (Oxford: Oxford University Press, 2005), pp. 357–70.

Majeed, Javed, *Autobiography, Travel and Postnational Identity: Gandhi, Nehru and Iqbal* (Basingstoke: Palgrave Macmillan, 2007).
Majumdar, Rochona, *Marriage and Modernity: Family Values in Colonial Bengal* (Durham: Duke University Press, 2009).
Mani, Lata, *Contentious Traditions: The Debate on Sati in Colonial India* (Berkeley: University of California Press, 1998).
Manjapra, Kris, *M. N. Roy: Marxism and Colonial Cosmopolitanism* (London, New York and New Delhi: Routledge, 2010).
Marks, Shula, 'What Is Colonial about Colonial Medicine? And What has Happened to Imperialism and Health', *Social History of Medicine*, 10 (1997), 205–19.
McGuire, John, *The Making of Colonial Mind: A Quantative Study of the Bhadralok in Calcutta, 1875–1885* (Canberra: Australian National University, 1983).
Mitra, Samarpita, 'Periodical Readership in Early Twentieth Century Bengal: Ramananda Chattopadhyay's Prabasi', *Modern Asian Studies*, 47, 1 (2013), 204–49.
Mukharji, Projit Bihari, 'Pharmacology, Indigenous Knowledge and Nationalism, Few Words from the Epitaph of Subaltern Science' in Mark Harrison and Biwamoy Pati (eds.), *The Social History of Health and Medicine in Colonial India* (London: Routledge, 2008), pp. 195–212.
Mukharji, Projit Bihari, 'Structuring Plurality: Locality, Caste, Class and Ethnicity in Nineteenth Century Bengali Dispensaries', *Health and History*, 9, 1 (2007), 80–105.
Mukharji, Projit Bihari, 'Symptoms of Dis-Ease: New Trends in the Histories of Indigenous South Asian Medicine', *History Compass*, 9 (December 2011), 887–99.
Mukharji, Projit Bihari, 'Vishalyakarani as E. Ayapana: Retro Botanizing, Embedded Traditions and Multiple Histories of Plants in Colonial Bengal, 1890–1940', *Journal of Asian Studies*, 73, 1 (2014), 65–87.
Mukharji, Projit Bihari, *Nationalizing the Body: The Medical Market, Print and Daktari Medicine* (London and New York: Anthem Press, 2009).
Mukherjee, Meenakshi, 'The Unperceived Self: A Study of Five Nineteenth Century Autobiographies' in Karuna Chanana (ed.), *Socialisation, Education and Women: Explorations in Gender Identity* (Delhi: Orient Longman, 1988).
Mukherjee, S. N., *Calcutta: Essays in Urban History* (Calcutta: Subarnarekha, 1993).
Mukhopadhyay, Bhaskar, 'Writing Home, Writing Travel: Poetics and Politics of Dwelling', *Comparative Studies in Society and History*, 44, 2 (2002), 293–318.
Mukhopadhyay, Bhaskar, *Rumours of Globalisation: Desecrating the Global from Vernacular Magins* (London: C. Hurst and Co, 2013).
Newbigin, Eleanor, *The Hindu Family and the Emergence of Modern India: Law, Citizenship and Community* (Cambridge: Cambridge University Press, 2013).
Nicholls, Philip, *Homoeopathy and the Medical Profession* (Beckenham: Croom Helm, 1988).
Niranjana, Tejaswini, *Siting Translation: History, Post-Structuralism and the Colonial Context* (Berkeley: University of California Press, 1992).

Palit, Chittabrata, 'Dr. Mahendralal Sircar and Homoeopathy', *Indian Journal for the History of Science*, 33, 4 (1998), 281–92.

Pande, Ishita, *Medicine, Race and Liberalism in British Bengal: Symptoms of Empire* (London and New York: Routledge, 2010).

Peacock, James and Dorothy Holland, 'The Narrated Self: Life Stories in Process', *Ethos*, 21, 4 (1993), 367–83.

Philip, Kavita, *Civilising Natures: Race, Resources and Modernity in Colonial South India* (Hyderabad: Orient Longman, 2003).

Pinney, Christopher and Rachel Dwyer (eds.), *Pleasure and the Nation: The History, Politics and Consumption of Public Culture in India* (Delhi: Oxford University Press, 2001).

Pollock, Sheldon, 'Cosmopolitan and Vernacular in History', *Public Culture*, 12, 3 (2000), 591–625.

Pollock, Sheldon, 'The Cosmopolitan Vernacular', *Journal of Asian Studies*, 57, 1 (1998), 6–37.

Porter, Roy, 'The Patient's View: Doing Medical History from Below', *Theory and Society*, 14 (1985), 175–98.

Porter, Roy, *Health for Sale: Quackery in England, 1660–1850* (Manchester: Manchester University Press, 1989).

Prakash, Gyan, 'Science "Gone Native" in Colonial India', *Representations*, 40, Special Issue: Seeing Science (Autumn 1992), 153–78.

Prakash, Gyan, *Another Reason: Science and the Imagination of Modern India* (Princeton, NJ: Princeton University Press, 1999).

Prasad, Sirupa, *Cultural Politics of Hygiene in India, 1850–1940: Contagions of Feeling* (Basingstoke: Palgrave Macmillan, 2015).

Quaiser, Neshat, 'Science, Institution and Colonialism: Tibbiya College of Delhi – 1889–1947' in Uma Das Gupta (ed.), *Science and Modern India: An Institutional History, c. 1784–1947* (Delhi: Pearson Longman, 2010).

Raheja, Gloria Goodwin, *Listen to the Heron's Words: Reimagining Gender and Kinship in North India* (Berkeley: University of California Press, 1994).

Raina, Dhruv and Irfan S. Habib, 'Ramchandra's Treatise through the "Haze of the Golden Sunset": An aborted Pedagogy', *Social Studies of Science*, 20, 3 (1990), 455–72.

Raj, Kapil, *Relocating Modern Science: Circulation and the Construction of Knowledge in South Asia and Europe, 1650–1900* (Houndmills and New York: Palgrave Macmillan, 2007).

Raman, Bhawani, 'The Familial World of the Company's Kacceri in Early Colonial Madras', *Journal of Colonialism and Colonial History*, 9, 2 (2008), www.muse.jhu.edu/article/246576 (last accessed 11 August 2018).

Ramaswamy, Vijaya and Yogesh Sharma (eds.), *Biography as History: Indian Perspectives* (Hyderabad: Orient Blackswan, 2009).

Ray, Rajat K., *Industrialisation in India: Growth and Conflict in the Private Corporate Sector 1914–47* (Delhi: Oxford University Press, 1979).

Ray, Tapti, 'Disciplining the Printed Text: Colonial and Nationalist Surveillance of Bengali Literature' in Partha Chatterjee (ed.), *Texts of Power: Emerging Disciplines in Colonial Bengal* (Minneapolis: University of Minnesota Press, 1995).

Rege, Sharmila, *Writing Caste, Writing Gender: Reading Dalit Women's Testimonios* (Delhi: Zuban, 1996).

Ricci, Ronit, *Islam Translated: Literature, Conversion and the Arabic Cosmopolis of South and South East Asia* (Chicago: University of Chicago Press, 2011).

Rocha, Leon and Robbie Duschinsky (eds.), *Foucault, the Family and Politics* (Basingstoke: Palgrave Macmillan, 2012).

Rogers, Naomi, 'American Homoeopathy Confronts Scientific Medicine' in Robert Jutte, Guenter B Risse and John Woodward (eds.), *Culture, Knowledge and Healing: Historical Perspective of Homoeopathic Medicine in Europe and North America* (Sheffield: European Association for the History of Medicine and Health Publications, 1998), pp. 31–65.

Rogers, Naomi, *An Alternative Path: The Making and Remaking of the Hahnemann Medical College and Hospital of Philadelphia* (New Brunswick: Rutgers University Press, 1998).

Sarkar, Sumit, 'Kaliyuga, Chakri, Bhakti: Ramkrishna and His Times' in *Writing Social History* (Delhi and New York: Oxford University Press, 1997), pp. 282–357.

Sarkar, Sumit, *Swadeshi Movement in Bengal, 1903–08* (Delhi: People's Publishing House, 1973).

Sarkar, Tanika, 'A Book of Her Own, A Life of Her Own: Autobiography of a Nineteenth Century Woman', *History Workshop*, 36, 1995.

Sarkar, Tanika, 'The Hindu Wife and the Hindu Nation: Domesticity and Nationalism in Nineteenth Century Bengal', *Studies in History*, 8, 2 (1992), 213–35.

Sarkar, Tanika, *Bengal 1928–1934: The Politics of Protest* (Delhi: Oxford University Press, 1987).

Sarkar, Tanika, *Hindu Wife, Hindu Nation: Community, Religion and Cultural Nationalism* (Delhi: Permanent Black, 2001).

Sartori, Andrew, 'Beyond Culture-contact and Colonial Discourse: "Germanism" in Colonial Bengal, *Modern Intellectual History*, 4, 1 (2007), 77–93.

Sartori, Andrew, 'The Categorical Logic of a Colonial Nationalism: Swadeshi Bengal, 1904–1908', *Comparative Studies of South Asia, Africa and the Middle East*, 23, 1&2 (2003), 271–85.

Savary, Luzia, 'Vernacular Eugenics? Santati-Sastra in Popular Hindi Advisory Literature (1900–1940), *South Asia: Journal of South Asian Studies*, 37, 3 (2014), 381–97.

Secord, James, 'Knowledge in Transit', *Isis*, 95, 4 (2004), 654–72.

Secord, James, 'Scrapbook Science: Composite Caricatures in Late Georgian England' in A. Shteir and B. Lightman (eds.), *Figuring It Out: Science, Gender, and Visual Culture* (Hanover, New Hampshire: Dartmouth College Press, 2006), pp. 164–91.

Sen, Sudipta, *Empire of Free Trade: East India Company and the Making of the Colonial Marketplace* (Pennsylvania: University of Pennsylvania Press, 1998).

Shaikh, Juned, 'Translating Marx, Mavali, Dalit and the Making of Mumbai's Working Class', *Economic and Political Weekly 1928–1935*, 46, 31 (2011), 65–72.

Sharma, Madhuri, 'Creating a Consumer: Exploring Medical Advertisements in Colonial India' in Mark Harrison and Biswamoy Pati (eds.), *The Social History of Health and Healing in Colonial India* (New York: Routledge, 2009), pp. 213–28.

Sharma, Ursula, 'Contextualising Alternative Medicine: The Exotic, the Marginal and the Perfectly Mundane', *Anthropology Today*, 9, 4 (1993), 15–18.

Singh, Dhrub Kumar, 'Choleraic Times and Mahendra Lal Sarkar: Quest for Homoeopathy as a "Cultivation of Science" in Nineteenth century India', *Medzin Geselschaft and Geschichte*, 24 (2005), 207–42.

Singha, Radhika, 'Making the Domestic More Domestic: Colonial Criminal Law and the Head of the Household, 1772–1843', *Indian Economic and Social History Review*, 33, 3 (1996), 309–43.

Singha, Radhika, *A Despotism of Law: Crime and Justice in Early Colonial India* (Delhi: Oxford University Press, 1998).

Sinha, Mrinalini, 'Lineage of the Indian Modern: Rhetoric, Agency and the Sarda Act in Late Colonial India' in Antoinette Burton (ed.), *Gender, Sexuality and Colonial Modernities* (London and New York: Routledge, 1999), pp. 207–19.

Sivaramakrishnan, Kavita, 'The Languages of Science, the Vocabulary of Politics: Challenges to Medical Revival in Punjab', *Journal for Social History of Medicine*, 21, 3 (2008), 521–39.

Sivaramakrishnan, Kavita, *Old Potions, New Bottles: Recasting Indigenous Medicine in Colonial Punjab, 1850–1945* (Hyderabad: Orient Longman, 2006).

Skaria, Ajay, 'Gandhi's Politics and the Question of Ashram' in Saurabh Dube (ed.), *Enchantments of Modernity: Empire, Nation, Globalisation* (Delhi and London: Routledge, 2009), pp. 199–233.

Spear, Percival, *Master of Bengal: Clive and His India* (London: Thames and Hudson, 1975).

Sreenivas, Mythili, 'Conjugality and Capital: Gender, Families, and Property under Colonial Law in India', *Journal of Asian Studies*, 63, 4 (2004), 937–60.

Srivastan, R., 'Concept of "Seva" and the "Sevak" in the Freedom Movement', *Economic and Political Weekly*, 41, 5 (2006), 427–38.

St Claire, William, *The Reading Nation in the Romantic Period* (Cambridge: Cambridge University Press, 2004).

Stewart, Tony K., 'One Text from Many: Caitanya Caritamrita as "Classic and Commentary"' in Wianad Callewaert and Rupert Snell (eds.), *According to Tradition: Hagiographical Writing in India* (Wiesbaden: Harrasowitz Verlag, 1994), pp. 231–48.

Stoler, Ann Laura, 'Colonial Archives and the Art of Governance', *Archival Science*, 2, 1–2 (2002), 87–109.

Stoler, Ann Laura, *Along the Archival Grain: Epistemic Anxieties and Colonial Common Sense* (Princeton, NJ: Princeton University Press, 2010).

Stoler, Ann Laura, *Carnal Knowledge and Imperial Power: Race and the Intimate in Colonial Rule* (Berkeley: University of California Press, 2002).

Stoler, Anne Laura (ed.), *Haunted by Empire: Geographies of Intimacy in North American History* (Durham: Duke University Press, 2006).

Sturman, Rachel, 'Property and Attachments: Defining Autonomy and the Claims of Family in Nineteenth Century Western India', *Comparative Studies in Society and History*, 47, 3 (2005), 611–37.

Sturman, Rachel, *Government of Social Life in Colonial India: Liberalism, Religious Law and Women's Rights* (Cambridge: Cambridge University Press, 2012).

Subramanian, Narendra, *Nation and Family: Personal Law, Cultural Pluralism and Gendered Citizenship in India* (Palo Alto: Stanford University Press, 2014).

Sujatha, V., 'Medicine, State and Society', *Economic and Political Weekly*, 44, 16 (2009), 35–43.

Sundd, Harvash Laal, *Sri Sankat Mochan Hanuman Charit Manas (Life of Hanuman, Preventer of Crisis)* (Delhi: Aravali Books International, 1998).

Taylor, Chloe, 'Foucault and Familial Power', *Hypatia: A Journal of Feminist Philosophy*, 27, 1 (2012), 201–17.

Teltscher, Kate, *India Inscribed: European and British Writing on India* (Delhi: Oxford University Press, 1995).

Terrell, Mary, 'Biography as a Cultural History of Science', *Isis*, 97, 2 (2006), 306–13.

Tilley, Helen, 'Global Histories, Vernacular Science and African Genealogics: Or Is the History of the Science Ready for the World', *Isis*, 101, 1 (2010), 110–19.

Topham, Jonathan, 'Publishing "Popular Science" in Early Nineteenth-Century Britain' in Aileen Fyfe and Bernard Lightman (eds.), *Science in the Marketplace: Nineteenth Century Sites and Experiences* (Chicago: Chicago University Press, 2007), pp. 135–68.

Topham, Jonathan, 'Scientific Publishing and the Reading of Science in Nineteenth-century Britain: A Historiographical Survey and Guide to Sources', *Studies in History and Philosophy of Science*, Part A, 31, 4 (2000), 559–612.

Wald, James, 'Periodicals and Periodicity' in Simon Eliot and Jonathan Rose (eds.), *A Companion to the History of Book* (Oxford: Wiley Blackwell, 2009), pp. 421–32.

Walsh, Judith, *Domesticity in Colonial India: What Women Learnt When Men Gave Them Advice* (Lanham: Rowman and Littlefield Pulishers, 2004).

Waltraud Ernst (ed.), *Plural Medicine, Tradition and Modernity, 1800–2000* (London and New York: Routledge, 2002).

Warner, J. H., 'Orthodoxy and Otherness: Homoeopathy and Regular Medicine in Nineteenth-century America' in Robert Jutte, Guenter B. Risse and John Woodward (eds.), *Culture, Knowledge and Healing: Historical Perspective of Homoeopathic Medicine in Europe and North America* (Sheffield: European Association for the History of Medicine and Health Publications, 1998), pp. 5–30.

Warner, John Harley, 'History of Science and Sciences of Medicine', *Osiris*, 10 (1995), 164–93.

Warren, Donald, 'The Bengali Context', *Bulletin of the Indian Institute of History of Medicine*, 21 (1991), 17–51.

Weatherall, M. W., 'Making Medicine Scientific Empiricism, Rationality, and Quackery in mid-Victorian Britain', *Social History of Medicine*, 9, 2 (1996), 175–94.

White, Paul, 'Darwin's Emotions: The Scientific Self and the Sentiment of Objectivity', *Isis*, 100, 4 (2009), 811–26.

Wilson, Jon E., 'Domination of Strangers: Time, Emotion, and the Making of Modern State in Colonial India', *Economic and Political Weekly*, 46, 30 (2011), 45–52.

Wilson, Kathleen, 'Re-thinking the Colonial State: Family, Gender and Governmentality in Eighteenth Century British Frontiers', *American Historical Review*, 116, 5 (December 2011), 1294–322.

Winter, Alison, 'Colonizing Sensations in Victorian India' in *Mesmerized: Powers of Mind in Victorian Britain* (Chicago: University of Chicago Press, 2000), pp. 187–212.

Wright, David, 'Translation of Modern Western Science in Nineteenth Century China, 1840–1895', *Isis*, 89 (1998), 653–73.

Wujastyk, Dominik, 'The Evolution of Indian Government Policy on Ayurveda in the Twentieth Century' in Dagmar Wujastyck and Frederick Smith (eds.), *Modern and Global Ayurveda: Pluralism and Paradigms* (Albany: State University of New York Press, 2008), pp. 51–66.

Wujastyk, Dominik, *Roots of Ayurveda: Selections from Sanskrit Medical Writings* (New Delhi: Penguin, 1998).

Yeo, Richard and Michael Shortland (eds.), *Telling Lives in Science: Essays in Scientific Biography* (Cambridge: Cambridge University Press, 1996).

Zachariah, Benjamin, *Developing India: An Intellectual and Social History c. 1930–50* (Delhi: Oxford University Press, 2005).

Index

Printed in the United States
By Bookmasters